Tobacco War

Tobacco War

Inside the California Battles

Stanton A. Glantz
Edith D. Balbach

UNIVERSITY OF CALIFORNIA PRESS
Berkeley · *Los Angeles* · *London*

University of California Press
Berkeley and Los Angeles, California

University of California Press, Ltd.
London, England

Library of Congress Cataloging-in-Publication Data

Glantz, Stanton A.
    Tobacco war : inside the California battles /
    Stanton A. Glantz, Edith D. Balbach.
        p. cm.
    Includes bibliographical references and index.
    ISBN 0-520-22285-7 (alk. paper)—ISBN 0-520-
    22286-5 (alk. paper)
    1. Tobacco—Law and legislation—California.
    2. Tobacco industry—Political aspects—Califor-
    nia.   I. Balbach, Edith D., 1953–   II. Title.
    KFC417.T6 G58 2000
    362.29'6'09794—dc21   99-037876

Printed in the United States of America
08 07 06 05 04 03 02 01 00 99
10 9 8 7 6 5 4 3 2 1

The paper used in this publication meets the
minimum requirements of ANSI/NISO Z39.48-1992
(R 1997) (*Permanence of Paper*).

And it ought to be remembered that there is nothing more difficult to take in hand, more perilous to conduct, or more uncertain in its success, than to take the lead in the introduction of a new order to things. Because the inventor has for enemies all those who have done well under the old conditions, and lukewarm defenders in those who may do well under the new. . . . Thus it happens that whenever those who are hostile have the opportunity to attack they do it as partisans, whilst the others defend lukewarmly.

N. Machiavelli, 1513

Life's like a movie. Write you own ending. Keep believing, keep pretending.

Kermit the Frog, 1993

Contents

List of Figures and Tables

FIGURES

Illustration section follows page 156

TABLES

Preface

Tobacco is in the news on a daily basis. Politicians from President Clinton down to members of local city councils are actively fighting the tobacco industry. The once-invincible industry has settled lawsuits for hundreds of billions of dollars. Many states are initiating major efforts to do something meaningful about the half-million needless deaths that tobacco causes in America every year.

It was not always this way. For over two decades a few activists did battle with tobacco interests in relative obscurity, usually with little support from the organizations and politicians who should have been helping them.

This is a book about the last quarter-century of tobacco politics in California. In the early 1970s a small band of activists were taken with the idea that people should not have to breathe secondhand tobacco smoke—an idea that was nothing short of bizarre at the time. Their efforts spawned hundreds of local tobacco control ordinances and, eventually, Proposition 99, the largest tobacco control program in the world. At every step of the way, these advocates had to confront the tobacco industry and its allies across the political spectrum. *Tobacco War* is their story.

The book draws heavily on work done by students and research fellows who have worked with Stanton Glantz to study tobacco politics and policy in California over the years: Michael Begay, Bruce Samuels, Mike Traynor, Heather Macdonald, Stella Aguinaga-Bialous, and Fred Monardi. We thank these individuals and our other colleagues whose work has made this book possible.*

We are particularly grateful to Attorney General Hubert Humphrey III of Minnesota. His dogged determination to get the truth out about the tobacco industry in Minnesota's case to recover smoking-induced costs and otherwise rein in the tobacco industry forced the release of millions of secret tobacco industry documents, including several important ones about California that we discuss in this book.

Over time, the research that formed the basis of this book has been supported by several agencies: the University of California Tobacco Related Disease Research Program (Grant 1RT520), the National Cancer Institute (Grant CA-61021), the American Cancer Society, and Edith and Henry Everett. We thank these agencies and individuals for making this work possible, particularly when the tobacco industry was making such support as difficult as possible. We also thank Annemarie Charlesworth for nailing down details and helping with final manuscript preparation and Lena Libatique for typing the index.

One of the authors of this book, Professor Stanton Glantz, participated in many of the events described here. While Glantz appears as a player, it is important to emphasize that this is *not* his personal memoir. Indeed, some of the key events in this story happened while Glantz was writing a statistics textbook on an out-of-state sabbatical.

The amazing thing about the California story is how many tobacco battles have taken place in the state over the past quarter-century. Indeed, we have omitted many important events to keep the book manageable and to focus on the California Tobacco Control Program. We do not discuss the liberation of the film *Death in the West,* which Philip Morris suppressed in England; or the development of the California En-

* Portions of this book draw heavily on the following research: B. Samuels and S. Glantz, The politics of local tobacco control, *JAMA* 1991;266:2110–2117 (copyright American Medical Association, 1991); M. Traynor, M. Begay, and S. Glantz, New tobacco industry strategy to prevent local tobacco control, *JAMA* 1993;270:479–486 (copyright American Medical Association, 1993); H. Macdonald and S. Glantz, Political realities of statewide smoking legislation: The passage of California's Assembly Bill AB 13, *Tobacco Control* 1994;4:1081–1085 (copyright BMJ Publishing Group); M. Traynor and S. Glantz, California's tobacco tax initiative: The development and passage of Proposition 99, *JHPPL* 1996;21:543–585; S. Glantz, J. Slade, L. Bero, P. Hanauer, D. Barnes, *The cigarette papers* (Berkeley: University of California Press, 1996); H. Macdonald, S. Aguinaga, and S. Glantz, The defeat of Philip Morris' "California Uniform Tobacco Control Act," *Am J Pub Health* 1997;87:1989–1996 (copyright American Public Health Association, 1997); E. Balbach and S. Glantz, Tobacco control advocates must demand high-quality media campaigns, *Tobacco Control* (1998; 7:397–408; copyright BMJ Publishing Group). We thank the copyright holders for permission to use this material.

vironmental Protection Agency report on secondhand smoke; or the fight by Glantz and his colleagues at the University of California to make the Brown and Williamson documents public; or the efforts by congressional Republicans to force the National Cancer Institute to cancel Glantz's research funding; or the lawsuits the tobacco industry filed against the university to try to stop Glantz's work; or the lawsuit that California filed against the tobacco industry; or the passage of Proposition 10 in 1998, which raised tobacco taxes by fifty cents a pack to fund child development programs. These stories will have to wait for the sequel.

California's story holds important insights for people everywhere who want to develop and implement—and to defend—meaningful tobacco control programs.

Stanton A. Glantz
San Francisco, California

Edith D. Balbach
Medford, Massachusetts

CHAPTER I

Introduction

New Year's Day 1998 was crisp and clear along the coast just north of San Francisco, a fine day for a hike. Stanton Glantz, a professor at the University of California, San Francisco, and longtime tobacco control advocate, joined a group of friends to hike from high on Mt. Tamalpais down to the ocean. At the end of the trail, the hikers would meet other friends at a bar in Stinson Beach for a drink and lunch. As they approached the bar, Glantz wondered what would happen there. On January 1, 1998, after all, every bar in California was to become smoke free. Glantz had actually opposed the state law making bars smoke free because he doubted that the state legislature would stand up to the tobacco industry and pass a strong law. He also believed that such matters were best left to local communities. The tobacco industry had already mounted a major campaign to encourage people to ignore the law. By then, however, most people thought Glantz was responsible for the law. He expected to walk into another smoky bar and hear comments from his friends that he had gone too far.

But he was pleasantly surprised. A couple of people stood outside the bar smoking cigarettes, but the air inside was smoke free. Bars, the last bastion of smoking, were smoke free. California had indeed come a long way since 1978, when attorneys Peter Hanauer and Paul Loveday had recruited Glantz for an ill-fated effort to pass a state law requiring non-smoking sections in restaurants. They did not even dare think about bars.

THE CHANGING ENVIRONMENT OF TOBACCO

The landscape surrounding tobacco was not changing merely in California. By New Year's Day 1998, tobacco was a highly visible issue in American politics. President Bill Clinton allowed his Food and Drug Administration to assert jurisdiction over tobacco products as drug delivery devices. Forty-one states had sued the tobacco industry for defrauding the public out of billions of dollars that taxpayers had spent to treat sick smokers; the states would soon force the tobacco industry to pay $200 billion to reimburse them for part of those costs.[1] Thousands of individuals sued the industry and some won. The industry was being forced to accept controls—albeit limited—on its advertising practices. Millions of pages of previously secret tobacco industry documents were made public, first in print,[2–7] then on the Internet and in a depository created from the documents that Attorney General Hubert Humphrey III of Minnesota forced the tobacco industry to make public. These documents showed that the tobacco industry had known for decades that nicotine is addictive and that smoking causes a wide variety of diseases. They also demonstrated how the tobacco industry used its considerable public relations, legal, and political muscle to hide this information from the public and the courts. Later in 1998 Congress had a rancorous debate over whether to enact national tobacco control legislation that put some restrictions on the tobacco industry in exchange for giving it legal immunity. In the end, Congress strengthened public health provisions of the proposed legislation to the point that the tobacco industry and its political allies killed it.

This burst of activity reflected the groundwork that had been laid over the previous two decades by tobacco control activists who had been working all over the United States to change how people viewed the tobacco industry and its behavior. Beginning in the 1980s, California activists, led by Hanauer and Loveday, created hundreds of city and county ordinances to protect nonsmokers from secondhand smoke and otherwise restrict the tobacco industry by working through their city and county officials. These local activists created strong public support for tobacco control policies. Even so, the tobacco industry continued to dominate the California Legislature, where tobacco control policies had scant support.

But in 1988 activists from the environmental movement and the American Lung Association and American Cancer Society reacted to this legislative impasse by creating the largest and most innovative program in the world through the initiative process, by which voters enact a law by popular vote. California voters enacted an initiative known as Proposition 99, which increased the tobacco tax by twenty-five cents a pack and devoted 20 percent of the money raised to fund a tobacco control program. Virtually overnight, California's investment in tobacco control went from almost nothing to over $100 million a year in schools, communities, and counties and at the state level. In addition, nearly $20 million a year was available to California researchers to conduct tobacco-related research. These programs dwarfed anything that any other state or the federal government had ever done on tobacco.

Far from running a traditional "smoking will kill you" campaign, the California effort viewed tobacco as a social and political problem and went after the tobacco industry directly and aggressively. The network of local tobacco control advocates that Proposition 99 created lit the afterburners on the nonsmokers' rights movement. Communities started passing clean indoor air and other tobacco control ordinances so fast that it was hard to keep track of them all. The culture around tobacco was changing. The initial results of the California campaign were nothing short of amazing: it tripled the rate of decline in tobacco use.[8] Unfortunately for the public health, the tobacco industry appreciated that this campaign was costing it billions of dollars in lost sales and mobilized to divert the money from tobacco control and to constrain the program to ineffective strategies. Nevertheless, the California experience shows that it is possible to rapidly reduce tobacco consumption if the political will is there to do it.

The tobacco industry was not alone in its efforts to divert money from tobacco control programs. Organized medicine and other constituencies that wanted more money spent on medical services for the poor spearheaded the lobbying effort to redirect money into medical services. Politicians in both parties were happy to do the industry's bidding in exchange for campaign contributions or because of a common ideological position.[9-11] In 1994, after several years of rapid reductions in tobacco use, the industry brought this progress to a halt.[12]

For public health advocates, success in political arenas required that they set aside the conciliatory tactics they had relied on in the past and learn to be more confrontational in dealing directly with the tobacco industry. However, they were less willing to confront the industry's surrogates, especially organized medicine or powerful politicians.

While the story of tobacco control in California reflects the individuals and organizations who were involved, the story is relevant every-

where. The tobacco industry's efforts to influence state and local programs are controlled nationally, and the patterns in California have re-
appeared wherever public health advocates try to clean the air or control
the tobacco industry. As a new century begins, more and more states are
implementing large-scale tobacco control programs, often through dedicated tobacco taxes or as parts of settlements of lawsuits with the tobacco
industry. Massachusetts was the first state to follow California, when
voters there passed Question 1 in 1992; Arizona was next in 1994, followed by Oregon in 1996.[13-17] Other states, including Wisconsin, Michi-
gan, and Maine, created tobacco control programs through the legislative process, and Florida, Minnesota, Texas, and Mississippi, among
others, did so through legal settlements with the tobacco industry.

RECURRING THEMES

The story of the battle over tobacco control in California has several re-
curring universal themes.

First, although health promotion and medical care have a logical connection, there has always been a tension between them in the allocation
of tax dollars. In the battles over the Proposition 99 revenues, the existence of an a priori agreement between those involved in health promotion and those involved in medical care did little to curtail these battles.
Moreover, the financial and political interests of organized medicine often had more in common with the tobacco industry than the public
health groups,[18,19] who had been marginal players in California politics
before Proposition 99 passed. Despite the fact that these groups successfully defeated the tobacco industry in a major electoral contest to pass
Proposition 99, it was hard for them to understand their power and wield
it after the election.

Second, it is easiest to make policy in areas where there is a clear consensus on how to achieve the program's goals. Before Proposition 99, no
one had ever run a large-scale tobacco control program and no one knew
exactly how to do it. In contrast, everyone knew how to spend money on
direct medical services. This difference, combined with the lack of precedent for mounting a prevention program of the magnitude of the one
created by Proposition 99, complicated the health advocates' task. The
absence of a proven approach to reduce tobacco use could have been
mitigated with a long time frame to develop and implement the program
and a careful evaluation process. Politicians, however, who tend to rely

on short schedules and temporary settlements, did not allow enough time for such a process, even though Proposition 99's tobacco control program was breaking new ground. This situation led anti-tobacco advocates to make early compromises that would come back to haunt them.

Third, programs tend to remain in place once established. Temporary agreements or one-time diversions of funds, as happened when tobacco control proponents agreed to allow some anti-tobacco education money to be used for medical services, become precedents in subsequent budget years because operating programs build their own constituencies.

Fourth, and finally, informed and activated public opinion is a powerful weapon in health policy generally and on tobacco policy specifically. When tobacco policy is left to the inside game played in back rooms, the outcome will favor the existing power structure. The tobacco industry is a tough, experienced inside player who has benefited from the existing power structure. In contrast, the public health groups' power is amplified in public arenas, where tobacco industry's power is sharply curtailed.

CONCLUSION

The California experience shows that it is possible to dramatically change how people think about tobacco and the tobacco industry and rapidly reduce tobacco consumption. Based on the initial results of the program, the state was on its way to reducing tobacco consumption by 75 percent in just ten years.[20-22] The California story shows that it is possible to run such programs successfully as long as the public health community exerts power effectively. It also shows that it is possible for the tobacco industry and its political allies to weaken or destroy these programs when the public health community is timid. The tobacco industry, faced with losing billions of dollars in sales, is highly motivated and aggressive. The controlling factor in the outcome is whether the public health community is willing to directly confront this reality and devote the organizational resources—both financial and political—to beating the tobacco industry. Victory is possible but not easy, and it requires constant, determined vigilance.

While Proposition 99 passed in 1988, it had its origins over a decade earlier, in the emergence of the nonsmokers' rights movement. In contrast to the large voluntary health organizations, the grassroots advocates of nonsmokers' rights saw political and policy interventions as the key to doing something about tobacco. Rather than convincing one person at a time to stop smoking, they fought to enact laws requiring smoke-free workplaces, public places, and restaurants.[23,24] Their efforts brought about systemic, environmental changes that had an impact on how citizens viewed the tobacco industry and their rights as nonsmokers. They made smoke-free bars not only possible but reasonable.

The California story begins with them.

CHAPTER 2

Beginnings: The Nonsmokers' Rights Movement

In the early 1970s a few people had the radical idea that nonsmokers should not have to breathe secondhand tobacco smoke. At that time it was considered impolite to ask people not to smoke. Smoking was not only acceptable; it was the norm. The executive director of the California division of the American Lung Association was a chain-smoker, and the American Heart Association distributed ashtrays and packs of cigarettes at its board meetings. Offering someone a cigarette was a way to open social discourse. Even the most ardent nonsmokers' rights advocates were only seeking nonsmoking sections in public places. No one dared even think of a smoke-free society.

Finding little support from the mainstream health organizations like the American Cancer Society, American Heart Association, and American Lung Association, nonsmokers' rights activists formed a loose network of grassroots organizations with various names, the most common being Group Against Smoking Pollution or GASP. The nonsmokers' rights activists viewed smoking and the tobacco industry as a social, environmental, and political problem; in contrast, the medical establishment—including most of the voluntary health organizations—viewed smoking as a medical problem in which individual patients (smokers) were to be treated (by telling them to stop smoking). The establishment's approach did not mesh easily with the tobacco control advocates' policy-oriented approach.

While the medical and health establishments did not take the non-smokers' rights movement seriously, the tobacco industry did. The industry recognized the issue of secondhand smoke as a major threat to the social support network that it had spent decades building around tobacco use. As early as 1973, the tobacco industry clearly identified the emerging nonsmokers' rights movement as a problem: "More and more, smoking is being pictured as socially unacceptable. The goal seems [to be] the involvement of others—non-smokers, children, etc.—in addition to health and government organizations. The main thrust of these zealots seems to be that 'smoking is not a personal right because it hurts others; that smoking harms non-smoking adults, children, and even the yet unborn.'"[1]

By 1978, the industry recognized the full dimensions of the threat represented by the nonsmokers' rights movement. A research report prepared by the Roper Organization for the Tobacco Institute (the tobacco industry's political arm) concluded:

> The original Surgeon General's report, followed by this first "hazard" warning on cigarette packages, the subsequent "danger" warning on cigarette packages, the removal of cigarette advertising from television and the inclusion of the "danger" warning in cigarette advertising, were all "blows" of sorts for the tobacco industry. They were, however, blows that the cigarette industry could successfully weather because they were all directed against the smoker himself.
>
> The anti-smoking forces' latest tack, however—on the passive smoking issue—is another matter. *What the smoker does to himself may be his business, but what the smoker does to the non-smoker is quite a different matter.* . . . Nearly six out of ten believe that smoking is hazardous to the non-smokers' health, up sharply over the last four years. More than two-thirds of nonsmokers believe it; nearly half of all smokers believe it.
>
> *This we see as the most dangerous development to the viability of the tobacco industry that has yet occurred.*[2] [emphasis added]

The nonsmokers' rights movement was growing and having some significant legislative successes. In 1973 the Arizona Legislature ended smoking in elevators, libraries, theaters, museums, concert halls, and buses. In 1975 Minnesota mandated separate smoking areas in restaurants, meeting rooms, and workplaces, in addition to the types of restrictions put in place in Arizona.[3] The Minnesota law was the last time that clean indoor air legislation would pass without vigorous opposition from the tobacco industry.

THE BERKELEY ORDINANCE

In the spring of 1973, lawyer and legal editor Peter Hanauer went to a meeting of Berkeley GASP after his wife saw a meeting notice on a community bulletin board. Hanauer recalled, "It was a fairly ineffective group at the time. I mean, we were busy grinding out leaflets and trying to get a few new members here and there."[4] While there were thoughts about some greater level of activism—two of the founders, Irene and Dave Peterson, had created a foundation to provide legal representation to people who were affected by secondhand smoke in the workplace—not much happened until they were joined by Paul Loveday, a former professional basketball player turned lawyer. Loveday brought a clear vision and strong leadership to the group and soon became president of GASP. The aggressive Loveday and studious Hanauer, who was elected treasurer, were the "odd couple" that became the backbone of the nonsmokers' rights movement in California.

Encouraged by the Minnesota Clean Indoor Air Act, GASP, led by Loveday, Hanauer, and Tim Moder, a chemist who turned his home into the group's headquarters,[3] decided to persuade the Berkeley City Council to pass an ordinance restricting smoking in public indoor spaces and requiring separate sections for smokers and nonsmokers in restaurants. Although they wanted a statewide law, they knew there was little chance of success without some preliminary steps. Passing a local law would show that nonsmoking sections were possible and would give them some experience in writing legislation. The proposed ordinance was introduced in the Berkeley City Council in April 1976.

After a year-long campaign, which included numerous city council meetings as well as meetings with restauranteurs and local merchants, the Berkeley City Council passed the ordinance by a 9-0 vote in April 1977. The Berkeley victory illustrated an important lesson for Hanauer: "At the local level, as we discovered over the years, we could beat the tobacco industry, because their lobbyists could not defeat grassroots organizations who had the ears of their neighbors and friends who were on the city council."[4]

PROPOSITION 5

Their Berkeley success encouraged Loveday and Hanauer to try to get the California Legislature to pass a state clean indoor air law. The tobacco industry, having learned its lesson in Minnesota, vigorously and successfully blocked GASP's attempt to replicate the Minnesota Clean Indoor Air Act in California. The bill did not even get out of committee.

After failing in the legislature, Loveday and Hanauer decided to take the issue directly to the voters through California's initiative process. The initiative, known as the California Clean Indoor Air Act, made smoking illegal in all public places unless they were specifically exempted. It required that partitions be erected in offices and public places, including restaurants, to separate smokers and nonsmokers. Violators were to be fined fifty dollars. In an effort to write an enforceable and reasonable law, Loveday and Hanauer included some exemptions, such as tobacco shops. Since the drug laws were not being enforced at rock concerts, they exempted rock concerts. This exemption, while reasonable from an intellectual point of view, was to become a major issue in the campaign. The idea of protecting nonsmokers from secondhand smoke was popular; polls (including those commissioned by the tobacco industry) showed support by a 3-1 margin.

Putting a proposed law before California voters as a statutory initiative requires proponents to collect valid signatures of 5 percent of the number who voted in the previous gubernatorial election,[5] which meant collecting 300,000 signatures in 1977. While most initiative campaigns rely on paid signature gatherers, the Proposition 5 advocates did not have that luxury because they had very little money. Moder became the paid campaign coordinator, working out of his house with his own printing press. By using campaign workers who were almost all volunteers, advocates qualified the initiative at a cost of only $50,000, the least amount of money per signature ever spent to qualify a statewide initiative.[4] The initiative appeared on the November 1978 ballot as Proposition 5.

Loveday and Hanauer formed a new organization to run the campaign, Californians for Clean Indoor Air. While nominally a coalition of many health and environmental groups, GASP provided the backbone of support. Loveday and Hanauer approached the voluntary health agencies for support, expecting them to be enthusiastic, but came away disappointed. Only the American Cancer Society (ACS) expressed interest in the initiative, and that interest was tempered. According to Hanauer,

> We did get the ear of Ray Weisberg, who was then the chair of the Public Affairs Committee of the California Cancer Society. He agreed with us . . . that the way to really get smoking reduced was to make it socially unacceptable. This was our whole rationale. We not only felt that eliminating smoking in

public places and the workplace was good for nonsmokers but that it also reduced smoking in the long run. Of course, the tobacco industry agreed with
us. We wished some of the health agencies had agreed with us as much as the
industry did. It took a long time. The Cancer Society came around mainly because of Ray Weisberg, but the other agencies at that time were very slow in
responding and gave sort of token support.[4]

The voluntary health agencies, particularly the ACS in California, supported the campaign with some money but were not heavily involved in
collecting signatures or conducting the campaign. Weisberg also convinced the California Medical Association (CMA) and the American
Lung Association (ALA) to support the initiative, which made Proposition 5 appear more mainstream. The CMA put its name on the letterhead
but, according to Hanauer, "wouldn't lift a finger during the whole campaign."[4] The CMA sent the "Yes on Prop 5" campaign a seven-dollar
invoice for some photocopying it had done for the campaign, which
Hanauer refused to pay.[4]

In addition to Weisberg, the other important recruit to the campaign
was Stanton Glantz, an assistant professor of medicine at the University
of California at San Francisco. Glantz, a Ph.D. in applied mechanics and
engineering economics, conducted research on the function of the heart
and was an expert in statistics. Glantz, who combined a background in
political activism with his scientific training, would serve as the campaign's technical expert. Unlike some scientists, he was willing to do public battle with the tobacco industry.

THE TOBACCO INDUSTRY JOINS THE BATTLE

The tobacco industry mobilized against Proposition 5 before it was even
written. According to Ernest Pepples, vice president for law at Brown and
Williamson Tobacco, the industry began planning its strategy

> before the terms of Proposition 5 were even known or concepts to combat it
> had been developed. Because of the early start a California Action Plan was
> presented to the chief executive officers [of the tobacco companies] within
> three weeks of the time the sponsors filed their "Clean Indoor Air Act" ini-
> tiative and its provisions became known for the first time. That Action Plan
> became the basic blue print of the campaign concepts, strategy, organization
> and tactics for the entire campaign to defeat Proposition 5. The Tobacco In-
> stitute made Jack Kelly a full time employee—he had been the paid executive
> of California's tobacco distributors group—to devote all his efforts to the
> campaign.[6]

The framing of the Proposition 5 debate was important to the tobacco industry, which wanted to avoid health issues and nonsmokers' rights to clean air. The industry's preferred framing was that voters should fight off government intrusion. Jim Stockdale of Philip Morris commented on the rights question:

> What troubles me is the danger of having the issue defined at the onset the way our opponents would like it to be defined, namely smoker vs. non-smoker. Our strategy should put us on the offensive. . . . Will the anti-smoking groups attempt to polarize the electorate into two groups—smokers vs. non-smokers—or will they attempt to broaden their appeal by coopting the individual rights argument (i.e., a non-smoker has an inalienable right to breathe "clean air")? We should have strategies for either situation. We have to clarify the thrust the campaign should take. The message should be to vote "no" to further governmental encroachment on individual rights.[7]

Using this thrust, the industry hoped to broaden its base of support to include groups such as Libertarians. The call to fight off government intrusion would persist for the next twenty years in the industry's battles over clean indoor air policies.

Ed Grefe, vice president for public affairs at Philip Morris, became actively involved in the Proposition 5 campaign and specifically blocked any mention of the health issue. According to Grefe, "the biggest argument I had internally throughout the entire campaign was to convince the other companies to keep their mouths shut about the health issue. They would say, 'Shouldn't we put out a little brochure?' I said, 'Forget it, we want no goddamn brochure on the health question. We can't win on the health question. We'll lose.' Legally, they could fight and win on the health question, they'd been doing it for years, but politically they couldn't. It's no use bucking public opinion."[8]

The industry, recognizing from its own polling that it had virtually no public credibility, decided to act through a nominally independent campaign committee known as Californians for Common Sense (CCS). Even though CCS was created, financed, and controlled by the tobacco companies through a closely coordinated effort, CCS attempted to minimize and even hide its industry connections. The industry wanted the public to believe that CCS was a group of concerned California citizens. As a result, several important guiding principles were established to keep the profile of the tobacco industry as low as possible. As Ernest Pepples of Brown and Williamson wrote in a secret Campaign Report,

> All campaign functions would be operated through the citizens committee, Californians for Common Sense.

> Tobacco company visibility would be confined to financial contributions to CCS. There would be no attempt to disclaim or discount the amount of tobacco contributions.
>
> Tobacco company personnel would not make campaign appearances, occupy campaign positions or make public statements relative to the campaign.
>
> No campaign events, programs or advertising would be directed to college campuses, specifically, or to youth in general.[6]

Although Pepples stated that there would be "no attempt to disclaim or discount the amount of tobacco contributions," the tobacco industry kept a low profile during the campaign, and campaign spokesmen denied the industry's financial role until legally required campaign disclosure statements proved the industry was financing the campaign. On one occasion, CCS issued a press release that misstated tobacco industry contributions to the campaign by leaving out $300,000 of in-kind campaign contributions. As in all similar campaigns everywhere since, more than 99 percent of the money came from the tobacco industry.

In spite of the prominent role given to CCS, however, the tobacco companies maintained tight control of CCS activities from behind the scenes. As Pepples noted in his Campaign Report,

> A group of 5 tobacco company representatives consisting of Jim Dowdell who was succeeded by Charles Tucker from RJR, Ed Grefe from Philip Morris, Arthur Stevens from Lorillard, Joe Greer from Liggett & Myers and Ernest Pepples from B&W kept in constant contact with the operation of CCS. Visits were made at least once a month by the group to the CCS headquarters in both San Francisco and Los Angeles. Also frequent telephone conferences were held between Woodward & McDowell [the firm hired to manage the campaign] and the five company people. During the final month of the campaign, almost daily conferences were held by telephone including Woodward & McDowell and Jack Kelly together with Lance Tarrance [the tobacco industry's pollster] in Houston conferring with the five company representatives.[6]

This tight control by the tobacco companies stood in sharp contrast with the industry's public position during the campaign: that Proposition 5 was a local California matter and that Californians for Common Sense was a campaign organization established by local citizens as a freestanding, autonomous organization. The industry's actual control also contrasted sharply with that of the national voluntary health organizations, which treated Proposition 5 as a local California matter and stayed out.

By the end of the campaign, Proposition 5's proponents had raised and spent $633,465, an amount dwarfed by the tobacco companies' $6.4 million—divided among the companies in proportion to their shares of the cigarette market. The justification for this level of spending was simple in terms of protecting industry sales. Pepples did the math:

> *If it is assumed that the passage of Proposition 5 would have caused a decline in volume of just one cigarette per California smoker per day, the chart attached to this letter shows the industry would have suffered an after tax loss equal to $5.9 million in the first year.* On that basis, it can be said that the industry will recover its "investment" [i.e., the $6.4 million spent to defeat Proposition 5] over a period of one year. If it is assumed that the passage of Proposition 5 would have caused a decline of 2 cigarettes per day per smoker, then the industry can expect to recover the $5.9 million expense in only 6 months.
>
> California represents about 10% of the population of the United States or 20 million people. *California is regarded as a trendsetter and theoretically if Proposition 5 had passed it would have had an impact on sales elsewhere in the United States.*[9] [emphasis added]

The spending by the tobacco industry exceeded the combined expenditures of both candidates for governor and for many years remained a record for election spending in California.

THE $43 MILLION CLAIM

The alleged high cost of implementing the initiative was one of the tobacco industry's key themes in its campaign against Proposition 5. In the previous election of June 1978, California voters had passed Proposition 13, which slashed property taxes and started the "taxpayers' revolt," and the issue of government waste was high on the public agenda. For months the tobacco industry's campaign hammered the claim that Proposition 5 would cost taxpayers $43 million to implement.

Proposition 5 proponents challenged this claim in letters to television and radio stations in early September, shortly after the tobacco industry began its massive advertising campaign against the initiative, asserting that the advertisements were "false and misleading." (Proponents argued that Proposition 5 would actually save money by reducing smoking and the associated costs.) The stations ignored this challenge. A couple of weeks later, someone leaked three important documents to the Yes on 5 campaign: a planning poll that Houston-based pollster V. Lance Tarrance and Associates had conducted for CCS in December 1977 and two reports presenting cost estimates for implementing Proposition 5 that provided the basis for the industry's advertising claims. These documents revealed yet another instance of the industry saying whatever it thought necessary to sway the public. The Tarrance poll in fact showed strong support for the idea of clean indoor air among all segments of California voters and tested the arguments that the industry was considering for its campaign to defeat the initiative. None of these arguments moved the voters save one: cost to taxpayers.

The pollster asked people three questions about how they would vote, depending on what the initiative would cost taxpayers to implement.[10] The initiative gathered a landslide 71.2 percent "yes" vote if it cost $0.5 million to implement. The margin of victory dropped substantially if the initiative cost taxpayers $5 million to implement; only 53.6 percent said they would vote "yes." If the initiative cost $20 million to implement, the "yes" vote fell to 41.4 percent and the industry won. The tobacco industry then hired the consulting firm of Economic Research Associates (ERA), which produced a report claiming Proposition 5 would cost taxpayers $19.7 million to post No Smoking signs in state buildings.[11] ERA produced a second report stating that enforcement would cost another $23 million, bringing the total alleged cost to $43 million, twice the amount that the tobacco industry needed to push voters toward a "no" vote.[12]

To obtain the $19.7 million cost estimate, ERA assumed that No Smoking signs would cost $27.50 each, even though hardware stores were selling them for less than $1.00. ERA made an even more fundamental error: they got the arithmetic wrong. In estimating the number of No Smoking signs that would be needed, ERA calculated the total square footage of office space in state buildings and then multiplied the square root of the office area by 4 to obtain an estimate of the number of linear feet of office walls in state buildings (it was assumed that signs would be placed at regular intervals). But the square root of 207.2 million square feet was miscalculated as 14.4 *million* feet whereas it should have been 14.4 *thousand* feet. Thus, even using the industry's own methods and $27.50 signs, the report overestimated the cost of signs by a factor of 1000. Simply correcting the arithmetic error brought the industry's cost estimate down to $19,700.

Loveday and Glantz thought they had caught the industry in a major scandal. They had the poll showing that a high cost claim was necessary to defeat the initiative and they had a flawed report that seemed designed to justify the number that the tobacco industry needed. On September, 19, 1977, they held press conferences in Los Angeles and Sacramento exposing the poll and the arithmetic error. Unfortunately, few members of the press understood what a square root was. According to Loveday, "What was really funny; I mean you look back on it and you say, 'God this was so aggravating, so frustrating.' The press didn't understand the math. Stan would try to explain at a press conference what had happened and that the press just couldn't . . . they didn't know a square root from a cigarette. . . . You can discover something like that but getting to the public with that information through the press when the tobacco industry is spending $6 million. . . . It was a pretty uphill battle." [13]

Even when the initiative's supporters thought they had a winning issue, the industry quickly recovered. On the way home from their press conference announcing the mistake, Loveday and Glantz heard a radio advertisement ridiculing the lower number. As Grefe observed, "All that square root stuff? The error is irrelevant. The whole strategy is to put the other person on the defensive. If I say, 'It'll cost a billion dollars' and you say, 'No, it'll only cost a million,' you've lost, you're dead." [8]

Even though the industry was successful in framing the election fight as a cost issue at this point, it continued to worry that the health issue could appear. According to Pepples,

> Lance Tarrance's organization kept a close watch on the effect of the pro-5 advertising. If other people's smoke became a dominant issue in the closing days of the campaign, we had an alternate ad campaign which was prepared and kept in the can in case it was needed. It had been tested in Madison, Wisconsin. It was based on work done by BBD&O [Batten, Barton, Durstine, and Osborne, an advertising firm with longstanding tobacco accounts]. The testing at Madison showed no perceptible improvement in attitudes about "other people's smoke," but it seemed to be bombproof. [6]

The industry never needed these advertisements because Proposition 5's supporters never succeeded in getting the campaign focused on health issues. In the end, the tobacco industry defeated Proposition 5, with 54 percent voting "no."

THE POSTMORTEM

The extent and intensity of the industry's efforts surprised Proposition 5's proponents. As Hanauer explained,

> I think we weren't prepared psychologically or politically for what hit us. I mean we were a bit naive in those days. We were just a bunch of citizens trying to get clear indoor air and who could be against that? If people want to smoke, they can wait and go outside. What's the big deal? We heard the first tobacco industry ads on the radio against us, months and months in advance.

They started advertising even before we qualified for the ballot. . . . They wanted to get the public questioning what we were doing as early as possible. . . . We laughed at the ads . . . we were naive in terms of just how sophisticated the industry really was and how they could turn the public against what the public had thought was a good idea.[4]

Proposition 5 did have some vulnerabilities that made it open to attack by the industry. In particular, the specific exceptions to the requirement that public places provide nonsmoking sections were ridiculed by the industry. For example, rock concerts, professional bowling and wrestling matches, pool halls, and gaming halls were exempted. The tobacco industry latched onto this distinction in a biting series of radio advertisements ridiculing the initiative.

Even in defeat Loveday believed that something had been accomplished. He observed, "Prior to Proposition 5, people who were concerned about nonsmokers' rights were looked on as real kooks; maybe you'd read something about it on the 42nd page. That's not true anymore; it's a very respectable issue. We have now gotten the point that people's cigarette smoke is harmful to the nonsmokers. And I think we've laid the groundwork where we can have something like this passed in the future in California and other places."[13] Indeed, since strategists for the tobacco industry knew that people did not approve of secondhand smoke, the campaign against Proposition 5 had to acknowledge that secondhand smoke was bad while claiming that Proposition 5 was worse. Pepples acknowledged the industry's vulnerability in California: "After election surveys show that 71% of the electorate say they would support 'some regulation' of smoking in public places."[6] In the process of defeating Proposition 5, however, the tobacco industry ran the largest public awareness campaign on secondhand smoke the world had ever seen.

While the tobacco industry did what it had to do to win, there were limits to the strategies it would pursue. Attacking the Legislature could have helped defeat the initiative, but this strategy was rejected because the industry was worried about offending its defenders in the Legislature, where it had historically been well protected. According to Pepples,

Woodward & McDowell very much wanted to carry a theme in the advertising which was a parody on the legislature. The opinion surveys indicated that the voters currently hold the legislature in very low esteem. The proponents had begun to respond to our original message that this was a bad law, poorly drafted. They conceded that it had some flaws but said not to worry, the legislature will take care of any flaw by amendment. Woodward & Mc-

Dowell, therefore, urged a direct attack on the legislature to take advantage of the negative voter attitudes toward the legislature and to crowd the proponents into a corner. The companies differed in their reaction but after internal discussion, it was agreed that the tobacco industry must live with the California legislature for years to come and should not damage its relations by supporting advertising which made fun of the legislature.[6]

This caution proved to be a wise move, since the California Legislature consistently supported the tobacco industry on a wide range of issues over the years, in particular with regard to diverting Proposition 99 funds away from tobacco control. As always, the tobacco industry was thinking in the long term.

Loveday would get a chance to try again in just two years, when he, Hanauer, and their compatriots presented California's voters with Proposition 10.

PROPOSITION 10

After the defeat of Proposition 5 in November 1978, its key proponents were exhausted, even though many supporters were urging them to try again. A few months after the Proposition 5 defeat, Glantz and his wife, Marsha, had dinner with Loveday and the inevitable subject of a second attempt came up. Loveday responded, "Are you nuts? I'm going to go out and make some money!" Two weeks later, Loveday called Glantz and asked him if he would join a new effort to try another statewide initiative.

What happened?

In the June 1978 election, California voters had overwhelmingly passed Proposition 13, the Jarvis-Gann Initiative, which drastically cut property taxes, despite the fact that most of the state's political and business establishment opposed it. The campaign to pass Proposition 13 was managed by a relatively new political consulting firm named Butcher-Forde.

A major electoral victory naturally attracts attention to a consulting firm, even if the victory is on a comparatively easy issue, such as getting people to vote to cut their own taxes. But Butcher-Forde also attracted attention within the California political community for the innovative way in which it managed and financed the campaign to qualify and pass Proposition 13. Rather than relying on volunteer or paid circulators to gather the necessary signatures along with a separate fund-raising campaign, Butcher-Forde combined these two operations. They ran a large direct mail campaign in which they sent petitions to prospective supporters with a request that they sign the petitions (and ask a few friends to sign), then return the signed petitions together with a donation. Thus, rather than costing money to collect the necessary signatures, the process of collecting the signatures became a fund-raising device. In the process, Butcher-Forde built a mailing list of supporters that could be sent subsequent fund-raising appeals to finance the election campaign. And, of course, Butcher-Forde took a commission on every piece of direct mail that was sent.

After winning Proposition 13, William Butcher and Arnold Forde were looking for another campaign to manage. Based on polling, they identified clean indoor air as a popular issue with the voters. They approached Loveday and Hanauer with a proposal that Butcher-Forde manage a campaign for a new clean indoor air initiative. Loveday and Hanauer would write the initiative and serve as spokesmen and Butcher-Forde would do the rest. They would raise the money, qualify the initiative, and run a winning campaign. It all seemed so easy.

Hanauer and Loveday drafted a new initiative, cleaning up some of the problems with Proposition 5 and calling it the Smoking and No Smoking Sections Initiative. The new initiative did not distinguish between rock and jazz concerts, eliminated the need for partitions, limited what government could spend on signs, provided for citations for violators, and gave nonsmokers fewer protections than Proposition 5 would have. Californians for Clean Indoor Air was renamed Californians for Smoking and No Smoking Sections to run the campaign, coalition partners were recruited, and the effort for a new initiative was formally started on August 24, 1979.

Unfortunately, Butcher-Forde found that getting people to give money to support clean indoor air was not as easy as getting them to support cutting their own taxes. The consulting firm dumped Californians for Smoking and No Smoking Sections two months into the signature drive. According to Hanauer,

> [Butcher-Forde] started organizing these fund-raising letter campaigns. They discovered early on what we had discovered during Prop 5, that this is not a pocketbook issue for people. That there are a lot of people who say, "Yes, we're with you," but if you get $10 out of them, you're lucky. . . . By the time we were halfway through the signature drive, the two of them came up to wine and dine Paul and me at a dinner at the airport, basically to kiss us off and say, "I guess you realize this is not a pocketbook issue and there's no way we can continue on this because we're losing our shirts." And we were happy to get rid of them because we didn't like them.[4]

Butcher-Forde's departure was a problem for tobacco control advocates, however. It was one thing to run a campaign and be defeated at the polls by a multimillion dollar advertising blitz from the tobacco industry. It was quite another to sponsor an initiative that did not even qualify for the ballot. Advocates felt that they could not back away from the initiative campaign.

Loveday, Hanauer, and their colleagues began a frantic effort to mobilize the old grassroots network and raise money. In the end, they managed to collect the necessary signatures, thanks in part to the opening of the *Star Wars* sequel, *The Empire Strikes Back*. The film was immensely popular and attracted long lines. Volunteers worked the lines to collect signatures. On June 26, 1980, the initiative qualified for the November 1980 ballot as Proposition 10.

The tobacco industry started detailed planning to defeat Proposition 10 well before it qualified for the ballot. On February 25, 1980, the tobacco industry's polling firm, Tarrance and Associates, presented a detailed analysis of Proposition 10, showing some changes in voter attitudes since 1978. According to the company's analysis, "These data suggest a strong feeling of 'fair' play and equal rights on the side of the anti-smokers that has not been apparent in previous campaigns."[14] Proposition 10 had the early support of 72 percent of the voters, up from the 68 percent that Proposition 5 had at the same time, primarily because nonsmokers felt that they had a right to clean indoor air. The report warned the industry that its successful campaign against Proposition 5 *"did not* lessen the public's desire for smoking regulation, it only convinced the public that Proposition 5 was a bad law" (emphasis in original).[14]

Tarrance and Associates suggested that Proposition 10 was more popular than Proposition 5 because it appeared to insure equal rights for smokers and nonsmokers and it lacked specifics about place, time, and enforcement methods. The report recommended these primary campaign themes to oppose the initiative: the ambiguity of the law and the power it would give to bureaucrats, the inequality of the bill because it gave preferential treatment to nonsmokers, the waste of police resources, the outrageousness of the fine, the adequacy of current law, and the undesirability of government intrusion in private lives.

The tobacco industry hired Robert Nelson and Eileen Padberg of the political consulting firm of Robert Nelson and Associates to run the campaign. Nelson incorporated Californians Against Regulatory Excess (CARE) on June 12, 1980, to serve as the front group to run the campaign. They then proceeded to recruit some prominent Californians to serve on the CARE's board of directors.[15] The fact that the campaign manager recruited the board (rather than the other way around) underscored the fact that the board was mere window dressing. Indeed, before the board ever held a formal meeting, Nelson had retained the advertising agency Woodward, McDowell & Larson, the same agency that had run the campaign against Proposition 5, to develop and run CARE's ads against Proposition 10.

While the tobacco industry's money bought them victory in 1978 in the Proposition 5 campaign, their spending started to hurt them toward the end of the campaign. Mervyn Field, head of the nonpartisan Field Institute, which conducts the California Poll, observed two years later: "Another negative aspect to disproportionately heavy advertising is that it becomes an issue in itself. For example, with Proposition 5, the fact that the tobacco industry was spending as much money as it was to defeat it, became an issue. There was a sort of a counter trend in the closing days of the campaign. *If the tobacco industry had spent a couple more million dollars, it might have lost the election*" (emphasis added).[16] Aware that the tobacco industry and its money had become an issue in the Proposition 5 campaign, CARE attempted to minimize tobacco industry involvement in the Proposition 10 campaign, despite the fact that the organization was established by and for the tobacco industry. On August 15, 1980, CARE distributed a letter stating, "Cost prohibits the No on 10 campaign from using media."[17] In September 1980, when an interviewer from the *Los Angeles Times* asked Padberg, "Do you need the cigarette companies to fight this measure?" Padberg responded, "We could do it without them. It certainly would be a lot easier with them. But we could do it without them."[18] In the end, the tobacco companies delayed their major advertising blitz until the weeks just before the election, pouring a relatively restrained $2.7 million into the CARE campaign against Proposition 10.

Although proponents of the initiative spent $707,678, it was not enough money to overcome the industry's saturation advertising. The voters rejected Proposition 10 by the same margin—54 percent "no," 46 percent "yes"—as they had Proposition 5 two years earlier.

GOING LOCAL

In December 1980, a month after losing the Proposition 10 election, Loveday, Hanauer, Glantz, Weisberg, and Chuck Mawson (a volunteer who had kept an industry "look-alike" bill bottled up in the state legislature during the Proposition 10 fight) got together in Hanauer's living room in the Berkeley hills to decide what to do next. After suffering their second defeat in a statewide initiative, they decided that it was time to change tactics. The Legislature was clearly under the thumb of the tobacco industry and, while the public supported the idea of clean indoor air, the nonsmokers' rights advocates recognized that they could not raise the money needed to counter effectively the tobacco industry's advertising campaigns against a state initiative. On the other hand, they knew from both polling and personal experience that the public supported clean indoor air.

They decided to work on local ordinances because the one clear success they could point to was the Berkeley local clean indoor air ordinance. They decided to focus the limited resources of the nonsmokers' rights advocates on one community at a time. They reasoned that, while the tobacco industry would almost certainly oppose every ordinance, their campaign contributions, lobbyists, and massive advertising campaigns would not work as effectively as well-organized residents who knew the members of the city council and favored the ordinance. To raise money, advocates decided to use the mailing list that had been developed during the campaigns for Propositions 5 and 10. Ray Weisberg promised to seek seed money from the American Cancer Society, and Chuck Mawson quit his job as a computer salesman to work full time on the effort, together with the campaign's part-time bookkeeper, Bobbie Jacobson. The campaign organization was renamed Californians for Nonsmokers' Rights (CNR), and the nonsmokers' rights movement entered a new phase.

Seven months later, on July 15, 1981, the first local clean indoor air ordinance was enacted when the city council of Ukiah, a small town 150 miles north of San Francisco, adopted an ordinance that was essentially identical to Proposition 10. Over the next three years, CNR continued to identify and work with local activists throughout California, and by May 1983 twenty-one cities or counties had passed local clean indoor air ordinances. CNR's local ordinance strategy was working.

THE SAN FRANCISCO ORDINANCE

Quentin Kopp, a powerful member of the San Francisco Board of Supervisors, had supported Proposition 5, and Hanauer knew him personally. Hanauer had approached Kopp on several occasions about the possibility of carrying a San Francisco ordinance, and in 1983 Kopp agreed to introduce a comprehensive clean indoor air ordinance for public places and workplaces. But before he could introduce his ordinance, another supervisor, Wendy Nelder, surprised everyone by announcing that she was going to introduce an ordinance limited to workplaces.

A week later Hanauer was on San Francisco radio station KCBS discussing smoking issues in general and CNR specifically, along with Michael Eriksen, who was in charge of health issues for Pacific Bell. (Eriksen subsequently became head of the federal Office on Smoking and Health at the Centers for Disease Control and Prevention.) Hanauer mentioned that CNR was working on a San Francisco ordinance without giving details. Nelder was angry that Hanauer had not mentioned her name and let him know that she wanted nothing to do with him or CNR. CNR was placed in the awkward position of working for an ordinance whose principal sponsor would not talk to the organization's members. Despite the personality problems and vigorous opposition from the tobacco industry, the Board of Supervisors passed Nelder's workplace smoking ordinance by a vote of 10-1 on May 31, 1983. San Francisco became the twenty-second locality in California to enact a clean indoor air ordinance when Mayor Dianne Feinstein signed it into law on June 3, 1983.

The ordinance required that all workplaces have policies on smoking that accommodated the needs of smokers and nonsmokers. If an accommodation acceptable to the nonsmoker could not be found, however, the work area would have to be smoke free. Using language suggested by the Bank of America, the ordinance gave flexibility to employers but established the right to a smoke-free environment for employees.

While the San Francisco ordinance was neither the first nor the strongest, it attracted national and international media attention.

THE TOBACCO INDUSTRY'S COUNTERATTACK

On June 14, 1983, less than two weeks after Feinstein signed the ordinance, several people who described themselves as a "group of union leaders and small businessmen" announced that they were organizing a petition campaign to overturn the ordinance at the polls the following November.[19] The group was nominally chaired by Jim Foster, a gay political activist and founder of San Francisco's Alice B. Toklas Democratic Club. The Chamber of Commerce announced that it was supporting the effort to overturn the ordinance, reversing an earlier agreement with

CNR to support the measure.[4] The campaign against the San Francisco Workplace Ordinance was initially called Californians Against Government Intrusion, but the name was changed to San Franciscans Against Government Intrusion (SFAGI), possibly because the acronym of the original name was pronounced "cagey."[20] The group had until July 1 (thirty days from the date of passage) to collect 19,000 valid signatures for suspending the law and forcing a referendum on the November ballot. David Looman, a political consultant and SFAGI committee member, said, "The tobacco industry has been asked for contributions, but no money has been received from any tobacco firm yet."[19]

The industry provided a substantial war chest—over a million dollars —and hired Nelson-Padberg Consulting (Eileen Padberg had been promoted to a full partnership with Robert Nelson since they had directed the Proposition 10 campaign) to run the San Francisco campaign. Over half the initial budget of $1,046,000, as of July 12, was for advertising, including direct mail, radio, and television. The money that the industry put into the campaign was only part of the effort; the cigarette companies planned to reach smokers with cigarette carton inserts or stickers and point-of-sale materials.[21] As the Nelson-Padberg campaign plan makes clear, Foster and SFAGI had very little to do with decision making for the actual campaign, all of which had been planned in July 1983.[22,23]

In order to collect over 19,000 valid signatures in the two weeks remaining before the July 1 deadline, the tobacco industry hired the Southern California firm of Bader and Associates to collect over 40,000 signatures.[24] The industry's use of paid signature-gatherers, at a cost of $40,000, made it difficult to hide the fact that the tobacco industry was financing the repeal effort.

For activists who had been involved in the campaigns for Propositions 5 and 10, the pattern over the next five months was predictable from previous industry behavior. A campaign manager would be hired to create a "grassroots" organization. The industry would then pretend that this organization was independent, vigorously denying industry involvement. In fact, the campaign would be funded by the industry and managed by the firm it had hired. When the campaign finance laws finally required disclosure of the fact that virtually all the money came from the tobacco companies, the anti-ordinance campaign would continue to assert that they were just "interested citizens" who approached the benign tobacco industry for help. As the tobacco industry has always done, the campaign against the ordinance would avoid discussing health dangers of secondhand smoke and focus instead on the costs of enforcement and the issue of government intrusion.[20]

TOBACCO CONTROL ADVOCATES MOBILIZE

While irritated with Nelder, ordinance proponents immediately mobilized to defend the ordinance at the polls. At a meeting in Weisberg's home in San Francisco's Seacliff district, Weisberg, Loveday, Hanauer, Glantz, and others decided to create a new independent political committee to raise the funds to run a Yes on Proposition P campaign to defend the ordinance. Since Hanauer and Loveday lived outside San Francisco and Glantz, a San Francisco resident, was president of CNR, none of them seemed an appropriate chair for the campaign. Weisberg accepted the chairmanship of the effort and pledged to use his connections with the ACS to obtain $15,000 to get the campaign off the ground. The San Francisco Lung Association also contributed $7,500. CNR committed its mailing list for fund-raising purposes, even though everyone recognized that diverting donations away from CNR would create severe financial problems.

From the beginning, the theme of local control was the centerpiece of the campaign to uphold the ordinance. On August 17 the proponents held a press conference on the steps of the San Francisco City Hall to announce formation of their campaign organization, San Franciscans for Local Control; Weisberg explained that the law "is to protect the health of people who live and work in San Francisco. . . . Our concern is the public welfare of San Francisco and the integrity of its legislative process. The tobacco companies' only concern is to sell more cigarettes."[25] The group hired Ken Masterton to manage the campaign and opened an office in San Francisco's Castro district.

Nelson-Padberg pointed out to the tobacco industry that "the campaign will be closely watched by major cities throughout America, and the conduct of the campaign—as well as the elections' results—will have major implications to attempts to adopt similar ordinances in other municipalities."[23] Tobacco control advocates thought it was remarkable that the tobacco industry considered the San Francisco ordinance so important; as a result, they also viewed the fight as nationally significant.

That summer, when Glantz and Hanauer attended the World Confer-

ence on Smoking or Health in Winnipeg, Canada, they found a strong
interest in the outcome of the Proposition P fight. Many tobacco control
advocates offered suggestions on how to win the campaign, to which
Glantz responded, "We don't need ideas, we need money. If we raise
$150,000, we'll win, if we raise $100,000, we'll lose."

THE PROPOSITION P CAMPAIGN

Polls showed that Proposition P was leading by a 2-1 margin at the beginning of the campaign, but in the face of the industry attack, the margin narrowed. The industry's strategy was based on its success in previous campaigns. According to Nelson-Padberg's planning document of
July 1983, the aim was to convince voters that the ordinance was "unnecessary, unworkable, or costly." [23]

The first objective of the Nelson-Padberg campaign was to secure a list
of voters from the most recent election—an effort to recall Mayor Dianne
Feinstein because of her support for gun control—and to sort them by approximately one hundred variables. A phone canvas of likely voters was
planned to identify those opposed to the ordinance; these voters would
then receive a thank-you letter and an application for an absentee ballot. Undecided voters were to get a "gentle push" argument as well as in-
tensive direct mail advertising. Nelson-Padberg planned for twenty paid
people to work five shifts for sixty working days to accomplish the phone
screen. The telephone canvas, which eventually reached 65,000 voter
households, formed the basis for the industry's direct mail campaign,
which was concentrated on likely voters, the relatively conservative western part of San Francisco, blacks, and gays.[26] The focus on the gay community was clear from the hiring of Foster and from the industry's effort
early in the campaign to raise the fear that Proposition P would set a
precedent that would be used to discriminate against people with AIDS.[20]

To make it difficult for Proposition P supporters to air their ads,
Nelson-Padberg planned to delay its radio and television advertising until the final four weeks before the election. Unlike the tobacco industry
with its essentially unlimited resources, the Yes on P committee had little
money. While the proposition's supporters hoped to buy some television
and radio advertising, they expected to get most of their advertising space
for free under the Federal Communications Commission (FCC)'s Fairness Doctrine. In 1983 the FCC still required that electronic media fairly
present both sides of controversial issues. Since the passage of Proposi-

tion P was obviously controversial, once the No side began running paid advertisements, the Yes side could approach the television and radio stations and ask for free time to respond. Nelson-Padberg recognized this possibility: "Earlier advertising would only stimulate additional Fairness Doctrine opportunities for our opponents, expose our advertising strategy to long scrutiny, and is not necessary due to the high voter awareness pre-existing the campaign."[23]

Exposing the tobacco industry's backing of the No on P campaign was the central thrust of the ordinance supporters. They attacked the industry at every turn and sought to capitalize on public distrust of the tobacco industry. They also made a concerted effort to reduce the effectiveness of the No on P advertising by forcing the television and radio stations that were broadcasting the advertisements to disclose the real sponsor—the tobacco industry, not San Franciscans Against Government Intrusion. The Federal Communications Act requires that advertisements identify the true sponsor, and the advertisements against Proposition P listed only San Franciscans Against Governmental Intrusion as the sponsor, with no mention of the tobacco industry. Volunteer lawyers, including Loveday, pulled together extensive documentation that the industry was really paying for the advertisements. They argued that it was the stations (not the sponsors) who were responsible for seeing that the "tag lines" on the advertisements identified the true sponsors. At a press conference Loveday and others announced that they were sending formal letters to all radio and television stations running the No on P advertisements to demand that the tag lines be changed to "Paid for by the tobacco industry"; they threatened to file complaints with the FCC against stations that refused.

A few days later, the NBC affiliates in San Francisco—KRON television and KNBR radio—required that the No on P campaign clarify the tag line in its ads to indicate tobacco industry involvement.[20] Rather than adding an oral tag line saying that the campaign was paid for by the tobacco industry, the industry pulled its advertisements off KNBR, one of the largest radio stations in San Francisco. After threatening to sue the stations, the industry decided to acquiesce on the television advertisements and changed the visual tag line to get them back on the air (visual tag lines are not as prominent as oral ones).[26] Even if other stations did not respond directly to the pressure to correct the tag lines, raising the issue had helped highlight the tobacco industry's efforts to hide its political activities.

Nelson-Padberg recognized the effectiveness of the Yes on P strategy surrounding the tag lines:

> Californians for Nonsmokers Rights did an excellent job of urging television stations to give them free television advertising time. Additionally, they were able to convince KRON-TV that the station should require our campaign to identify our advertising as having been "paid for by San Franciscans Against Government Intrusion which is financially supported by companies in the tobacco industry." This requirement by KRON-TV stimulated extensive discussion by other television stations, radio stations, and daily newspapers in the city. In fact, this action by KRON served as a kind of a catalyst to the "money" issue, driving this issue into very sharp focus in the final days preceding the election.[26]

The favored campaign theme of the proponents got an important shot in the arm just three weeks before the election.

The Yes on P forces, having learned from the Proposition 5 and 10 campaigns to make the tobacco industry the issue, managed to maintain a consistent message throughout with the central theme "Tell the Tobacco Industry to Butt Out of San Francisco." Working with a small advertising agency run by Edgar Spizel, they prepared two television advertisements making this point. One advertisement involved several well-known San Francisco politicians and other figures of varying political persuasions; they all agreed on one thing—that the tobacco industry should butt out of San Francisco politics. The other, which won an Addy award, showed a cowboy on horseback riding up a San Francisco street and urging people to tell the tobacco companies to "butt out" and "vote yes on P."

While the Yes on P forces believed from the beginning that they had a real chance to win because an election contest against the tobacco industry in San Francisco would take less money than one throughout the entire state, they grew increasingly frustrated by the way city politicians were allowing personalities to interfere in running an effective campaign. According to Hanauer,

> It was very exciting because we knew we were in the race this time. The polls showed that we had a good chance, that we weren't losing ground rapidly like we had in the other two campaigns. And we had support that we didn't have before, both editorially and [among] some business people. What we didn't have was Wendy Nelder's assistance. . . . She wanted to run her own campaign. She insisted on making her own television spots. They were atrocious. They were the epitome of the bad talking head . . . "Please vote 'yes' on P because I say so." . . . She was driving everybody crazy. . . . And we kept trying to persuade her, "Don't waste your money on these, as we have this wonderful advertising campaign."

> She had her heart in the right place. She was genuinely concerned about secondhand smoke, but she didn't know much about the health issue. And she didn't know the politics of tobacco.[4]

Quentin Kopp, who had a substantial constituency, was another source of frustration because of his reluctance to back a Nelder ordinance.[4] San Franciscans for Local Control wanted to use Kopp's name on a flyer being mailed to the Sunset district, the conservative neighborhood (at least by local standards) in western San Francisco where Kopp lived and his name would carry weight. Kopp refused, even though he supported the ordinance.

On November 3, 1983, six days before the election, Tarrance and Associates reported that Proposition P was still on the way to passing: 50 percent planned to vote "yes," 38 percent "no," and 12 percent was undecided. The Tarrance report added, "On the YES side, there are three main arguments: non-smokers' rights, health hazard, annoyance/irritation. Not only do these three messages hold together well, they are unanswerable and seem to be dominating the campaign."[27] Even before the election results were known, the tobacco companies were beginning to worry about the fallout. On November 4, 1983, Gene Ainsworth of RJ Reynolds forwarded the Tarrance poll to Ed Horrigan (an RJR executive), with this comment:

> Passage of the tough Workplace Smoking Ordinance in San Francisco, with all its attendant press coverage, will trigger a rush to pass similar legislation in many areas of the nation—especially in California. In light of these probable developments the industry needs to consider, on a priority basis, the preparation of a Model Ordinance . . . as a "stop-gap" measure which can be used if the situation in any particular area gets out of control. . . . The long term counter to San Francisco type legislation is the implementation of an effective industry program to address the issue.[28] [emphasis added]

The win in San Francisco was not only national but international news. ABC's *Nightline* devoted its election-evening program to the Proposition P victory, and CBS's *60 Minutes* did a segment on the campaign. The margin of victory was narrow—1,259 votes—but it was a victory nonetheless and it set the stage for other localities to pass ordinances.

LESSONS FROM THE PROPOSITION P CAMPAIGN

The early and prominent role of the industry turned out to be an important election issue. In analyzing their loss, a Nelson-Padberg report concluded, "If signatures could have been gathered through volunteers, that would have delayed the issue and perhaps prevented it from ever becoming central. If money could have been raised from non-tobacco interests in the city of San Francisco, that would have prevented it from becoming a key issue; or if some other issue could have been made more important to reporters, that might have shifted or softened the focus, perhaps preventing the money issue from being so critical later in the campaign."[26] Tobacco control advocates had learned how to frame the issue as one of outside interference by the tobacco industry.

Nelson-Padberg's report also complimented the Yes on P campaign: "The Yes on Proposition P campaign was well managed, tightly focused, selected the issues appropriate to the problem and made efficient use of their limited resources . . . unlike prior campaigns [for Propositions 5 and 10], they focused clearly on the health issue in the final days of the campaign, bringing the public's attention to the most devastating argument available to them."[26]

Hanauer believed that at least part of the reason for the proponents' success lay in the growing sophistication of the press: "The industry had a little more unsavory reputation by this time. And I think the press was much more sympathetic by the time Prop P came around and much more attuned to questions about finance, tobacco industry lies, and the health issues."[4]

On the other hand, Nelson-Padberg called proponents "unscrupulous" because of their last two mailers—one detailing tobacco industry lies and one featuring stars who had died of lung cancer, thus implying that "Proposition P would somehow fight lung cancer."[26] About the former mailer, the Nelson-Padberg report said, "Although all of their allegations were fabrications, the piece was very effective in hammering home their message."[26] The report also identified other problems that the tobacco industry had failed to overcome. For example, the Bay Area was home to the leadership of the Proposition 10 campaign, Loveday, Hanauer, Glantz, and Weisberg, who "could dedicate all of their efforts to the 380,000 registered voters in San Francisco, rather than the 11,000,000 registered voters statewide. Additionally, 10 of the 11 members of the Board of Supervisors and the Mayor were publicly committed to support the smoking control ordinance, creating a most difficult political dynamic to overcome."[26] Operating in a more limited media market, proponents could present their message—in news stories as well as paid advertising—more effectively than they had done in the statewide Proposition 5 and 10 efforts. Hanauer agreed: "Certainly $125,000 in one city and county went a lot further than a half a million statewide."[4]

The report on Proposition P prepared by V. Lance Tarrance outlined for the industry three of its key problems. First, the tobacco industry's involvement was not a strong reason for people to vote for the proposition, but the amount of money spent by the industry was. According to Tarrance, "Future campaigns should work to minimize this issue."[27] When respondents were asked to evaluate the industry campaign contributions, 52 percent disapproved and 27 percent approved, compared with 45 percent and 37 percent, respectively, during the Proposition 5 campaign in 1978. The campaign contribution issue was becoming a more salient one for voters. Second, the health effects of secondhand smoke were considered a serious threat. Again, comparing the two elections, the report found that in 1983 59 percent thought secondhand smoke was harmful, up from 49 percent in 1978. Third, the message that people should be allowed to work things out themselves did not get through to people as effectively as the government intervention issue did, and the "accommodation" message might have been a more powerful argument in converting votes.

Among specific voter subgroups, the gay vote was "disappointing." In early polling gays were one group who appeared to be prepared to vote against the proposition, but in the end their voting pattern was virtually identical to those of other groups. This fact particularly pleased the Yes on P forces, for they perceived the tobacco industry concentrating on winning the gay vote.

In 1991, when the Tobacco Institute drafted a report titled "California: A Multifaceted Plan to Address the Negative Environment,"[29] the passage of Proposition P was listed as the first "important event" among those that had raised the level of acceptability of smoking restrictions. Hanauer could agree with the industry on this point: "This was a landmark. I've always said that this was the whole key to the national nonsmokers' rights movement. If we had lost Prop P, it would have set us back ten years or more."[4] In 1989 the US Surgeon General's report *Reducing the Health Consequences of Smoking: Twenty-Five Years of Progress* identified the San Francisco victory as a stimulus to further ordinance activity.[30]

CONCLUSION

Passing local ordinances rapidly became the preferred strategy for tobacco control advocates; at the local level they were able to neutralize the industry's power and portray the industry as "outsiders." Local grass-roots advocates were a powerful voice.[30] In 1984 CNR changed its name to Americans for Nonsmokers' Rights and formally began working to spread the local ordinance strategy nationwide. By the end of 1986, 112 California cities and counties (of 192 nationwide) had enacted tough worksite ordinances of their own; by October 1988, this number had grown to 158 in California (and 289 nationwide).

The tobacco industry also recognized the power of the local ordinance movement. In a 1986 speech, Raymond Pritchard, chairman of the board of Brown and Williamson Tobacco, explicitly recognized this fact:

> Our record in defeating state smoking restrictions has been reasonably good. Unfortunately, our record with respect to local measures—that is cities and counties across the country—has been somewhat less encouraging. San Francisco provides a stark example of what this industry and its customers can face at the local level. We must somehow do a better job than we have in the past in getting our story told to city councils and county commissions. *Over time we can lose the battle over smoking restrictions as decisively in bits and pieces—at the local level—as with state or federal measures.*[31] [emphasis added]

The defeats of Propositions 5 and 10 contributed in important ways to the California tobacco control movement. First, the campaigns educated voters about the dangers of secondhand smoke as well as the rights of nonsmokers to breathe clean indoor air. Second, the devious nature of the tobacco industry became also more recognized by politicians, the ordinary voter, and the media. Third, tobacco control activists learned how to be effective in the political process. Proposition P represented the first big public defeat that the tobacco industry had ever suffered, and it laid the foundation for Proposition 99.

CHAPTER 3

Proposition 99 Emerges

In November 1988, in spite of a massive statewide campaign by the tobacco industry, California voters enacted Proposition 99. The proposition, which increased the tobacco excise tax by twenty-five cents per pack of cigarettes and comparable amounts on other tobacco products, financed the largest, most ambitious tobacco control program in the world. Using the Proposition 99 tax revenues, the state spent as much as $100 million annually fighting tobacco, which dwarfed the federal government's activities. At its most effective, in the early 1990s, the Proposition 99 anti-tobacco education program tripled the rate of decline in tobacco consumption. It spawned an unprecedented effort at passing local ordinances and led to smoke-free public places and workplaces, followed by smoke-free restaurants and bars. Yet the idea for Proposition 99 did not come from the nonsmokers' rights activists who had defeated the tobacco companies in San Francisco's Proposition P campaign, the voluntary health agencies, or the medical establishment. It came from an environmentalist.

The leaders of Americans for Nonsmokers' Rights (ANR), in the aftermath of Propositions 5, 10, and P, decided to concentrate on passing local ordinances because they understood that cities and counties presented a forum in which the grassroots organizations' power was amplified and the tobacco industry's power was muted. They had no interest in another bruising election, much less a state-level campaign. The voluntary health agencies—the American Lung Association (ALA), American Cancer Society (ACS), and American Heart Association (AHA)—were slow to embrace policy interventions to protect public health, sticking to the medical model of pursuing health one patient at a time. The medical establishment was preoccupied with increasing the amount of money available to pay for the delivery of medical services and with making it harder to sue doctors.

THE IDEA

Early in 1986 Gerald Meral, executive director of the Planning and Conservation League (PCL), a statewide California environmental group based in Sacramento, approached his friend Curt Mekemson, who worked for the ALA, to discuss his idea of increasing the tobacco tax by five cents and using the proceeds for environmental programs. Such a tax would raise the price of cigarettes and reduce smoking, a goal of Mekemson's, while raising money for environmental programs, one of Meral's goals. Meral knew that Mekemson, in his previous job as executive director of the Alaska Lung Association, had spearheaded the successful effort to double Alaska's cigarette tax from eight cents to sixteen cents.

Mekemson put Meral off: "I told Gerry, no, I wasn't interested. I was going backpacking for six months, but I might talk to him afterwards. So I went off and did my backpacking trip."[1]

Meral did not take no for an answer. In September 1986, when Mekemson returned from backpacking to work as the legislative director of ALA's Sacramento Emigrant Trails affiliate, Meral cornered him again with the same question.[1] This time Mekemson said yes.

Mekemson and Meral recruited two other legislative advocates: Tony Najera, director of government relations at ALA, and Betsy Hite, director of public issues at ACS. The four began conducting research and planning strategy. Although Meral had originally proposed an increase of only five cents per pack, Mekemson felt that the increase should be larger and that revenues should also support tobacco prevention and education programs. In an October memorandum to Najera, Mekemson stated that "the majority of the funds should go toward supporting health related programs, [and] that within health related programs our greatest focus should be on prevention [with] a portion of the funds directly related to the smoking issue."[2]

THE COALITION FOR A HEALTHY CALIFORNIA

Several events in September and October 1986 gave the tax effort additional momentum and legitimacy. Mekemson persuaded Assembly Member Lloyd Connelly (D-Sacramento) to join the effort. Connelly, a highly respected figure in the Assembly, brought a significant leadership presence to the tobacco tax effort, both organizationally and politically. He was drafted into the effort over a breakfast. According to Mekemson,

> Lloyd was along. Connelly was a longtime friend and acquaintance of mine and he called me up and said he wanted me to tell him Alaskan bear stories because he's into all this wilderness stuff. . . . So we had breakfast at the Fox and the Goose and I told Lloyd all the bear stories. And he wanted to know what I was doing. And I said, "Well Lloyd, I think I want to take on this tobacco tax issue." . . . What caught Lloyd's attention . . . was the impact that increasing the tobacco tax would have on reducing tobacco use among kids. Bringing Lloyd on brought in a lot of credibility to the effort, and his own incredible energy and ability to organize things. . . . And he committed one of his staff people to working with us.[1]

Over breakfast, Connelly said it was hopeless to get a tobacco tax increase through the Legislature. He was willing to be involved only if the groups were willing to press ahead with an initiative.[3] Proposition 99 was born.

Meral used his political skills to broaden the range of groups interested in increasing the tobacco tax. He convinced the Senate Office of Research to hold an informal meeting on October 14, 1986, with representatives from the PCL, ALA, ACS, ANR, California Teachers Association, Senate Revenue and Taxation Committee, California Medical Association (CMA), Connelly's office, and the Senate Office of Research itself. This informal meeting served several purposes: it increased the tax effort's legitimacy, defined the potential participants of a coalition, and provided a forum in which to discuss strategies and goals early in the process.

Most of the research and organization, however, was still done by the ALA, ACS, PCL, and Connelly's office. Mekemson and Najera set the agenda for the meeting by preparing a draft paper that identified the specific issues and requirements for passing a tobacco tax increase.[4] Their paper raised the following questions.

   1. *What was the case for increasing the tax?* There were three distinct supportive arguments: the impact on smoking and health, the po-

tential benefits from programs supported by the new revenues, and the high economic costs of smoking. In addition, the time was ripe. California's cigarette tax of ten cents had not been increased since 1967. Every other state except Virginia had increased its tobacco tax since 1967; only six other states had lower taxes than California, and four of those were tobacco producing states.

2. *Which is the best approach for increasing the tax—an initiative or the Legislature?* Because of the tobacco industry's lobbying power in Sacramento, enacting a tax increase through the Legislature seemed hopeless since it had defeated thirty-seven bills to do so since 1967. Although an initiative meant mounting a major election campaign against the tobacco industry, it seemed to be the only way to increase the tax. In spite of the failure of previous statewide initiatives—Propositions 5 and 10—conditions seemed favorable for this one. Public attitudes toward smoking were changing and there was a large societal cost associated with smoking. In addition, by using the initiative process, the proponents could decide the amount of the tax increase and how the money would be spent. Proponents felt that, with careful crafting of the initiative, it would be possible to build public support for the tax.

3. *How much should the tax be increased and how should the new revenues be allocated?* Early discussion considered an increase of twenty cents to forty cents per pack. A high tax was favored because it was felt that it would have the largest impact on tobacco consumption and generate the most revenues, but too high a tax might invite criticism and loss of public support. The ALA estimated that a 10 percent increase in the price would lead to a 14 percent drop in tobacco consumption and that every one-cent increase would generate $25 million in new revenues. Three important points were raised regarding revenue allocation: How could the money be used to have the greatest impact on tobacco consumption? How could the money be allocated to gain support from interest groups whose backing would be necessary to win? How could the money be used to generate the broadest public support?

4. *What are the technical aspects involved in running an initiative?* Qualifying the initiative would be a difficult task, followed by an even more difficult election campaign. This process would require employing a professional campaign director, conducting polling to determine campaign strategy, and hiring professional signature-gatherers, all of which represented substantial financial and organizational commitments.

From the beginning, the public health and environmental advocates had problems with the CMA. Jay Michael, CMA's vice president for government relations, tried to limit participants in the planning effort. From the beginning he tried to exclude the more politically sophisticated Connelly and the PCL so that he would have to deal only with the voluntary health agencies, which lacked the political muscle and sophistication that Connelly and Meral had. According to Mekemson, who was trying to help organize the coalition,

> What we ran into with the CMA was they were concerned about the breadth of the coalition that we were developing. In other words, they didn't want Lloyd [Connelly] involved in it; Jay didn't want Lloyd involved in it. They didn't want the environmentalists involved in it. It seemed to be okay as long as it was Heart, Cancer, Hospitals, so forth and so on.
>
> And of course, I insisted on continuing to involve Gerry [Meral], I mean it was Gerry's initial idea. And obviously Lloyd. Lloyd brought in his power and wonderful ability to analyze things from a political perspective, and his experience with initiatives as well as Gerry. . . .
>
> One day we had an incredible meeting. Jay called me up, and he said he didn't want Lloyd or Gerry at the meeting, and I insisted on it. And he insisted right back. So finally I had agreed that I would show up with Tony [Najera of ALA] and Betsy [Hite of ACS] and we could all sit down and work it out but they are going to be involved. Well, I just beat Gerry there. I waited outside CMA's offices on a hot day. I said, "Gerry, here's the situation." Then Lloyd came along and I said, "Lloyd, here's the situation."
>
> And Lloyd just got that look in his eyes and said, "No way," he marched in, left us standing outside. I don't know what he said to Jay, but when we walked in, Jay was pissed. Obviously absolutely infuriated. Because Lloyd comes back out and says, "Come on in, Gerry. I worked it out." . . . That was the last meeting we had at the CMA building because I . . . put them right over here [at ALA of Sacramento–Emigrant Trails], not on neutral ground, on *our* ground.[1]

On November 20, 1986, Connelly sent a letter inviting potentially interested organizations to join the effort to increase California's tobacco tax and cited three objectives of the tax: to reduce teenage smoking, to raise revenues to fund public awareness campaigns, and to reduce the overall suffering and financial burden caused by tobacco.[5] On December 4, 1986, Connelly hosted a meeting to identify organizations that might support the tobacco tax effort.

Prior to this meeting, George Williams, executive director of the ALA of California, and the ALA board of directors set the standard of commitment by providing $50,000 to support the tobacco tax effort. This very large (for a voluntary health agency) financial commitment showed the ALA's dedication to the effort and forced other agencies to be ready to make the same financial commitment. Mekemson saw this early and substantial commitment as a key factor in establishing a significant anti-tobacco education component of the emerging initiative. He observed,

> It said to everybody out there, "This is really a serious proposition," and that's what we had to accomplish. In other words, we had to show . . . that this was something that's going to happen. But the other important thing that the $50,000 does is that it really bought the American Lung Association a seat at the table. For any negotiations that took place or happened, we would be a key player. That became important, especially when we decided to divide up the pie . . . we kept running up against CMA, who would say, "Certainly some money should go into education. How about five percent [of tobacco tax revenues]?" . . . So between having the $50,000 contribution from ALAC, and the fact that we started the whole process, and the fact that the poll supported it, those were the chips I needed to get 20 percent set aside for prevention in that very intense battle that we had.[1]

The California Association of Hospital and Health Systems (CAHHS) and the CMA, both major political forces in the Legislature, were now willing to join the tobacco tax effort. The support of these two medical organizations was viewed as significant because of their credibility, their potential to provide money, and their link to individual hospitals and doctors throughout the state. Hite remembered that Jim Nethery, a dentist who was president of the ACS California Division, worked to involve the CMA.

> There was a lot friction with all of the groups and CMA. Categorically it was the groups and CMA. The CMA changed their direction a number of times. We had verbal promises from their president [Dr. Armstrong] at the time. . . . He and Dr. Nethery, who was the president of the American Cancer Society at that time, had a number of discussions that CMA was completely behind us, they'd spend whatever it would take to get it through; it was a really good public health policy to try and discourage smoking by raising the tax and by dedicating some of those funds to education. As we went further and further along in the drafting over the next eight months, CMA became less willing to commit resources and more willing to take the benefits.[6]

The health groups did not know that key CMA leaders were actively working with tobacco interests on economic issues that were important to organized medicine, particularly malpractice and tort liability issues, at the same time as they were meeting with the health groups.[7] In the end, common economic interests with the tobacco industry would dominate the CMA's decision-making process. In the meantime, it was in the

CMA's interests to push the tobacco tax initiative, both as a way to increase the pool of money available to pay for medical services and as a bargaining chip with the tobacco industry in negotiations over malpractice reform and tobacco products liability.

Mekemson and others had approached ANR and the other leaders in the fights for Propositions 5, 10, and P, but they declined to get actively involved. As Hanauer explained, "We were deathly afraid that we couldn't win a statewide initiative. . . . I got snake bitten twice and I wasn't in the mood to try a third time . . . Fortunately there were other people who were willing to do that, and were able to bring fresh blood into that kind of campaign. Stan Glantz and I and Paul [Loveday] shuddered at the thought of even getting involved, much less working forty, fifty hours a week at that point on a statewide campaign."[8]

ANR supported the concept of a tobacco tax but did not think it could pass.[1,9] ANR took the position that any new state-level initiative would meet the same fate as Propositions 5 and 10: the public's strong early support would wither in the face of the tobacco industry's expensive counter-campaign. ANR was also offended that the large, wealthy organizations that were setting up the campaign demanded a contribution of $25,000 from ANR (at the time, a four-person operation with a budget under $200,000) for the privilege of sitting on the Executive Committee.[10] In addition, the local ordinance strategy adopted by ANR and other grassroots organizations was producing important successes at the local level. As already noted, by the end of 1986, 263 local tobacco control ordinances were in place, 117 of which were in California, and ANR did not want to put its energies into a statewide campaign.

By early January 1987, an informal coalition was ready to attempt to increase California's tobacco tax. The Coalition for a Healthy California consisted of the ALA, AHA, ACS, CMA, PCL, CAHHS, and Lloyd Connelly.

THE LEGISLATIVE EFFORT

The next step in the tax effort was to attempt to pass a tobacco tax increase through the Legislature. Connelly's invitation letter to the December 4, 1986, meeting of the Coalition stated, "While we are planning to make an initial effort at the Legislature, we frankly expect the tobacco lobby will defeat us there. After all, they've been doing so for 20 years."[5] Still, a legislative attempt was necessary to develop the Coalition further, to test the various arguments for a tobacco tax increase, and to educate the public regarding the desirability of an increase. The process also was designed to improve the drafting of the initiative by exposing it to public comment. In addition, the process of going through the Legislature provided some hope of a compromise with the tobacco industry before an initiative battle had to be faced.[3] It was also necessary, before going to the voters, to try the legislative approach and demonstrate that it simply would not work.[11]

As predicted, the Coalition had to contend with the tobacco industry's lobbying power in the Legislature. Despite the industry's very low public credibility and the popularity of the tax increase on cigarettes, the industry had been very successful in defending its political agenda within the Legislature through large campaign contributions to legislators and its organized and politically influential lobbyists.[12–14] According to Hite, the Coalition tried to persuade the tobacco industry to let the bill go through, but without success: "We did our best to tell the tobacco folks, 'We're going to do this, we're going to do an initiative on this, and we've got right on our side and you know we've got the numbers on our side, you know we're right, we're going to win this. Cut your losses and let's do legislation.' And they wouldn't."[6]

The Coalition decided to seek a constitutional amendment rather than a simple statute for two reasons. First, proponents of the tax increase wanted to avoid spending limits that the voters had enacted in 1979 when they passed Proposition 4, known as the Gann Limit (after Paul Gann, its primary sponsor). This constitutional amendment, which was passed the year after Proposition 13, limited the growth of state government expenditures to the rate of inflation and population growth. While the Gann Limit did not prohibit an increase in the cigarette tax, it could have prevented the state from spending the money raised by the tax.[15] Second, proponents wanted to protect the tax-funded tobacco education programs from the Legislature, and only the voters can change a voter-passed initiative. Assembly Member Tom Hayden (D-Santa Monica) realized that protecting Proposition 99 would be an ongoing battle. Hayden had gained fame as a leader in the antiwar movement of the late sixties and early seventies as a member of the Chicago Seven. He eventually channeled his energy into mainstream politics and, in addition to becoming a member of the Legislature, founded Campaign California, which pushed a variety of liberal, environmental causes, including several ballot initiatives.[16] Hayden would become one of Proposition 99's defenders in the Legislature.

Since the proponents of the tax increase were certain of defeat in the

Legislature, they wanted to craft the proposed tax initiative to draw maximum public support. With money from the CMA, ACS, and ALA, they hired Charlton Research to conduct a public opinion poll in January 1987 on the topic of raising the tobacco tax.[17] The Coalition sought public input in five major areas: the amount of the tax, the breadth of the tax, the distribution of the new revenues, the issue of whether to adjust for inflation, and ways around the Gann Limit.[18]

The poll found substantial public support for a cigarette tax increase of twenty-five cents a pack (to a total of thirty-five cents): 73 percent supported the increase (57 percent strongly, 16 percent somewhat) and only 23 percent disapproved of it. Even after hearing the arguments for and against a cigarette tax increase, support remained high—at 68 percent. Nearly two-thirds of the respondents said they would be likely to vote for the tax increase for the following reasons: tobacco use costs society billions of dollars, increasing the tax would discourage smoking among young people, and tobacco use is the single most preventable cause of death in America. And 42 percent said they would be more likely to vote in favor of a tax increase if they knew large out-of-state cigarette companies would contribute millions of dollars to oppose the initiative. Arguments against the tobacco tax were less persuasive. The most popular argument against the tax—that increased cigarette taxes mean another government bureaucracy and more bureaucrats spending more tax money—made 46 percent of the respondents less likely to vote for the tax.[17]

The poll provided the Coalition with public feedback and helped to influence how to allocate new revenues from the tax increase. Funding education programs to prevent drug and tobacco abuse was the most strongly supported (72 percent), followed by health research on tobacco-related disease (60 percent), MediCal (Medicaid in California; 42 percent), and increased funding for parks and wildlife (20 percent). The results of the poll were significant for two reasons. First, they clearly demonstrated that the tobacco tax had overwhelming public support. Second, they clearly showed that funding prevention and education was more popular than funding health care services. The Coalition decided that the bill would allocate revenues to three major types of programs: reducing smoking, mitigating the health impact of smoking, and mitigating the nonhealth impact of smoking.

On February 23, 1987, Connelly introduced Assembly Constitutional Amendment 14 (ACA 14), cosponsored by Assembly Member William Filante (R-Greenbrae), a physician, to increase the tax on cigarettes from ten cents to thirty-five cents per pack, with comparable taxes on other tobacco products. By April 1987, ACA 14 addressed the Gann Limit and the allocation of revenues. ACA 14 stipulated that the new revenues raised by the tax would be allocated as follows: tobacco use prevention (47.5 percent, with 27.5 percent for school health promotions aimed at reducing cigarette smoking and substance abuse and 20 percent for community-based smoking prevention activities); augmentation of MediCal funding for the treatment of lung cancer, chronic obstructive lung disease, heart disease, and other tobacco-related illnesses (27.5 percent); clinical research on the diagnosis and treatment of tobacco-related diseases (15 percent); and efforts by various local and state jurisdictions to mitigate the nonhealth impact of tobacco use such as fires and litter (10 percent). The allocation of revenues roughly paralleled the Charlton Research poll results: education and prevention were favored over health care services, and environmental programs were given the lowest priority. Only the research allocation did not reflect the public's preferences as shown in the poll (being placed third instead of second).

The bill's proponents were not the only ones planning strategy in the spring of 1987. By March, the tobacco industry, far from considering a compromise with Connelly, was actively planning its opposition. The Tobacco Institute had commissioned Houston-based V. Lance Tarrance to conduct a private poll to measure public opinion regarding a tobacco tax increase and to develop the tobacco industry's political strategy to defeat it. In the polling results, the initiative was winning 63 percent to 30 percent, with 6 percent undecided.

Like the Coalition poll, the Tobacco Institute poll tested various arguments and issues to determine potential weaknesses and strengths of the tobacco tax increase. The results were not encouraging for the tobacco industry:

> The data strongly indicate that a campaign for fighting the tax increase will not be received well by voters. Convincing voters that the tax level is already too high, and stressing the importance of the Gann Spending Limit law may be possible, but the bottom line is that people *do not like smoking or smokers*. Therefore, anti–cigarette tax support should not be expected to rise substantially from the levels they are now. The single chance the anti-tax campaign has *is to move this issue away from smoking*. These data show moderate levels of support for a campaign constructed around the following themes: (1) Increased taxation—*any tax* increase is bad; (2) Government mismanagement of tax money; (3) Scheme to "bust" the Gann Spending Limit [and] get around state spending law; (4) 25 cents a pack is *too much on a single prod-*

uct—unfair. Realistically, these themes could win, if backed by a broad coalition of anti-tax people. . . . Even with such a coalition, the "no" campaign
would be expensive and difficult given the *very negative* feelings against
smoking.[19] [emphasis in original]

Many of these themes were to appear in the tobacco industry's election
campaign against Proposition 99.[20] In fact, the industry named its front
group Citizens Against Unfair Tax Increases.

Although Coalition leaders doubted that the Legislature would approve ACA 14, they mounted a genuine effort to build public support.
Mekemson outlined their strategy: "We could generate a lot of media
around it, and that would be the beginning of our sort of push to the public. We also felt that it would be an opportunity to take some of the concepts and ideas that we had developed and throw them out on the table
to see whether they would float or not. We also felt that it would be a way
of beginning to sort of feel the tobacco industry out and take a look at
what their strategy would be and arguments."[1]

In late April, the Coalition held a series of press conferences about
ACA 14, the Coalition, and the tobacco tax effort. The Coalition released
its poll data showing overwhelming support for the tobacco tax,[21] and
Assembly Members Connelly and Filante held a press conference in Los
Angeles at which Patrick Reynolds (grandson of R. J. Reynolds) testified
in support of ACA 14.[22] In early May the independent California Field
Poll showed that two-thirds of those surveyed supported increasing the
cigarette tax by as much as thirty cents per pack.[23] The ALA and ACS
were also active throughout the spring of 1987, sending action alerts to
local affiliates and urging legislators to vote for ACA 14.[24,25] Connelly
was cynical about the likelihood of legislative action but pushed it so as
to move the initiative process forward.

The tobacco industry took ACA 14 more seriously than Connelly did.
A discussion of how to defeat ACA 14 consumed most of a meeting of
the Tobacco Institute's State Activities Policy Committee on April 3,
1987, in Washington, DC. According to Gene Ainsworth of RJ Reynolds, ACA 14 received this extensive attention because "given the size
of the California cigarette market (9.7 per cent of total domestic vol-
ume), and California's political bellwether position, the specter of a
state-wide initiative to increase the cigarette excise tax is a most serious
situation."[26] The Tobacco Institute State Activities Policy Committee
gave specific directions to its lobbyists to keep the tax issue off the ballot through both the legislative and initiative processes. The group also

clearly identified the CMA as an important player to be neutralized if the industry was to avoid an initiative fight over the tobacco tax. Ainsworth observed, "It is clear that the money machine for the Coalition's California tax proposal is the California Medical Association. Without the promised $1 million from the CMA, the tax initiative would be difficult to qualify and we could possibly avoid a costly and extremely difficult state-wide tax battle in 1988."[26]

Between April 15 and May 18, a Sacramento lobbying firm representing the tobacco industry, A-K Associates, mounted a major and wide-reaching campaign behind the scenes to stop ACA 14. The firm's report to Roger Mozingo, head of the Tobacco Institute's State Activities Division in Washington, catalogued these activities.

> The California Chamber of Commerce, California Taxpayers Association, California Retailers Association and California Manufacturers Association all were recruited and went on record as being opposed to ACA 14. This allowed us the opportunity to meet with and brief the "key" people within each of these groups in order to educate them about ACA 14 and the possible statewide initiative. These groups are now on record and can be expected to be a valuable resource if needed to actually fight an initiative.

> Hispanic Lobbying Associates was retained to generate Hispanic opposition to ACA 14. The Mexican American Political Association, American G.I. Forum, Latino Peace Officers Association, California Hispanic Chamber of Commerce, California Hispanic Women's Forum and the Latin American Pacific Trade Association all officially went on record in opposition to ACA 14. These groups are still with us awaiting our signal to be turned loose against the tax Initiative.

> A very successful letter writing campaign to "key" legislators by companies and TI [Tobacco Institute] was orchestrated and effectively carried out.

> Personal lobbying of organized medicine began even during the lobbying efforts on ACA 14 in the Legislature. These included personal meetings with the following California Medical Association leaders:

> > Bob Elsner, Executive Director.
> > Jay Michael, Director of Government Relations.
> > Dr. Gladdin Elliott, Immediate Past President.
> > Allen Pross, CALPAC Director.
> > Dr. Kai Kristensen and Dr. Phillips Gausewitz, San Diego area.
> > Frank Clark, Executive Director of the Los Angeles Medical Society.
> > Dr. Manny Abrams and Dr. David Olch, Los Angeles area.
> > Dr. Frank Glanz and Dr. Marshall Ganns, Orange County area.
> > Dr. Ed Hendricks and Dr. Pierce Rooney, central valley area.

> Dr. Michael Lopiano, Santa Barbara area.
> Dr. Paul Dugan, northern California rural area.
> Dr. Tom Elmendorf and Dr. James Moorfield, Sacramento area.
> Dr. Fred Achermann and Dr. Roberta Fenlon, San Francisco area.

Met with "key" black political leaders to solicit and begin solidifying black support among state legislators for the anti-initiative campaign. We met personally with the following black state legislators or legislative staff:

> Willie Brown, Speaker of the Assembly.
> Maxine Waters, Majority Whip.
> Curtis Tucker, Chairman of the Assembly Health Committee.
> Dodson Wilson, Staff to Speaker Willie Brown.

Met with David Kim re Korean community and advise [*sic*] re other possible Asian consultants.

Met with Assemblyman Dick Floyd, Tommy Hunter (Calif. State Pipe Trades) and Jack Henning [secretary-treasurer of California AFL-CIO] regarding the proposed tax initiative.

Met continuously with Jack Kelly [regional vice president of the Tobacco Institute] to coordinate testimony and lobbying activity.[7]

The tobacco industry got its way in Sacramento. When ACA 14 came before the Assembly Revenue and Taxation Committee on May 18, only seven of the committee's sixteen members showed up (two short of the necessary quorum), precluding any action on the bill.[27] Committee chairman Johan Klehs (D-San Leandro) did not even allow supporters of ACA 14 to testify.[15] Assembly Member Dick Floyd (D-Wilmington) marched up and down the aisles blowing cigar smoke at supporters of ACA 14. The tobacco industry's contract lobbyist, A-K Associates, declared victory:

> In order to accomplish our anti-initiative strategy to discourage support for the pro-initiative coalition, we felt it was imperative to attain a decisive victory in the first committee to show strength and resolve on the part of the opponents to the proposed tax increase. In fact, when these two bills were heard before the Revenue and Taxation Committee, they were dealt a "crushing" defeat. Neither received a motion, much less a single affirmative vote.
>   Our major goal of weakening potential support and showing strong opposition was certainly accomplished. The California Medical Association was shocked that their intense lobbying effort could not receive one "aye" vote in the Committee, considering their campaign support for the members

of the Revenue and Taxation Committee (Organized Medicine—$80,300 vs. TI—$17,750 during 1986). The minutes of the proponents' June 17, 1987 organizational meeting even makes reference to this defeat.[7]

The motion to propose ACA 14 died for lack of a second.

THE CMA AND THE TOBACCO INDUSTRY

Initiative proponents wanted the CMA involved because, unlike the voluntary health agencies, it had significant political muscle and it was rich and accustomed to spending money for political purposes, including initiative campaigns. The tobacco tax was also appealing to the CMA because it created a new pool of money—$600 million a year—to pay for medical services. From the beginning, however, the relationship between the health groups and the CMA was rocky. Indeed, in 1993, Connelly reflected, "If I had to do it over again, I wouldn't have had CMA in the room, because they were more trouble than they were worth."[3]

The tobacco industry was also interested in the CMA's deep pockets and saw that keeping the CMA out of the upcoming fight over the initiative was crucial. The industry knew that it would be difficult and expensive to beat the tobacco tax initiative at the ballot box and decided that the best strategy was to block proponents from collecting enough signatures to qualify the initiative in the first place.[7] Since it costs money to run a signature drive and the CMA was the most likely source of big money, the tobacco industry turned its attention to convincing the CMA to stop supporting the tobacco tax effort. An A-K Associates report explained strategy this way:

> Recognizing that the most effective approach to any such battle is to contain and, if possible, take away potential resources from the proponents, our initial goal was to contain the California Medical Association, who had already pledged $1 million to qualify the initiative. With this kind of resources, there is no way the initiative could be kept off the ballot. *A game plan was formulated to discourage and keep the CMA out of the initiative. This included possible counter anti-medicine initiatives and legislation,* as well as the use of A-K's considerable contacts within organized medicine. *Having already expended considerable effort in this area during the Legislative phase of the program we turned our attention almost full time to dissuading the CMA from joining the fray.*
>
> *We were immensely successful in this regard. CMA, after considerable pressure, decided to "tokenize" the tax initiative campaign* with, at best, a $25,000 contribution and the possible use of their mailing list for a solicitation letter. To date CMA has not actually given the proponents any campaign

money. *The decision was made that no punitive action would be taken in regard to anti-medicine initiatives or legislation as long as the CMA maintained this non-participatory attitude toward the tobacco tax initiative.* Following are the major activities that have taken place to date:

Met with key organized medicine leaders to continue to dissuade them from actively participating in the proposed tobacco tax initiative.

Generated some well placed and vocal complaining from organized rank and file membership throughout the state to the CMA's Council (organized medicine's governing body in California).

Arranged for the Council to take the policy position that all requests for political issue contributions of either staff or resources must first go to their Finance Committee for approval before the Council can take action. This effectively took the tobacco tax initiative issue out of the hands of the current CMA leadership and placed it in the hands of the "old guard." This placed a huge roadblock in front of people like Dr. Armstrong, the current CMA President, who is an avowed anti-tobacco crusader and was one of the major witnesses in support of ACA 14 in the Assembly Revenue and Taxation Committee hearings.

Made multiple trips to San Francisco to meet with "key" CMA executive staff to firm up their opposition to CMA's participation in the initiative.

Arranged for the Golden State Medical Society (statewide black physicians organization) to object to the CMA's participation in the initiative.

Met with several legislators who are anti-medicine for various personal and political reasons to have anti-medicine legislation drafted and leaked to the right CMA leaders.[7] [emphasis different from original]

Initiative proponents complained that the CMA was not enthusiastically supporting the initiative effort, but they had no idea of the depth of the connections between the CMA and the tobacco industry.

THE NAPKIN DEAL

Tort reform was an active issue before the Legislature at the same time as ACA 14, and the CMA needed to protect its Malpractice Insurance Compensation Reform Act (MICRA). In 1975 the CMA had persuaded the Legislature to pass MICRA, which capped medical malpractice judgments and the size of trial lawyer contingency fees. MICRA had launched an ongoing fight about product liability among doctors, trial lawyers, insurance companies, manufacturers, and others, with everyone willing to make substantial campaign contributions to block everyone else from getting what they wanted through the Legislature.

The manufacturers and insurance companies, tired of dealing with the Legislature, had used the initiative process to pass Proposition 51 in 1986. Proposition 51 ended the legal doctrine of "joint and several liability" whereby the wealthiest defendants in multi-defendant lawsuits paid the vast majority of the damages if other defendants did not have the resources. The insurance companies were willing to go to the ballot again to pass an even more favorable law. On the other side, the trial lawyers and consumer groups were willing to try to pass their own initiative that would make it easier to sue and recover damages.

On September 10, 1987, Assembly Speaker Willie Brown (D-San Francisco), who had by the end of the 1988 election cycle received $125,900 in campaign contributions from the tobacco industry, hosted a dinner meeting at Frank Fat's, a Sacramento restaurant popular with Capitol movers and shakers.[28,29] He invited the trial lawyers, the CMA, and the insurance companies to work out a tort reform deal that would accommodate all of their interests and avoid a very costly initiative battle. They were joined by the tobacco industry.

The dinner guests (public health and consumer groups were excluded) worked out a nonaggression pact in which everyone at the table got something. Insurance companies got protection from lawsuits and avoided regulation of their industry, doctors kept their existing liability protections and got a higher standard of proof that a victim had to meet to receive damages, and trial lawyers got larger contingency fees to compensate them for the fact that the cases would be harder to win. The tobacco industry (and producers of castor oil, butter, sugar, and alcohol) got virtual immunity from lawsuits based on consumer use of its "inherently" unsafe product.[29]

The deal was written on a napkin; the "Napkin Deal" emerged as a legendary political deal in Sacramento.[29,30] The resulting bill, introduced by Senator Bill Lockyer (D-Hayward), was the subject of a perfunctory one-hour committee hearing, went to the floor (where it was blocked from amendment by the leadership), and passed by a wide margin.

The tobacco industry clearly understood the intimate connection between MICRA and the tobacco tax initiative insofar as it related to the CMA. In its report to Mozingo of the Tobacco Institute, dated September 24, 1987, shortly after the Napkin Deal was enacted into law, A-K Associates analyzed the CMA's position:

> To date organized medicine has stayed out of the [tobacco tax] initiative fight. In all honesty, luckily, the CMA's primary objective was tort reform and they planned to use the bulk of their resources in sponsoring a tort reform Initiative at the same time as the tobacco tax Initiative would be on the ballot if it

should qualify. Obviously, we used this to our great advantage in convincing CMA to stay out of the tax initiative. During the last day of the 1987 California legislative session, the trial attorneys and the proponents of tort reform came to a political compromise which was subsequently enacted by the legislature. As part of this compromise there was an agreement to a five year moratorium on tort reform initiatives agreed to by all parties, including the CMA. This could potentially open up the CMA to re-thinking their position in regard to the proposed tobacco tax initiative. We are duplicating all of our previous efforts to assure that this does not happen.[7] [emphasis in original]

The industry understood how central the malpractice insurance reform issue was to the CMA, more central than Proposition 99. The CMA would be willing to make some trades to get the tobacco industry's support. When Roger Kennedy, a Santa Clara County physician who was active in both tobacco control and the CMA, was asked whether he was surprised when the CMA signed off on the Napkin Deal, he said, "I think that it was something that was so important to the leadership at that time. . . . In order to preserve that MICRA . . . they probably would have done almost anything. Because that was number one."[31]

CONCLUSION

Meral and Mekemson's idea of increasing the tobacco tax and allocating some of the money to public health and environmental programs had matured and developed a committed constituency, led by the ALA and ACS. After documenting public support for their idea, they made the obligatory attempt at getting the Legislature to act. Following the bill's defeat, the proponents of the tax increase were poised to start their initiative campaign and hoped, vainly, that they would receive substantial support from organized medicine. They had no idea how deeply the tobacco industry had already neutralized the CMA as they moved into the battle to qualify the tobacco tax initiative for the ballot campaign for voter support.

CHAPTER 4

Beating the Tobacco Industry at the Polls

Having laid the groundwork for going directly to the voters with their proposal to increase the tobacco tax, proponents still had to finalize the initiative and develop the necessary political and financial resources to withstand the huge campaign that everyone knew the tobacco industry would mount.

LOCKING IN MONEY FOR PREVENTION

By mid-May 1987, Curt Mekemson (ALA), Tony Najera (ALA), Betsy Hite (ACS), and Assembly Member Lloyd Connelly (D-Sacramento) had begun discussing the transition from the legislative to the initiative process.[1,2] Tim Howe, Connelly's chief of staff, took responsibility for writing the initiative. His goal was to present something clear and understandable to the public that was as impervious to industry attack as possible. Mekemson, Hite, Najera, and Connelly were Howe's primary sources of feedback during this initial drafting.

As the details of the initiative began to take shape, Mekemson was adamant that some of the revenues go toward funding tobacco prevention programs. Even before the Legislature defeated ACA 14, he predicted,

> I think we have three major arguments for dealing with the tobacco problem: health impacts, kids, and economic impacts. While we may need to substantiate each of these in greater detail, they are real and extremely difficult for the tobacco industry, or others, to challenge. In these arguments lies the justifica-

tion for increasing the tax and for focusing the tax revenues on the problem. Most important *is prevention*. Everything else pales in relation to persuading kids not to smoke and helping smokers to quit. This is our justification for demanding that a substantial portion of the funds go for school and community health education. *Without this guarantee, prevention funds will be eliminated whenever short term crises emerge.*[2] [emphasis in original]

Mekemson's early insistence that money for prevention be tied to the initiative proved critical in fights over implementation years later. Even with this strong language, public health proponents would face an uphill fight to maintain the prevention elements within Proposition 99 against strong opposition in the Legislature from the tobacco industry and the CMA.

Connelly wanted some legislative discretion to make the proposition less vulnerable to attack as an instance of "ballot-box budgeting." In a May 13, 1987, memorandum, Mekemson was worried about not including some restrictions. He wrote, "I continue to feel that we need to set percentages. I know it isn't nice not to trust the infinite wisdom of the legislature, but I don't. If it comes down to dealing with immediate crises as opposed to funding long term solutions, the pressure for the immediate is tremendous."[1] Mekemson, Najera, Hite, and Connelly decided to hold a "high-level/high-stakes" meeting of leaders from the participating organizations and other interested groups. The meeting occurred in San Francisco on June 17, 1987, with the CMA, California Association of Hospitals and Health Care Systems (CAHHS), Planning and Conservation League (PCL), Blue Cross of California, California Dental Association, California Thoracic Society, and the Health Officers Association of California attending. The following revenue allocation was presented at the meeting: 25 percent to medical care (which included 5 percent for research), 20 percent to education, 5 percent to the environment (non-health), and the remaining 50 percent to established accounts, to be allocated by the Legislature.

In writing the initiative, the Coalition tried to select language that would broaden public support. One important instance of this approach was the titling of the initiative. The polling conducted for the Coalition (by Charlton Research) as well as for the tobacco industry (by Tarrance and Associates) had showed that Proposition 99 was viewed more positively when framed as a health issue. So Connelly pushed the Coalition to come up with a title that emphasized the health message; this title would help define the issue in the campaign, in the literature mailed to all voters, and in the voting booth where voters were reading the ballot items. According to Hite, "We submitted for title and summary with this real great encouragement from Lloyd about how it needed to be the 'Health Protection Act, Health Protection Act!' And the opponents were just scared to death that was how it was going to get titled. And guess what? We got it titled. Attorney General Van de Kamp was very good to us."[3]

A seemingly minor clause in Proposition 99, as it was eventually finalized, was to cause great problems for tobacco control advocates. The drafters of the initiative specified that it could be amended by a four-fifths vote of both houses of the Legislature if the amendments to the initiative were "consistent with its purposes." This clause was included to avoid criticism that the initiative would be inflexible; as a practical matter, the authors felt that only technical amendments would be able to garner this level of support. Pro-tobacco forces would eventually use this clause to loot Proposition 99 revenues.

ORGANIZING THE CAMPAIGN

The ALA's original $50,000 contribution defined the financial standard for Executive Committee membership of the Coalition for a Healthy California. From June through September, the Executive Committee consisted of the ALA, ACS, PCL, and Connelly. The AHA, which did not consider political issues like the tobacco tax initiative a priority,[4] did not participate on the Executive Committee, nor did the CMA or CAHHS.

The effort by the tobacco industry to "tokenize" the CMA's participation was only one part of the industry's strategy to deny resources to the Coalition. In its report to the Tobacco Institute, A-K Associates noted, "Connelly, being a strong and respected member of the liberal political community, personally sought help from the Hayden/Fonda machine and organized labor."[5] The industry hoped to block the participation of these groups, too.

Campaign California, a liberal statewide political organization founded by Assembly Member Tom Hayden (D-Santa Monica) and his wife, actress Jane Fonda, had approached the Coalition in the spring and expressed interest in participating in the tobacco tax effort. While Campaign California had money to help finance the effort, a full-time campaign staff, and statewide volunteers, some Coalition members were concerned that Hayden, Fonda, and Campaign California's liberal politics would have a negative impact on the Coalition and the tobacco tax effort. By July, however, they let Campaign California join the Executive

Committee because the Coalition needed their help. The industry countered this move by approaching Campaign California through the polling firm Fairbank, Bregman and Maullin (which also did a lot of work
for Democrats) to convince Hayden "that there is little advantage to him
personally or politically to get involved in the Connelly tobacco tax Initiative. Hayden/Fonda has pledged a modest $25,000 to the tax initia-
tive." [5] This amount was the same as that pledged by the CMA, enough
to support the effort without providing it with sufficient resources to succeed. But in contrast to the CMA, Campaign California was to make a
significant contribution to the campaign that went well beyond monetary
value.

Connelly tried to attract organized labor by offering to incorporate
into the tobacco tax initiative the provisions of a pending union initiative designed to strengthen Cal-OSHA's worker protections. Jack Henning, secretary-treasurer of the California AFL-CIO, turned him down.
(Organized labor had sided with the tobacco industry in opposing
Propositions 5, 10, and P.) The tobacco industry, working through Paul
Kinney of A-K Associates, had already made a deal to keep organized
labor out of the tobacco tax effort.[5]

In September 1987, W. James Nethery, a dentist and the immediate
past president of ACS, was elected chair of the Coalition, which reinforced ACS's involvement. The Coalition hired Jack Nicholl as full-time
campaign director. Nicholl, the past executive director of Campaign
California, brought essential statewide political and campaign expertise
to the Coalition. Nicholl set up the campaign headquarters in Los Angeles. When later asked why he had chosen Los Angeles over Sacramento,
he answered, "If you listen to most of the griping that's going on, it's the
Sacramento crowd that's griping. . . . They were always tied in these
knots of conflict and contradiction among themselves. . . . That's why I
insisted that the headquarters had to be in LA. Because that's where
people are, that's where the money is, and that's where you get away
from this crap." [6] The Coalition also hired Ken Masterton to coordinate
the signature campaign. Masterton, who had managed the winning campaign for Proposition P in San Francisco in 1983, was not only experienced on the tobacco issue but also willing to work with both voluntary
and paid circulators.

Nicholl tried once again to interest some of the veterans of the Propositions 5, 10, and P campaigns and was rebuffed as others had been.
Nicholl approached Stanton Glantz of the University of California, San

Francisco, whose expertise in anti-smoking legislation he respected. Glantz declined to get involved: "I told them I thought they didn't have a prayer of winning. And even if they did, it was a stupid idea because the only thing that mattered was the tax and they may as well take the money out and dump it off the Golden Gate Bridge, because the health department would never run the kind of gutsy program it would take to do any good. And so I had basically nothing to do with it because shortly thereafter I went to Vermont on sabbatical to write a statistics textbook. I'm pleased that I was wrong."[7]

THE INDUSTRY CAMPAIGN

As the Coalition was gearing up in September 1987, the tobacco industry was also moving ahead with its plans to oppose the initiative. Fairbank, Bregman, and Maullin conducted a statewide poll for the Tobacco Institute. The results were not encouraging for the industry:

> In putting together a campaign on an initiative, whether for or against it, one usually looks for how the issue polarizes different segments of the population. Some of these are often in the form of Democrats vs. Republicans, men vs. women, liberals vs. conservatives, more affluent vs. less affluent. . . . These common voting divisions do not exist as readily on this issue. On most questions in the study there are few or no differences in the larger voting groups. . . . the only consistent group against the initiative is that of current smokers, who comprise just 20% of the electorate.[8]

As revealed in the industry's poll conducted six months earlier by Tarrance and Associates, the greatest vulnerabilities for the initiative appeared to be in the issues of taxation and government regulation. The most persuasive arguments against the initiative were the following: "this law would create another state bureaucracy with a large budget" (43 percent said this argument made them less likely to vote for the initiative) and "government will have more money to mismanage and waste" (41 percent said this argument made them less likely to vote for the initiative).[9]

Echoing the strategies used successfully by the tobacco industry in opposing Propositions 5 and 10, the industry's pollsters advised the "no" campaign to take this approach: Proposition 99 is a flawed solution to a real problem. They reasoned that "if the debate remains one of pro-smoking vs. anti-smoking, the American Cancer Society/Heart Association/Medical Association vs. the tobacco industry, then the measure will pass easily. If, however, the debate can be turned to the defects in the particular initiative, conceding the 'good intentions' of the authors, then the voters may decide the issue in terms favorable to the 'no' side." [8] To win, the industry had to focus attention away from the health issue and toward the flaws in the initiative.

GETTING THE MEDICAL PROVIDERS TO BUY IN

After repeated invitations, CAHHS representatives finally attended an October 1, 1987, meeting of the Coalition's Executive Committee. They expressed an interest in the initiative but raised concerns about its language and revenue allocations. The Executive Committee agreed that CAHHS, as a medical provider organization, should meet with the CMA to discuss the initiative language as well as the organization's involvement in the tax effort.

The Executive Committee recognized that the initiative had to amend the Gann Limit so that its spending provisions could withstand a legal challenge. To qualify a statute initiative for the ballot in California, supporters were required by state law to collect valid signatures amounting to 5 percent of the number of votes cast in the last gubernatorial election (372,178 valid signatures in this instance); but a constitutional amendment initiative, which was needed to address the Gann Limit, required signatures amounting to 8 percent of the votes cast in the last gubernatorial election, or 595,485 valid signatures.[10,11] Assuming a 65 percent validity rate, the Coalition had to collect over 915,000 raw signatures.

The need for extra funds as well as additional organizational and political support to collect the additional signatures was the main reason why the Executive Committee sought to enlist the participation of the CMA and CAHHS. The CMA was clear about its price for entry: it wanted more money for medical services. Carolyn Martin, a volunteer with the ALA who would play a leading role in the battles over Proposition 99, recalled the meeting years later: "My most vivid memory of the meeting was how shocked I was that the CMA proposed eliminating the Research Account completely and using the money for medical services. Since the American Lung Association includes the California Thoracic Society [a physicians' organization of lung specialists], I said, 'absolutely not.' I couldn't believe doctors would oppose money for basic medical research on tobacco-related diseases! Yes, I was naive." [12]

The CMA got its money.

According to the minutes of an October 26 meeting, the Executive Committee agreed to qualify a constitutional amendment and to allocate an additional 25 percent of tax revenues toward medical services in exchange for CMA and CAHHS participation and financial assistance to the tobacco tax effort. The minutes stated that "The Coalition is relying on pledges from CMA/CAHHS that between the two they can guarantee $250,000 in cash or signature equivalents and if they cannot make such guarantees in good conscience, they must tell us [the Executive Committee] so." [13] Duane Dauner, president of CAHHS, and Fred Armstrong, president of CMA, accepted these conditions.

Unbeknownst to the participants at the October 26 meeting, however, the tobacco industry had already created procedural changes to return power to the "old guard" at the CMA and to neutralize Armstrong's authority on the initiative. The CMA had no intention of producing $250,000 in cash or signatures. In fact, when he was interviewed in 1993, CMA vice president and chief lobbyist Jay Michael did not remember that the CMA had made any commitments. He said, "I was the point person. If anyone would know, I would know, and I don't remember. I'm not sure we would ever say we would bring X amount. I don't think we ever did that." [14]

In contrast to the CMA, CAHHS fully intended to keep its commitment and did so after finally deciding to get involved. According to Doug Hitchcock, the vice president and counsel for government relations at CAHHS, "We made a very heavy organizational commitment that we followed through on. And because we had done initiatives before, I think we brought some experience to the Coalition on ballot initiative campaigns. . . . Where hospitals were comfortable doing the signature-gathering campaign, they did signatures; where they weren't, they wrote a check, and most hospitals, as I recall, did some signature-gathering and then wrote a check for the balance of their commitment." [15]

The new revenue allocation was not based on the results of the February 1987 Charlton Research poll, as ACA 14 had been, but rather on political and monetary considerations within the Coalition (figure 1). Funding for medical services was given higher priority than education and prevention. Medical services received the greatest share of revenues— 45 percent—much more than the original legislative proposal of 27.5 percent. The allocation for education and prevention was reduced from 47.5 percent to 20 percent. The share for research was reduced from 15 percent to 5 percent. (The research money was given its own ac-

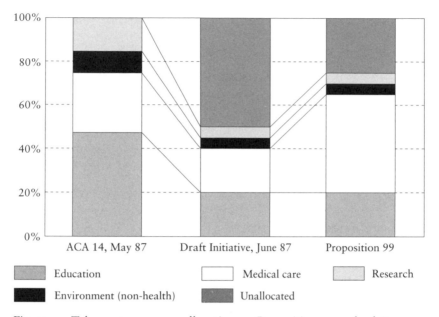

Figure 1. Tobacco tax revenue allocations as Proposition 99 evolved. In order to attract support for the initiative, proponents moved money out of anti-tobacco education and research into medical services. ACA 14, the attempt to enact the tax through the Legislature, had more closely followed public opinion.

count so that it would not be the first money to be cut or redirected.) The allocation for nonhealth (environmental) programs was cut from 10 percent to 5 percent. The 25 percent to be allocated by the Legislature, down from 50 percent, could be appropriated for the uses specified for the other accounts.

COLLECTING THE SIGNATURES

On December 4, 1987, volunteers and paid circulators began collecting signatures throughout the state. The Coalition held statewide press conferences on December 16 to launch the petition drive, and it received extensive media coverage.[16,17] The tobacco industry, which had hired the Sacramento-based political consulting firm Townsend and Company to conduct its campaign activities, formed Californians Against Unfair Tax Increases (CAUTI) and immediately denounced the initiative.[17]

The financial status of the Coalition was extremely important to the success of the ongoing signature drive. Chronically short of money, the Coalition depended almost entirely on the financial contributions of its Executive Committee members.[18] According to Nicholl,

> We tried to work the corporate self-interest angle and the medical industries. Tried to work all the professional associations, and the suppliers, and people who would benefit by more money being pumped into the service delivery end of the health care system. . . . None of it worked; it was a complete failure. . . . The only things that worked were the institutional interests that were built into the text of the initiative. That's what worked. The hospitals primarily, because they were going to get millions and millions, hundreds of millions of dollars a year. And the Cancer Society, because this was its mission statement. Lung Association, same way."[6]

In addition, Americans for Nonsmokers' Rights (ANR), while not actively participating in the campaign, allowed the Coalition free use of its mailing list as well as access to its large network of politically oriented grassroots volunteers.[19]

The Coalition experienced several problems during its signature-gathering campaign. The start of the petition drive in the middle of December coincided with the holiday season, and bad weather during the winter months caused an initial low return in signatures. After the first month and a relatively slow start, Campaign California and its grassroots network of volunteers joined the signature-collecting effort as additional paid circulators.[20] Other initiative campaigns, also aimed at the November 1988 election, were paying professional petitioning firms forty-five cents to seventy-five cents per signature; Masterton was paying only thirty cents to thirty-five cents per signature, which reduced the number of paid circulators working for the Coalition.[21] As it had planned the previous September, the tobacco industry even began circulating its own petition, entitled "The Tobacco Tax Ripoff."[5,22] This petition was not an official one approved by the secretary of state to qualify an industry-sponsored initiative; it was solely designed to reduce the pool of available paid circulators (by paying them as much as fifty cents per signature) and to confuse voters about the tobacco tax issue.

The voluntary health agencies had an overly optimistic view of the commitment and effectiveness of their local units in gathering most of the signatures. Their inability to get signatures surprised Nethery:

> I anticipated that the volunteers, mainly meaning Heart and Lung and Cancer, would collect two-thirds of signatures. In reality they probably collected less than a third. What the truth of the matter was, and maybe I was naive, was that voluntary health agency volunteers are not psychologically and men-

tally equipped to get involved in political campaigns. They're out to do good and be nice people, and raise funds for other people. But they're not there to go toe to toe with anybody, whether it be on television or whether it be in the media, or anything.[23]

Those who had observed the ability of the Propositions 5 and 10 campaigns to gather signatures through an all-volunteer effort failed to take into account the difference between the ANR and the voluntary health agencies. ANR had its roots in political activism. The voluntary health agencies had their roots in medical practice and middle-class charity. For ANR, political involvement was assumed; for the health agencies, it was often a dubious enterprise. The health agencies' ambivalence about political involvement would continue throughout the Proposition 99 battles, including the efforts to secure implementing legislation that reflected the initiative.

The CMA was not of much help to the signature-gathering campaign. A confidential report, dated March 29, 1988, and entitled "Tobacco Tax Initiative," summarized the weaknesses of the Coalition campaign and expressed qualms about backing the initiative. The author, "JM" (probably Jay Michael), reported:

1. The campaign is broke, and the signature effort is slowing down,

2. Campaign owes American Lung Association $25,000

3. Jack Nicholl, the campaign director, is an unknown quantity and Gilanto—the ad man is also unknown. If the initiative qualifies it is uncertain that this team has the expertise to carry off the campaign.

4. A minimum of $2 million is needed to conduct the most basic campaign. Nobody has the slightest idea of how the money might be raised.

5. The tobacco industry has in its possession the most sophisticated data attainable on which to develop strategy and is prepared to spend whatever is necessary to defeat the proposal. They have bought options to retain the best campaign management available. Campaign strategy is beginning to jell.

6. The proponents possess only fragmentary data, thin expertise, no strategy and is broke.

7. The tobacco industry is planning a "doctor/hospital bashing campaign."

Watershed Decisions Faced by CMA

1. Do we want the initiative to qualify?

2. Do we want to attempt to gain some measure of control over the direction of the campaign?

3. Do we need to protect physicians from a doctor-bashing campaign?

4. What will be CMA's financial involvement in the campaign?[24]

The CMA proposed to work with CAHHS to gain some control over the campaign. It also proposed to "Meet with industry representatives in an attempt to circumscribe the type of campaign each side might wage."[24] The CMA was apparently continuing to work both sides of the fence, participating minimally in the Coalition while consulting with the tobacco industry. Whatever the results of the meetings with tobacco industry representatives, the industry eventually appeared to pull its punches somewhat on the doctor-bashing theme once the campaign began.

In the end, 73 percent of the signatures were gathered by paid circulators (66 percent from Masterton and 7 percent from Campaign California), 9 percent from ALA, 5 percent from ACS, 6 percent from CAHHS, 2 percent from the CMA, and the rest from mail efforts and miscellaneous sources.[25] The Coalition collected 1,125,290 raw signatures by the May 4, 1988, deadline, and the initiative qualified for the November 1988 election as Proposition 99.[26]

LAUNCHING THE ELECTION CAMPAIGN

On May 2, 1988, the Coalition held a series of press events across the state when the signatures were delivered for validation.[27] Some signatures were delivered in ambulances to attract press coverage. The same day, CAUTI held a press conference arguing that the tobacco tax was just another way that special interests and doctors would get richer. Even though the election was six months away, the battle promised to be long and controversial.

In late April, the Coalition had commissioned Charlton Research to gauge public opinion on the tobacco tax initiative and determine campaign themes and strategy. Support for the tobacco tax increase remained between 61 percent and 65 percent before and after various arguments for and against the initiative had been presented (table 1). The most popular argument for supporting the initiative was that 20 percent of the revenues were allocated to health education and tobacco-use prevention; 82 percent of the respondents said they would be likely to support the tax for this reason. The next most popular argument was that 45 percent of the revenues went for people who could not afford health care; 72 percent reacted favorably to this argument. But when the argument was restated—that 45 percent of the money would benefit doctors and health providers—it received the highest negative reaction; 58 percent of the respondents said they would be less likely to support the tax in re-

TABLE I. STATEMENTS TO GAUGE WHETHER RESPONDENT WOULD BE MORE LIKELY OR LESS LIKELY TO SUPPORT A CIGARETTE TAX INCREASE

	More Likely to Support Tax %	Less Likely to Support Tax %	No Difference %	Don't Know %
Statements Classified as Positive				
20% of the tax revenues will pay for programs to teach children about the dangers of smoking.	82	11	6	1
45% of the tax will go toward caring for the growing number of people who cannot afford health care.	72	18	8	2
Only smokers will pay this tax.	68	21	10	1
5% of the tax would go to protecting wildlife and improving and protecting parks.	68	18	13	2
Smoking costs all of us millions of dollars each year through increased insurance premiums and lost productivity, and smokers should pay more for the hidden costs of smoking.	66	24	9	1
California has not received its fair share of tax revenues because it has lagged behind the rest of the nation by not raising its cigarette tax since 1967.	57	21	17	5
Statements Classified as Negative				
A handful of special interests benefit from this initiative, particularly doctors and health providers who receive 45% of the funds for purposes unrelated to smoking.	21	58	15	6
Experience in other states has demonstrated that such a large tax increase will lead to bootlegging and other crime problems, yet the measure provides no new money to assist law enforcement.	24	49	20	7
Only 5% of the tax revenues would go to research on tobacco-related diseases.	41	43	12	4
The cigarette tax is a regressive tax that hits hardest at blue-collar working men and women.	29	37	31	3
This 250% tax increase would make California's tobacco tax one of the highest in the country.	44	30	22	4

Data from C. F. Rund and K. O'Donnell. *The attitudes and opinions of California voters toward a cigarette tax increase*, San Francisco: Charlton Research, Inc., April 1988. Table originally appeared in M. P. Traynor and S. A. Glantz, California's tobacco tax initiative: The development and passage of Proposition 99. *J. Health Politics, Policy, and Law* 1996;21(3):543–585. Reproduced with permission of the *Journal of Health Politics, Policy, and Law*.

sponse to this statement.[28] Although the Coalition effectively used all of these themes, limited resources did not allow statewide advertising on the same scale as the tobacco industry's.

The industry had already geared up for the campaign. It hired the public relations firm of Ogilvy and Mather to provide spokespersons for the CAUTI campaign. Staff members in both Northern and Southern California were designated to handle media requests. Kimberly Belshé joined the tobacco industry team as its Southern California spokesperson and helped the tobacco companies organize their in-house mailings to smokers.[29] In 1993, when asked where to find Belshé, Nicholl commented, "She's not with them anymore. I saw her turn up somewhere else. She became an aide to a politician."[6] By November 1993, everyone would know where to find Belshé because Governor Pete Wilson had appointed her to be the director of the Department of Health Services, the state agency charged with implementing the Proposition 99 health education programs.

The industry's polls indicated that, although the tobacco companies were in trouble, several messages might play well with the voters. Jeff Raimundo, an account executive at Townsend and Company and communications director for CAUTI, later described the tobacco industry's use of the polling data in its campaign against Proposition 99:

> Our polling told us that doctors were . . . almost as unpopular as the tobacco industry. Doctors per se, not your own doctor. . . . Our polling also told us that the public was generally opposed to tax increases [and] that the public was generally opposed to using the initiative process to accomplish social policy . . . and that the public by and large thought individual rights were something that ought not to be trampled by initiative. Having said all that, the poll results showed us going in [with] public support of this initiative, like 75 percent to 20 percent. And I think their polls were about the same. It was huge. . . . And using all of our strategy to try to attack the soft spots in the initiative, even in our polling we could only pull it down to about 58 percent to 42 percent. Which is where it ended up.[29]

By June, the tobacco industry was broadcasting radio advertisements using the theme that rich doctors would get richer with this tax while the poor would pay the most for it. The industry had considered running advertisements during the signature-gathering phase but did not want to give the circulators extra publicity. After the initiative qualified, these advertisements were designed to counter the free publicity that had surrounded the proponents on filing day. According to Raimundo, "There had been a lot of publicity around the qualifying of the initiative. And we didn't want that to go unresponded to for months. . . . They were getting all kinds of positive publicity. We had to do something to . . . plant the seeds of doubt about the initiative."[29]

The two campaigns shared a similar approach—designing a message around polling data—but they used the data in very different ways. CAUTI had the money to saturate television, radio, and print media with paid advertising that promoted the tobacco industry's position. The Coalition, with its limited resources, relied on free publicity to define the issue and to get its message to the public. The Coalition used the grassroots network it had established during the signature collecting campaign.[30] Members held coordinated press conferences throughout the state using local volunteers who were assisted by press materials and information that Nicholl and his campaign staff provided. They established speaker bureaus, trained volunteers to debate the opposition, and secured endorsements.[31] All this activity received widespread media coverage. Some of the more effective press conferences in early July featured children helping to promote the tobacco tax.[32] During the campaign, only three major newspapers in California ran editorials opposing the tobacco tax.[31]

Although the Coalition used the name and credibility of the American Heart Association (AHA) throughout the tobacco tax effort, the AHA had not contributed significant organizational, staff, or financial resources.[4] Nicholl summarized the attitude of the voluntaries:

> Here's the way I describe it. Cancer is Republican, Lung is Democrat, and Heart is nonpolitical. They can't stand it. They don't like politics, they're not comfortable with it. It's like walking on nails for them. So they were not really there until the end. Cancer is controlled by all these docs. This is just the lay person's view of things. And Lung Association, boy, if they were better trained, they'd be better, but their heart is out on the streets and, you know, kind of a democratic approach. But Heart, it is just not comfortable with politics.[6]

However, on July 11, 1988, the AHA Greater Los Angeles Affiliate finally contributed $25,000 to the Coalition, and the California Affiliate (which included all of California outside Los Angeles County) gave $25,000 in early September.[33,34] AHA had never even had representation in Sacramento until August 1988, when it hired Dian Kiser to be its first lobbyist. AHA worried that its name would be linked with radical organizations like Campaign California or ANR.[4]

PUTTING THE ISSUE BEFORE THE VOTERS

On July 20, the tobacco industry sued to stop the initiative. Two weeks before the deadline to submit ballot arguments, which the state mails to all voters, tobacco distributors filed a petition for a writ of mandamus and request for stay in the attempt to keep the initiative off the November ballot.[35] The distributors maintained that Proposition 99 violated California's 1978 property-tax–cutting initiative (Proposition 13), which they claimed allowed only the Legislature to increase taxes, and then only by a two-thirds vote. They also claimed that the collection of taxes for multiple purposes violated the "single subject" rule, a constitutional provision requiring that an initiative only deal with one subject. The tobacco industry's challenge failed, and the Coalition held press conferences labeling the suit as an "outrageous misuse of the legal process."[35] The Coalition used the free media opportunity to further educate the voters about Proposition 99 and expose the tactics and misleading advertisements of the tobacco industry.

By early August 1988, Proposition 99 had established a substantial lead. The California Field Poll, released on August 10, revealed that 72 percent of the voters supported Proposition 99, 24 percent opposed it, and 4 percent had no opinion.[36] An August 11 memorandum from Charlton Research to Nicholl stated, "After several months of the opposition's paid media and our own free media exposure, voters favor the initiative more than ever before."[37] Encouraged by the poll results, the Coalition launched another series of press conferences to generate free publicity.

In addition to the free media coverage that Proposition 99 was receiving, the Coalition also acquired a significant amount of free time for airing television and radio advertisements through the Fairness Doctrine, primarily because of the efforts of Campaign California. During the 1988 election, the Federal Communications Commission (FCC) Fairness Doctrine still required stations to broadcast both sides of controversial issues, even if only one side could pay for the advertisements.[38] Campaign California, which already had regional offices and staff throughout the state in all major media markets, negotiated with television and radio stations with the goal of acquiring one free pro–Proposition 99 advertisement for every three paid tobacco industry advertisements.[39] While not every station agreed with these terms or acknowledged the legality of the Fairness Doctrine, by the election campaign's end, Campaign California had negotiated approximately $1.5 million in free television and radio time using the Fairness Doctrine—in addition to the money and services Campaign California had already contributed to the effort.[31,40] The Coalition's use of the Fairness Doctrine was even more impressive in light of the FCC's stringent limitations on the application of the Fairness Doctrine, although the agency did not explicitly repeal it for ballot initiatives until later.[40,41]

Nicholl deliberately downplayed Campaign California's role during the campaign, in the interest of making Proposition 99 look very health-oriented and not political. As Nicholl explained,

> You rarely saw Campaign California, you rarely saw Lloyd Connelly, you rarely saw the environmentalists, you only saw the health side, and that was conscious, that was my decision—to profile what was our primary selling point, which was a health measure. But I mean you shouldn't necessarily single out Campaign California in that regard, because the environmental thing was in a sense a weak link for us . . . and Lloyd, who was just absolutely instrumental in making this whole thing. But we didn't play him up either. And he was really wise in making sure that we didn't. But wise beyond our wisdom, I think.[6]

The Coalition spent what it could on paid advertising. One of the Coalition's more effective television commercials, produced by its media and public relations consultant, Sid Galanty, depicted James Almon, a smoker who later died of emphysema. The commercial showed a noticeably frail Almon, his labored breathing assisted with oxygen, admitting that it was too late for him. He went on to say that he wished he had known more about the dangers of smoking when he was younger and that Proposition 99 would help prevent people from starting to smoke. Almon had died by the time the commercial aired. Another effective commercial portrayed actor Jack Klugman asking voters which side they believed in the debate about Proposition 99—the tobacco industry or groups like the ALA, ACS, and AHA.

In August the Tobacco Institute's polls likewise showed that voters overwhelmingly supported Proposition 99—by 74.5 percent. Even after respondents were presented with every possible argument against Proposition 99, public support remained as high as 61.5 percent. This poll also showed the popularity of Proposition 99's anti-tobacco and education programs, which received the strongest approval rating (56.9 percent, compared with only 15.4 percent who somewhat or strongly disapproved), followed by wildlife habitats (55.9 percent), hospitals (49.1 percent), and tobacco-related health research (45.1 percent). Money for doctors' services was much farther behind all other allocations, receiving the support of only 11.4 percent (48.5 percent somewhat or strongly disapproved).[42] The tobacco industry's commercials were affecting the public.

The Proposition 99 campaign also benefited from a reinvigorated ACS effort in September. ACS volunteers and staff had been assured that their principal contribution would be to gather signatures and that the campaign would be conducted by others. John Bailey, the new ACS executive vice president, was deeply offended by the tobacco industry's advertisements against Proposition 99 but discovered that, except for a few individuals, ACS was not involved in the campaign. Bailey, who had a background in politics, convinced the ACS volunteer leadership that "we won't have a chance like this one for the rest of the century and we better get off the sidelines and into the play."[43] Bailey thereupon made passage of Proposition 99 the primary goal of ACS staff members throughout the state. When the PCL suggested a gimmick in the important Central Valley, "99 for 99," a road tour of the major cities along Highway 99 from Redding to Chessfield, Bailey made sure ACS offices in Marysville, Stockton, Modesto, Fresno, and other valley communities got on board. The tour succeeded in gathering media coverage in this crucial vote-rich region.

THE CMA'S QUIET WITHDRAWAL

As the campaign progressed, the proponents' efforts continued to be hamstrung by the CMA for two reasons. The CMA had not come through with the money it had promised, and as a part of the Coalition, the CMA was a target for the tobacco industry. David Langness, a CAHHS board member who served on the Coalition's Executive Committee as the AHA representative, offered an explanation for the CMA's behavior: "At that point, the allocations were set, the language was cast in stone [and] it was a done deal. . . . They [the CMA] knew that if we lost, it was no skin off their nose. . . . The doctors committed to a large amount but never paid it, which is funny in a way, because they are who are reaping the greatest reward now. Maybe they were smarter than all of us."[44]

Despite the CMA's low level of participation, the tobacco industry remained concerned that the CMA might move in with serious money for proponents and held off on its doctor-bashing campaign to insure that this did not happen. The doctor-bashing tactic came late and was not a central focus of the campaign. According to Raimundo, "We had been holding back a little, hoping that they [the CMA] wouldn't get involved in the campaign, not wanting to do anything to piss them off and send them in . . . we had run out of things to talk about. We had to come up with another issue. So we started in on the docs."[29] At a Tobacco Institute planning meeting, held on July 6, 1988, to discuss Proposition 99, participants discussed three basic messages to be used in their advertising campaign against the initiative: police burden/crime increases, tax money into doctors' pockets, and government interference/fairness. Roger Mozingo, director of state activities for the Tobacco Institute, observed, however, that "how we address the doctors issue is obviously sensitive; thus, our approach will have to be carefully positioned."[45] The doctor issue had likely tested well in focus groups, but the industry was clearly not embracing this as a major strategy, perhaps as a result of its conversations with the CMA.

Nonetheless, the CMA used the anticipated tobacco industry opposition to Proposition 99 as its excuse for not making more of a commitment to the campaign. Langness observed,

> They [CMA] said, "Oh they're [the tobacco industry] going to spend 40–50 million dollars and they're going to defeat you with sheer money and no matter how much money we put in, it's going to be going down a rat hole." So what's unfortunate was, we based our campaign on the eventuality of CMA money and it never came. And we weren't able to do a lot of things that we would otherwise have been able to do had it come. And also, during the second period after their "guns and gangs" campaign failed to do anything in the polls, the tobacco industry really hit the doctors. I don't know if you heard any of their ads about the golf clubs dropping in the trunk of the Mercedes. But they were obviously the most visible target. And frankly had we bounced them at that point, had we just kicked them out, it probably would have been smarter. Because it would have removed that target from the campaign.[44]

In June 1988 the CMA Council, in fact, had formally decided to back off in its support for the campaign. It agreed

> not to contribute additional funds to the tobacco tax initiative campaign. *The CMA believes it is not in the best interest of physicians to battle the tobacco industry,* which has pledged to defeat the November ballot measure with a multi-million-dollar campaign that is likely to single out physicians as personal beneficiaries of the revenues generated. Part of the revenue from the increased tobacco tax will be used for health education and to offset the uncompensated care problem. The CMA will support the initiative by providing physicians with information about the initiative through *California Physician* magazine and possible all-member mailings.[46] [emphasis added]

This decision was not made public at the time, however, and Jay Michael continued to press for more of the Proposition 99 monies to go into health care.

There were even official conversations about kicking the CMA out of the Coalition. According to Langness,

> We talked about it in meetings. People were angry as hell. Because basically what the docs did was played an end game on us. They committed to a certain amount of funds, we based the campaign on those funds, then when we look forward to such a point where the campaign was locked in, they said, "Oh gee, sorry, we ran out of money." They know that if we lost, it was no skin off their nose. And if we won, great! They'd get a cheap victory. I think all of us got an education in extremely cynical coalition politics at that point.[44]

The Coalition did not act on these feelings, however; the CMA remained in the coalition.

THE FAKE COP FIASCO

The tobacco industry's polling data did not suggest that the theme of cigarette smuggling and crime would have a major influence on voters' opinions. Only 32.6 percent of those polled thought that Proposition 99 would lead to an increase in crime.[42] Still, according to Raimundo, CAUTI's task was to move the Proposition 99 debate away from the health issue.[29,47] And when the tobacco industry began its advertising blitz in mid-August, the crime theme worked especially well. In addition, very early in the campaign, CAUTI secured the endorsements of the California Sheriffs' Association and the California Peace Officers' Association, two organizations that gave credibility to the tobacco industry's claim that the tobacco tax would result in cigarette smuggling.

In August and September, CAUTI's most effective commercial showed an undercover police officer stating that if Proposition 99 passed, he would have to spend all his time chasing cigarette smugglers and that the illegal bootlegging would lead to a massive crime wave. He also claimed that the money obtained from cigarette smuggling would be used to buy guns and drugs. After the tobacco industry's August media blitz on cigarette smuggling and crime, support for Proposition 99 began to decrease. The tobacco industry was surprised at the success of this campaign, but the success had a downside. As Raimundo observed,

> We were so successful, the success blinded us to the downsides of sticking on an issue too long. And as a result I think it gave the other side time to rally a response. But we caught them off guard on the crime issue. They did not an-

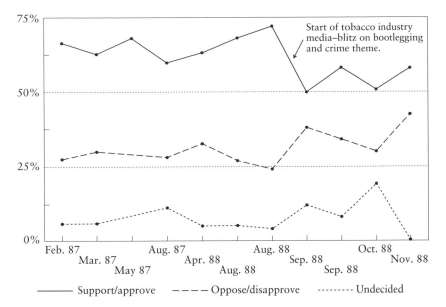

Figure 2. Public support for Proposition 99 through the election campaign. Support for the initiative remained high before the tobacco industry began its advertising campaign against the initiative. But despite a massive campaign against the initiative by the tobacco industry, support never dropped below 50%. Proposition 99 passed with 58% of the vote. *Source:* M. P. Traynor and S. A. Glantz, California's tobacco tax initiative: The development and passage of Proposition 99, *J Health Policy, Politics, and Law* 1996;21(3):543–585. Adapted with permission of *Journal of Health Politics, Policy, and Law.*

ticipate that we would drive it so hard, and they didn't anticipate that the public would respond to it as much as they did. . . . The best world for me as communications director for this campaign would have been to stay on it for two, three weeks, catch them off guard, they're scrambling to come up with a response, and by the time they come up with a response, we're already on to a different issue. We're talking about the doctors' rip-off. So when the reporters come to us and say, "They just held a press conference with [Attorney General] John Van de Kamp saying it's a bunch of baloney about the crime issue," we can say, "That's not the issue here; the issue is the doctors' rip-off." I mean we'd just do our spin-doctoring on the campaign as much as possible.[29]

Charlton Research confirmed the decline in support for Proposition 99 in a memorandum to Nicholl. The measure's 27-point lead in April (61 percent for, 34 percent against) was down to a 13-point lead (51 percent for, 38 percent against).[48] On September 22, 1988, another California Field Poll showed that voter support for Proposition 99 had sharply dropped—from 72 percent in August to 58 percent (figure 2).[49]

The Coalition nonetheless benefited from several key events in late August and early September, which helped slow and ultimately stop Proposition 99's decline in support. Attorney General John Van de Kamp released a report based on state and federal data showing that cigarette smuggling was negligible even in states with high tobacco taxes. Van de Kamp criticized CAUTI's advertisements, calling them "a scare tactic of the worst and baldest kind. . . . [and] utter nonsense, fabricated by people who represent the tobacco industry."[50] As a result of this and other Coalition efforts, the two law enforcement associations dropped their opposition to Proposition 99 and took a neutral position.[51,52] The report and Van de Kamp's position gave the Coalition and Proposition 99 free media coverage and damaged the tobacco industry's most effective campaign argument.

Nicholl also discovered that the undercover cop who appeared in the tobacco industry's advertisement, Jack Hoar, actually had a desk job at the Los Angeles Police Department and was a part-time actor. In spite of this, Hoar had signed a sworn affidavit, which he submitted to KGO-TV in San Francisco, declaring "under perjury and the penalties therein" that he was not an actor.[53] More important, in the movie *To Live and Die in LA* Hoar had played a criminal who killed two secret service agents and spit a chaw of tobacco on one of the dead bodies. Nethery described how the Coalition had stumbled onto this information:

> Jack [Nicholl] was at a party one night and . . . the topic was 99, and these ads came up, and one of the actors said, "Oh. I know that guy." So Jack's antenna just went right up, and we found out immediately that this guy had been in movies, he was a cop, he was assigned to the studios for security. Once in a while they need a cop quick, they'd drag him in. Well, one thing led to another, and he had finally gotten film credits on this movie, *To Live and Die in LA*.
>
> Jack rushed out that night, rented the movie, and the next day we were talking to everybody in the state practically, but we were talking and trying to figure out what to do. We had the evidence that this was a lie.
>
> We had a written affidavit to KGO in Jack Hoar's handwriting, and so . . . I approached some of the lawyers involved with the Cancer Society, and they said, "You'll just get your ass sued off . . . you can't dare touch it. Can't use it any way, shape, or form." Well, Sid Galanty, and here's where he really earned his money, he says, "Bull." He says, "That's news." He said, "We'll send it to the news media." And we made up enough for every TV station in the state . . . .
>
> Basically we showed the written statement to KGO, we showed clips from the tobacco spots, and then we showed clips from *To Live and Die in LA,* including the credits with Jack Hoar. . . . The TV people just blew them out of

the water on that. And within a day they were gone. . . . They pulled those ads so fast you couldn't believe it.[23]

The Coalition held press conferences throughout the state, distributing the affidavit and showing the industry's commercial and a clip of Hoar's scene in the movie. Television, radio, and newspaper press coverage of the event saturated every media market in California.

CAUTI tried to argue that Hoar was not a full-time actor and that the desk job was only temporary. As Raimundo explained,

> They [the proponents] used heavy-handed techniques, just as the tobacco industry has over the years. I don't want to say they lied, but they certainly manipulated facts in a way that was untruthful. . . . What they did was, they take a set of facts and then miscast what those facts represented. The perfect example of that was when they had Jack Hoar, . . . they said he was an actor, he's not a cop. And that was horseshit! He was an undercover cop temporarily on the desk assignment in LA. He's a Los Angeles police sergeant. He had only acted in two bit parts in his entire life, and didn't have enough time to have a Screen Actors Guild card. He was not an actor. And if you watch *To Live and Die in LA,* I guarantee you he was no actor. If you watch our commercials, he's not much an actor. . . . It was like he was like a stiff cop, because that was what he was: he was a stiff cop.[29]

But it was too late. The plausibility of the bootlegging and crime argument was destroyed and CAUTI stopped running the undercover cop commercials. The Coalition damaged the credibility of the theme and at the same time highlighted the tobacco industry's misleading campaign tactics.[54]

On November 2, less than one week before the election, the Coalition and Proposition 99 gained additional positive media coverage. Dr. Ken Kizer, Governor George Deukmejian's director of the Department of Health Services (DHS), released a report at a press conference organized by the Coalition which included an examination of the financial cost of smoking and smoking-related deaths in California in 1985. The total economic burden to Californians during that year totaled more than $7.1 billion—$4.1 billion for direct medical costs, $2.2 billion for lost future earnings due to premature death, and $800 million for smoking-caused lost productivity.[55] Because the governor had recently announced his opposition to Proposition 99, Kizer was quick to state that he was not advocating support for Proposition 99, but simply presenting DHS findings. CAUTI responded, "This was obviously timed to be released in the final week of a political campaign. If the timings and the motivations

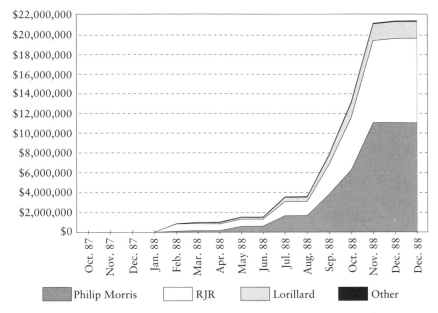

Figure 3.   Expenditures to oppose Proposition 99. Virtually all the $21.4 million spent to oppose Proposition 99 came from the tobacco industry (Other = Brown & Williamson Tobacco Company, Smokeless Tobacco Council, Tobacco Institute, and individual contributions). *Source:* M. P. Traynor and S. A. Glantz, California's tobacco tax initiative: The development and passage of Proposition 99, *J Health Politics, Policy, and Law* 1996;21(3):543–585. Adapted with permission of *Journal of Health Politics, Policy, and Law.*

become suspect, obviously the statistics must become suspect."[56] Nevertheless, the Coalition capitalized on the report to generate more free publicity for Proposition 99.

By election day, the tobacco industry had spent $21.4 million on the campaign, compared with the Coalition's $1.6 million (figures 3 and 4).[57,58] The use of free media, the Fairness Doctrine, coordinated statewide press conferences, and local volunteers were all invaluable to the campaign. In addition, the undercover cop fiasco, the Attorney General's report, and the dropped opposition of law enforcement groups all contributed to undermining the tobacco industry's bootlegging and crime theme. The release of the DHS report in the final days of the campaign also helped. While the Coalition campaign was smaller than the tobacco industry's campaign, it was large enough to permit the Coalition to communicate these messages effectively to California voters.

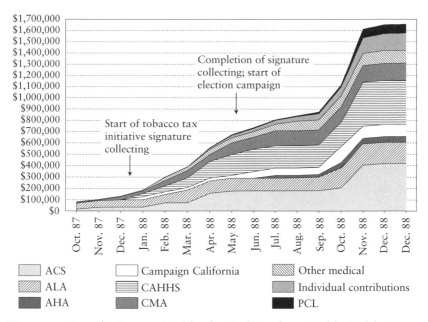

Figure 4. Contributions received by the Coalition for a Healthy California to support Proposition 99. Despite expenditures of only $1.6 million, the Coalition successfully passed Proposition 99. The health groups contributed 45%; the medical groups, 40%; environmental groups, 5%; and others, 9%. *Source:* M. P. Traynor and S. A. Glantz, California's tobacco tax initiative: The development and passage of Proposition 99, *J Health Politics, Policy, and Law* 1996; 21(3):543–585. Adapted with permission of *Journal of Health Politics, Policy, and Law.*

On November 8, 1998 the voters of California passed Proposition 99 with 58 percent of the vote.[59]

REFLECTIONS ON THE INDUSTRY'S DEFEAT

In his postelection analysis prepared for the tobacco industry, Ray Mc-Nally, whose firm Ray McNally and Associates coordinated the industry's direct mail campaign, wrote, "In retrospect, I believe we overplayed the crime issue. We came on too hot, trying to sell the argument that California streets would run red with blood if Proposition 99 were enacted. Had we turned the heat down, focusing less on the potential for violence and more on the actual economic loss and added strain on law enforcement caused by smuggling, then used actual experiences and spokespersons from other states as 'proof,' we would have preserved our credibility and alienated fewer opinion leaders at the start of the campaign."[60] Nicholl substantially agreed with McNally and thought that the key mistake the "no" side made was dropping the crime theme after the Hoar controversy. If the pro-tobacco forces had merely dropped the Hoar advertisement, apologized, and continued the general crime theme, Nicholl thought the proponents of the initiative would have been in trouble. He said, "The victory was getting them to stop playing the ad, because that ad took us from over 70 percent down to 55 percent. And if they kept going, they would have kept taking us down. . . . The voters walking into the polls in November, if they had stuck with that thing, they couldn't see beyond it."[6]

Hanauer's initial skepticism about victory turned out to be wrong. He observed, "It showed that the tobacco industry could be beaten on a statewide campaign. Beyond that, and probably the reason why it was beaten, it showed once and for all that the people hated the industry."[61]

CONCLUSION

Proponents invested over two years to pass Proposition 99, conducting essential polling, planning strategy, gaining media exposure, developing a coalition, and running a successful campaign for enactment of the tax directly by the voters. The tobacco industry's large war chest worked for it in the campaigns against Propositions 5 and 10, but failed in the campaigns against Propositions P and 99. The popularity of using a tobacco tax to fund education and prevention programs as well as the unpopularity of the tobacco industry meant that public health activists did not have to match the tobacco industry dollar for dollar. They needed only a budget sufficient to take advantage of the tobacco industry's low credibility. Proponents of Proposition 99 effectively made the very size of the industry war chest an issue because they had enough money to publicize it. The initiative proponents had learned a lot in ten years, as had the public and the media.

In California it was clear that the industry was the enemy. What was less clear was the extent to which the CMA was also a problem. While the political and financial support of medical organizations, particularly the hospitals, helped pass the initiative, their presence in the pro–Proposition 99 camp presented a threat to public health programs. Actions and statements made by the CMA before, during, and after the tobacco tax effort showed that the CMA considered the tobacco tax solely as a source of revenue for medical services, which foreshadowed the subsequent pressure for diversion of funds from health education into medical services once Proposition 99 arrived at the Legislature. Although health education programs received the greatest public support during the campaign in both Coalition and Tobacco Institute polls, this support provided no guarantee that public health priorities would dominate the organizational interests of the other Coalition members. The difficulties that arose at the initiative stage were to be amplified when the issue of implementing legislation came before the California Legislature.

CHAPTER 5

Moving to the Legislature

Proposition 99 raised over $600 million a year in new tobacco taxes, over $150 million of which was allocated by the voters to anti-tobacco education and research, creating the largest tobacco control program in the world. The public health groups turned to the initiative process to secure the tax increase because the tobacco lobby had successfully blocked at least thirty-six attempts to pass a tax increase in the Legislature since 1967.[1] Unfortunately, after winning at the polls, the health advocates had to return to the same Legislature to pass implementing legislation to turn the promise of Proposition 99 into a reality.

Proposition 99 specifically assigned the money raised by the new tax to six accounts: Physician Services (35 percent of revenues), Health Education (20 percent), Hospital Services (10 percent), Research (5 percent), Public Resources (5 percent), and Unallocated (25 percent). Curt Mekemson wrote these allocations into the initiative to shield the prevention (Health Education and Research) programs from the Legislature and the powerful special-interest groups that dominated it. Protecting the integrity of the initiative in the Legislature would not be easy. As the *Los Angeles Times* editorialized on November 10, two days after the election, "Now comes the really hard part: negotiating the Legislature's special-interest steeplechase to make sure that the estimated $600 million to be raised annually by the tobacco tax increase is allocated as the sponsors intended and spent as they promised voters it would be spent."[2]

Proposition 99 went into effect on January 1, 1989. Since the state's fiscal year begins in July, the first state budget to appropriate Proposition 99 revenues would be the 1989–1990 budget. As a result, there would be eighteen months' revenues—about $900 million—to spend in the first budget year, which began on July 1, 1989. Of this amount, $180 million was to go toward health education. This money attracted a lot of attention and many new "friends" for the Coalition for a Healthy California.

THE TOBACCO INDUSTRY'S PRICING STRATEGY

Following its defeat at the polls on November 8, 1988, the tobacco industry immediately adopted marketing, political, and legal strategies to counter the effects of Proposition 99 on its sales. It developed marketing strategies to blunt the effect of the price increase brought about by the tax increase so that people would not quit smoking. It also intervened politically to try to get the Board of Equalization, the state agency that collects the tobacco tax, to set a low tax rate on tobacco products other than cigarettes. It also sued to try to overturn Proposition 99.

The tobacco companies knew that smokers were sensitive to the price of cigarettes. (Indeed, the fact that price increases reduce consumption was one of the arguments that the ALA and others used to justify creating Proposition 99 in the first place.) After losing the election, RJ Reynolds decided to push its lower-priced brands, especially Doral and Magna, because "we do plan to capitalize aggressively on business shifts that will undoubtedly occur as a result of the California tax increase."[3] The company's marketers told management, "We will be developing and recommending programs on DORAL that include newspaper advertising, direct mail, on-carton coupons, and pack purchase incentives. On MAGNA, we will be looking at additional pack purchase incentives to help generate trail for this brand."[4] Philip Morris planned strategies to protect all of its brands, including such premium-price brands as Marlboro.[5] Specific promotions consisted of packaging lighters with Marlboro two-packs at the beginning of January, coupons to reduce the effective price for cartons of Marlboros at the end of December and for the Benson & Hedges, Merit, and Virginia Slims brands, a two-for-one promotion for Merit Ultra Lights at the end of December, coupons to reduce the effective price of Cambridge cigarettes during January, and the launch of Alpine cigarettes, a lower-priced brand, at the beginning of that month.

In late November 1988, the tobacco distributors mounted an effort to establish a low tax rate on non-cigarette tobacco products. The initiative had established a tax increase of twenty-five cents on each pack of cigarettes (1.25 cents per cigarette), but had left other tobacco products to be taxed at a rate "equivalent to the combined rate of tax imposed on cigarettes" established by the State Board of Equalization. Proposition 99 proponents wanted a high rate while the tobacco industry and tobacco distributors wanted a low rate based on weight rather than wholesale price.

On November 30 the Coalition presented its case to the board, which decided to establish a tax rate of 42 percent on the wholesale price of tobacco products, calculated by dividing the per pack tax on cigarettes (thirty-five cents) by the average wholesale price of cigarettes (eighty-four cents). Tobacco distributors had lobbied for 19 percent, using a complex formula that Assembly Member Lloyd Connelly said would "befuddle Albert Einstein."[6] The Board of Equalization agreed with the Coalition and established the higher rate.

The tobacco industry then took its case to the Legislature, and in February 1989 Senator William Campbell (R-Industry) introduced a resolution urging the Board of Equalization to adopt an alternative method of computing the tax rate on tobacco products, one favorable to the tobacco industry, whereby one cigarette "is the equivalent of one cigar, one-twentieth of a can of snuff, or one bowl of pipe tobacco." The bill died in the Senate Revenue and Taxation Committee, representing a victory for the Coalition.

The tobacco industry sued to void Proposition 99 after it passed. On January 17, 1989, Kennedy Wholesalers, Inc., a tobacco distributor, filed a lawsuit claiming that Proposition 99 was unconstitutional. The distributor claimed that Proposition 99 violated Proposition 13, needed approval by a two-thirds vote of both houses of the legislature, restricted the appropriations power of future legislatures, burdened one class of persons with a tax that benefited the public generally where no rational relationship exists, and violated the rule that required initiatives to cover only one subject. The arguments were identical to those in the suit filed by the tobacco industry in July 1988 in their failed effort to keep the initiative off the November ballot. The Coalition opposed the industry in court, and on March 17, 1989, Sacramento Superior Court Judge Anthony DeCristoforo denied the motion to declare Proposition 99 unconstitutional.

The industry appealed, and the suit eventually went to the state Supreme Court, which in 1991 upheld the lower court and unanimously rejected the claim that Proposition 13 required any new tax, including one passed by citizen initiative, to be approved by two-thirds of the legislature. The court found that Proposition 13 was designed to limit the power of the legislature but not the public's power. The court also rejected claims that the initiative violated the single subject rule.[7] All the industry's legal maneuvering, although unsuccessful, hurt the Coalition, which had to raise money to pay the legal fees incurred in fighting the tobacco industry in court.[8]

CONFLICTING VIEWS OF HEALTH EDUCATION

The wording of Proposition 99 creating the Health Education Account stated only that funds were to be available "for appropriation for programs for the prevention and reduction of tobacco use, primarily among children, through school and community health education programs." No agency was given responsibility for the Health Education program, and one of the important questions to be addressed was how much money would go to health departments and how much would be given to schools.

A broad outline for tobacco education was available. At the urging of public health activists, in February 1988, prior to the Proposition 99 election, Senator Diane Watson (D-Los Angeles) had introduced Senate Bill 2133, the Tobacco Use Prevention Act, to begin planning the implementation of Proposition 99 tobacco education programs. The bill required that the Department of Health Services (DHS) develop a program to reduce tobacco use in California through a multifaceted approach that, for the first time, combined mass media advertising with community-based interventions on a large scale. John Miller, Watson's primary staffer on the bill, was particularly committed to an anti-smoking media campaign. Miller "wanted to hire the same guys who sold cigarettes to unsell them."[9]

The voluntary health agencies and ANR supported the bill. Proponents clearly did not understand the tobacco industry's well-developed strategy of working through intermediaries. Miller even wrote Watson, "It does not appear that the tobacco lobby will try to kill 2133."[10] The tobacco industry maintained a low profile, preferring to let the California Chamber of Commerce, California Manufacturers' Association, and the California Taxpayers Association lead the formal opposition, although the Tobacco Institute formally opposed the bill late in the legislative process.

Although Governor George Deukmejian vetoed the bill after the Legislature passed it, SB 2133 provided health groups with an early opportunity to assert their vision of what the state's anti-tobacco education program should look like if Proposition 99 passed. Had it been signed into law, a program to implement Proposition 99 would have been in place when the initiative passed, which might have avoided the problems that arose when its proponents returned to the Legislature to seek implementing legislation after they passed Proposition 99 at the polls. As it was, several different organizations advanced competing plans for how to spend this money after the election.

The ALA wanted to see the Health Education Account spent in accordance with the basic elements of SB 2133 but with three changes: (1) at least 50 percent of the Health Education Account should target students eighteen or younger, (2) there should be no "sunset clause," which ended the spending authority for the current provisions on July 1, 1999, and required further legislative action, and (3) a provision should be added to make anti-tobacco education a mandated program, meaning that the Legislature would require local public agencies to participate and they would receive money for doing so.[11]

The California Department of Education (CDE) wanted to broaden the focus of the program beyond direct anti-tobacco education, arguing that "the same pressures and reasons which cause young people to smoke are those which cause them to use drugs and alcohol, become sexually active, consider suicide or adopt obsessive eating habits. The skills needed to prevent drug abuse, improve nutritional selections, abstain from sexual activities, and engage in lifelong physical activity are the same skills needed to prevent tobacco use."[12] CDE's specific plan was to have the funds administered by the new Office of Healthy Kids, Healthy California, which had been set up to concentrate health education programs within CDE. CDE wanted the money distributed in five ways: (1) award grants to all districts on an entitlement basis to implement comprehensive health education programs with a smoking prevention component, (2) make available effective smoking prevention curricula and materials, (3) provide training on implementing smoking prevention education in the context of a comprehensive health education program, (4) design and implement a media campaign for the classroom and public media, and (5) establish an advisory committee.

DHS, on the other hand, proposed a program completely inside DHS, with grants going to local agencies, including schools, to implement programs for the target populations.

The California Association of School Health Educators (CASHE) suggested a program that was prepared by Ric Loya, executive secretary of CASHE, and Alan Henderson, board member of CASHE. The program had six major components: (1) an independent commission to oversee program implementation with its own staff and budget appointed by the governor, Legislature, and CDE, (2) funding based on applications for school and agency programs run by credentialed health educators, (3) training support, (4) demonstration projects, (5) educational research, and (6) an incentive program to encourage smoke-free schools.[12]

ACS, in conjunction with CASHE, proposed that $30 million of the Health Education Account go toward funding mandatory health education. The remaining money was to fund block grants to the County Offices of Education to carry out education programs.

AHA recommended that at least half of the money go to mandating and implementing comprehensive school health programs in public and private schools. The remainder of the money was to go to other education outreach programs. AHA made no recommendations about program administration.[13]

Those outside the education establishment worried that money given to schools might not be used for tobacco education, and the early proposals advanced by CDE and CASHE, the school health educators, did little to alleviate this concern. When he was interviewed in 1995, Steve Thompson, who was head of the Assembly Office of Research in 1989 and a key agent for Speaker Willie Brown in the Proposition 99 negotiations, remembered that "there was a great deal of skepticism, based on previous performance, that putting money into the school systems was going to have much impact."[14] Miller and Najera were similarly disenchanted with the CDE proposal, advanced by Robert Ryan, head of the Office of Healthy Kids, Healthy California, and Bill White, his deputy, to put the money into "healthy kids, healthy this, healthy everything." Miller recalled, "We kept saying, 'How are you going to account for what the hell you're doing with tobacco?' And that became a real sore subject and concern of those of us who wanted to make sure that that money bought tobacco control programs in school systems in California."[15]

In submitting different proposals on how to implement the Health Education Account, the three voluntary health agencies were clearly not cooperating on implementation of the initiative. Tensions between the three agencies continued to build over the next several months and weakened their political position in the coming legislative debates.

A HOSTILE LEGISLATIVE ENVIRONMENT

Proposition 99 arrived at the Legislature with some controls in the form of specific accounts, each with a percentage allocation. Even so, the Legislature was still responsible for deciding which agencies would run the programs, the forms those programs would take, and the allocations to those programs. The text of Proposition 99 had been worded as simply as possible to build support with the voting public. This brevity and simplicity, while keeping the initiative clear for the voters, meant that the initiative was not written to withstand the special-interest lobbying and legislative manipulation that would greet it at the Legislature.

Five realities about the California Legislature were particularly relevant to Proposition 99.

First, the tobacco industry was a major political player in the Legislature. There had been no tax increase on tobacco for over twenty years, reflecting the power of the industry and the weakness of the voluntary health groups. The tobacco industry had spent $21 million in its unsuccessful bid to defeat Proposition 99 and was not likely to turn a blind eye to its implementing legislation. The industry responded to Proposition 99 by increasing its already substantial lobbying presence and campaign contributions to members of the California Legislature. In the 1985–1986 election cycle, before Proposition 99 passed, the industry had spent only $274,394 on campaign contributions and lobbying in California. In 1987–1988, when ACA 14 (Proposition 99's legislative predecessor) was being considered by the Legislature and when Proposition 99 passed, expenditures for industry lobbying and campaign contributions increased to $2,818,534 (excluding the $21 million the industry spent trying to defeat Proposition 99 at the polls); in 1989–1990, when the Legislature was considering the legislation to implement Proposition 99, they jumped to $4,077,264.[16]

Second, no health organization with a California lobbying presence was dedicated solely to tobacco issues, which meant that every organization lobbying for Proposition 99 programs had to consider how its stance on Proposition 99 might affect its relationship with the governor and the Legislature on other matters. The primary organizations with an interest in tobacco control (ALA, ACS, and AHA) had only a limited lobbying presence in Sacramento, consisting of one or two full-time lobbyists, and these organizations had not traditionally been willing to adopt strong positions or risk making enemies.[17,18]

Third, the California Medical Association (CMA) and the California Association of Hospitals and Health Systems (CAHHS) were powerful players in Sacramento as a result of their large campaign contributions and extensive information resources. While these organizations paid lip service to anti-tobacco activities, these activities were of minor importance compared to economic issues affecting their members. The dominance of economic issues over public health issues was starkly illustrated by the CMA's collaboration with the tobacco industry in 1987 to pass the Napkin Deal, with the attendant "tokenizing" of support for Proposition 99.

Fourth, within the Legislature, led by Assembly Speaker Willie Brown (D-San Francisco) and his longtime aide, Steve Thompson, there was a core of liberal Democrats who were committed to funding health care for children and who were likely to see new monies as a route to doing this.[19] As of 1988, the tobacco industry had given Willie Brown $124,900 in campaign contributions, more than any other member of a state legislature in the United States and more than the tobacco industry had given many members of Congress. Moreover, contributions to Brown from the industry increased rapidly after Proposition 99 passed; by the time he left the Legislature in 1996, Brown had accepted $635,472 in tobacco industry campaign contributions.[16,20] There was a natural confluence of interests between Brown, Thompson, the CMA (another major source of campaign contributions to Brown), and the tobacco industry in shifting anti-tobacco education money into paying for medical services for poor children. This axis was continued after Thompson left Brown's staff in 1985 to become the head of the Assembly Office of Research. According to Thompson, in 1989 he "basically was representing the position of the Speaker's office. . . . I did most of the health advising for their office. So I was basically speaking for them on this issue [Proposition 99]."[14] The ties between Brown, Thompson, and the CMA became even stronger in 1992, when Thompson left the Legislature to become vice president and chief lobbyist for the CMA.[19,21]

Joining the CMA, CAHHS, and Brown in their interest in health care for children was the highly regarded lobbyist Peter Schilla, of the liberal advocacy group Western Center for Law and Poverty, whose priority was to increase health care for poor people. Although the Western Center was not involved in the initiative campaign, Schilla was very influential with liberal members of the Legislature, particularly on issues related to health care for the poor. John Miller, chief of staff for Senator Diane Watson (D-Los Angeles), and Mary Adams, the AHA's lobbyist, shared the opinion that Schilla was one of the major forces behind Proposition 99's implementing legislation. Miller later recalled that Schilla "never cared much about health education, but he did care about funding the other programs. And he was putting it all together and knew we needed to be placated and so he did some of that." Adams agreed, saying, "I recall personal conversations that I had with John Vasconcellos [D-San Jose, a prominent liberal member of the Assembly] about the overarching Prop 99 accounts. I was really surprised at the information that he had and asked him where he got it. And he said from Peter Schilla . . . it was already very clearly thought out, not just that but then one step more." [15]

Fifth, the Legislature was hostile toward Proposition 99 because it earmarked money; it represented voters' restrictions on legislative decisions concerning the funds and thus limited the Legislature's fiscal prerogatives. As John Miller commented, "They despise it. And it is a built-in antagonism. A serious one." [22]

Within this hostile environment, the answers to three key questions would determine the fate of Proposition 99 in the Legislature.[23] First, would Proposition 99 advocates be able to maintain the source of their power—public opinion? Second, would they be able to advocate sound proposals for spending the tax revenues and to keep the issue framed as "following the will of the voter"? Third, would program advocates find a leader for their cause, an "entrepreneur" who could recognize opportunities to act and who had a commitment to challenge the status quo? Without an entrepreneur to identify opportunities to act, to guide legislation, and to be confrontational within the process, Proposition 99 was likely to have difficulties surviving in the Legislature.[24]

CALIFORNIA'S FISCAL PROBLEMS

California's fiscal situation had become increasingly grim since the passage of Proposition 13 in 1978, which limited local government's ability to raise property taxes and forced the state to take over funding for many locally provided services, and of the Gann Limit (Proposition 4) in 1979, which limited yearly increases in government spending. The two measures passed during a period when the state had built up a substantial financial surplus, which buffered their effects. By the time Proposition 99 was before the Legislature in early 1989, the situation had changed: the state was facing a deficit. Elizabeth Hill, the Legislative Analyst, said that she expected the state to end the 1988–1989 fiscal year as much as $126 million in the red and that the subsequent year's budget problems might be "even worse." [25] The Legislative Analyst is a widely respected nonpartisan official who has a reputation for objectivity and is charged with preparing an analysis of the governor's budget for the Legislature.

Proposition 99 brought in new money whose expenditure was not restricted by the Gann Limit, and there was nothing requiring that the money be used only for the programs that the Coalition wanted. The CMA, CHHS, and the Western Center wanted more money for medical services for poor people. The Service Employees International Union (SEIU), a labor union representing county employees, particularly in the health care field, and the County Supervisors Association of California (CSAC), an organization representing California county governments, saw Proposition 99 as a new source of jobs and money for their constituents. Governor George Deukmejian had many cash-starved programs under his administration's Health and Welfare Agency. So did the CDE, which reported to the State Superintendent of Public Instruction, not the governor. The Research Account initially attracted the attention of California's research universities, especially the University of Southern California, Stanford University, and the University of California, which saw it as a new source of money. None of these new players had any particular commitment to tobacco control.

DOWN THE LEGISLATIVE PATH

The primary challenge faced by the voluntary health agencies was that the tobacco education program would be the first and largest of its kind, and no one knew a sure way to reduce smoking. In the absence of a proven model, the public health groups had to argue their case as trying something new and carrying out the will of the people.

The voluntary health agencies recognized their vulnerability. When he was asked about the effort to implement Proposition 99, ALA lobbyist Tony Najera commented, "We were vulnerable for two reasons. We didn't know what the heck was needed. . . . and second, we had so much money. We had accumulated so much money before any action plan was even looked at." [15] Thompson also recognized the vulnerability of the new program: "There were some [existing] programs being defunded or not fully funded competing against things that didn't exist. So, in a traditional budgetary context, it's not as difficult to take money from something that hasn't happened and give it to something that's being reduced." [14] The existing health care programs with established constituencies also provided a clear mechanism by which the money could be spent. According to the Senate Health Committee's John Miller, "The hospitals and the doctors and the others who got big lump sums of money from this tax had a system in place to just plug it in and spend it. I mean, it was gone within minutes of arriving, because their distribution network was already there. We didn't have that." [15] The voluntary health agencies were thus arguing for a new program for which there were no existing bureaucracy, no proven approaches, and no constituency to defend it against established programs with well-developed financial and political infrastructures.

The CMA, after extracting as much money as possible from Proposition 99, had walked away from anything but token participation in the initiative, even before it qualified for the ballot. After Proposition 99 passed, the CMA struck out on its own almost immediately. At a Coalition meeting on December 28, 1988, the CMA told the other members present of its intent to go after the entire Unallocated Account to fund health insurance for workers who lacked health insurance.

The interest of the voluntary health agencies in continuing a relationship with the CMA, in spite of CMA's increasingly adversarial actions toward prevention programs, would prove to be characteristic of their behavior throughout the Proposition 99 allocation discussions. ANR co-director Julia Carol observed: "I think [the voluntaries] view the CMA as somebody they have to have. All three agencies work with the CMA on issues other than tobacco. Their boards are made up of doctors who are also members of the CMA. The CMA has tremendous clout in the Legislature and they see them as allies that they cannot have a permanent rift with. . . . they see the CMA as indispensable to who they are and how they have to work." [26] Despite the CMA's failure to deliver its promised support for the initiative (creating debate over removing it from the Coalition before the initiative passed) and the CMA's repeated raids first on the Health Education Account and then on the Research Account, the voluntary health agencies would cling to the CMA.

THE COALITION'S DISINTEGRATION

In contrast to its clear and consistent strategy during the two-year effort to develop and pass Proposition 99, the Coalition had not developed a coordinated plan to implement Proposition 99 after the election victory. On December 15, 1988, in its first meeting after the election, the Coalition met and briefly discussed whether it should be the lead organization in securing the legislation to implement Proposition 99. Jack Nicholl, who had managed the election campaign, sent a memo to the Coalition Executive Committee arguing that the Coalition should remain together and proposing a budget for doing so: "The Coalition is the guardian of Proposition 99 as it was written. Individual organizations will use their quite substantial lobbying resources to pursue implementing legislation. The Coalition's mission is to preserve the framework of Prop 99 which the voters passed by a margin of 58%–42%. If we don't do it, no one else will. . . . Our principle [sic] objective will be to generate grass roots pressure on the Governor and the Legislature to head off attempts to change the direction or intent of Proposition 99." [27] Nicholl proposed a budget of $8,000 per month to insure that over $100 million a year was spent wisely on new tobacco control programs.

The Coalition said no. Instead of maintaining a budget and staff for the Coalition, the Executive Committee decided that "each member agency could rely upon its own staff and resources from this point on, and that a core staff from key agencies (especially related to legislative activity) could provide a focus." [28] The Coalition would be a mechanism for cooperation among the individual agencies. Money for an ongoing effort was an obstacle for the voluntary health agencies. According to Carolyn Martin, a volunteer with ALA who was active in the campaign to pass Proposition 99, "Money was a big problem. The non-profit agencies, ACS and ALA, had spent an astronomical amount of money on the Proposition 99 campaign. Obviously, CMA and CAHHS would not contribute to this effort." [29] The Coalition met to discuss issues during the legislative session, and it was listed as a supporting organization for several bills. But it ceased to function as an effective body. Each organization pursued its own strategy and lobbied for its own bills with its principal legislators.

On January 5, 1989, the now resourceless Coalition hosted a press conference to present its Program for a Healthy California, which outlined its plans for disbursing funds from the various accounts of Proposition 99. The program recommended that at least 70 percent of the Health Education Account go toward school-based programs, with grantees to include not only school districts but also clinics, community-based organizations, local health departments, colleges and universities, voluntary health agencies, and hospitals. The remainder of the account was to be used for an Oversight Committee, which would be responsible for program planning, implementation, and evaluation, and for the media campaign, which would be designed to reinforce the school-based program. The Research Account was to be administered using the federal National Institutes of Health model and was to include biomedical, behavioral, social, and epidemiologic research. The Unallocated Account was to be used to fund a fire prevention program and other funding categories.[30]

The CMA was already moving to gain control of as much of the money as possible. The day before the Coalition's press conference, CMA executive vice president Robert H. Elsner sent a letter to Coalition chair Jim Nethery asking the Coalition to refrain from making statements about the Unallocated Account. He specifically urged that the press conference and the supporting materials "not include any specific recommendations or proposals for use of the unallocated funds. In the press conferences it should be made clear the Coalition has not adopted any policy on specific proposals for implementing Proposition 99. . . . However, if after the various proposals have been discussed by the Coalition and a consensus cannot be reached, various organizations ultimately may have to go their own way."[31] Nethery and the Coalition ignored him. The press conference was the last major coordinated effort of the Coalition for a Healthy California as it was constituted during the election.

The decision not to stay together formally with a paid staff meant that there would be no changes in the existing institutional patterns that might disrupt the existing legislative patterns related to tobacco policy making. In particular, it meant that there would be no lobbying presence in Sacramento dedicated solely to the tobacco debate or to maintaining the integrity of the Proposition 99 programs. Ken Kizer, the director of DHS and a strong supporter of the Proposition 99 program, described the problem created by the lack of a unified coalition:

> Passage of [Proposition 99] really came about because everybody worked together. It was one of the few instances where the health constituencies actually got together on the same team and worked in a coordinated way. But that Coalition seemed to unravel relatively quickly, being superseded by self-interest. . . . In the absence of a concerted pressure driving it in one direction, then it reverted back to the Legislature to arbitrate the disparate views of the folks who wanted to get more for themselves. . . . *Everybody in the Legislature knows how easy it is to fracture the health community and how they are largely their own worst enemy and how they can capitalize on that.*[32] [emphasis added]

Kizer understood that with each organization following its own insider strategy in the Legislature, consensus was going to be difficult to achieve in implementing Proposition 99.

Nicholl was not the only person who felt the need for a continuing organizational presence focused on implementing Proposition 99. In 1989 the federal Centers for Disease Control and Prevention in Atlanta offered to give the Coalition $9,000 to help with public relations activities, and the money was eventually given to the Western Consortium for Public Health through Lester Breslow. (The Western Consortium was a nonprofit organization that allowed the schools of public health in California to cooperate on grants and contracts.) Breslow, a professor at UCLA, was a former director of health services and the former dean of the UCLA School of Public Health.

The Western Consortium, apparently at Nethery's request, wanted to use the money to hire Betsy Hite, who had recently left ACS.[33] According to Nethery, who continued to chair the Coalition, "I got a little heavy-handed. I didn't have a staff, and they put me in a position which I shouldn't have agreed to in the first place of operating the Coalition without a staff. And so at one point in time the public health people came along and offered me this money, and I was going to use it to hire Betsy. And I made a really dumb statement. I said, 'Now I have my lobbyist' . . . I could have thought that and it would have been okay. But you know, keep your stupid mouth shut."[34] Other members of the Coalition did not trust Hite because they felt she put her personal views ahead of the consensus position. ALA opposed the decision to hire Hite;[35] ALA executive director Williams wrote a strong letter to Nethery, saying, "Surely you understand that Betsy is thought controversial by some members of the Coalition. To bring her back into the fray at this date without careful preparation was I think insensitive. . . . why does the Western Consortium want to hire her and then expect the Coalition to take her on as a partner? The three lobbyists for the voluntaries are working well; what would the addition of Betsy contribute?"[36] In the end, Hite was not hired to work with the Coalition. Instead, the Western Consortium prepared a case study of the effort to implement Proposition 99.[37]

Nethery was in the minority in believing that a campaign-style effort would be necessary to see that the Legislature properly implemented Proposition 99. For most of those who were involved in passing Proposition 99, the degree to which the political fight would continue in the Legislature came as a surprise. David Langness, who worked for CAHHS but represented the American Heart Association on the Coalition, commented, "The 99 Commission was a little fractious at times before the election. But after the election, we didn't anticipate the necessity for long-term post-election work. And that was one of the big lessons that I learned during that campaign. And it's one of the lessons that I'm trying to transmit to the other people I'm consulting with, like the Arizona [Heart] Association. [Arizona passed a Proposition 99 clone in 1994.] And that is: The campaign doesn't stop on election day."[38] When asked if she was surprised at how fast the Coalition split apart, Jennie Cook, a longtime ACS volunteer and, in 1989, immediate past chair of the board of ACS California, replied, "As soon as it was passed, we figured, 'Okay, we walk away and do something else.' What a joke! . . . We all figured that there was no more to do, it was done. It was a law. What more could we do? . . . We had spent months coming up with how we wanted the money designated and we figured that that was in the initiative, so that would make it law."[39] The voluntary health agencies assumed that because the voters passed Proposition 99, the Legislature would simply implement it as the voters wanted.

They were wrong.

THE GOVERNOR'S BUDGET

In January 1989 Governor Deukmejian issued his budget for the 1989–1990 fiscal year, the first budget to include the Proposition 99 revenues. He recommended that the Health Education and Research Accounts be funded in accordance with the initiative. The Health Education programs received their full 20 percent—$175.6 million—for a new smoking prevention program administered by DHS. The Research Account received its full 5 percent—$43.9 million—for a research program administered by the University of California. The voluntary health agencies did not want to have the entire Health Education Account within DHS or have the university administer the Research Account, but the funding allocations at least followed the initiative.[40]

The controversial part of the governor's budget lay in his proposal to use Proposition 99's Hospital Services and Physician Services Accounts to pay for county medical services. His budget called for a $358 million reduction in state revenues to fund county programs to treat the medically indigent (a General Fund obligation) and then allocated $331.3 million of Proposition 99's tobacco tax revenues back to the counties for a supposedly new program, the California Health Indigent Program. Several individuals saw the governor's plan as supplanting already existing levels of service, a violation of the "maintenance of effort" requirement in the initiative.

The governor also proposed using Proposition 99 funds to finance $54 million in unavoidable state obligations, such as health care costs associated with caseload increases, $14 million for various state prison programs, $18 million for capital outlay improvements in state mental hospitals, and $7 million for caseload increases in several categorical health programs. He also proposed expanding community mental health and drug treatment programs for female drug addicts. Some of these expenditures, such as those for prisons and for capital improvements in the state mental hospitals, were not consistent with Proposition 99, which required increases in medical services.

The governor's budget drew an immediate negative response from the press, the Coalition members, the Legislative Analyst's Office, and members of the Legislature. The CMA described the governor's proposal as a "shell game."[41] A *Los Angeles Times* editorial labeled the Governor's action "The Big Raid," stating, "This is not a pie for the health-care sponsors of that successful proposition to carve up for the benefit of each and every health-care provider. It must be used to address the priorities for which it was intended, to supplement and not to replace the existing resources. *To do otherwise would betray the trust of the voters and violate the rule of law*" (emphasis added).[42]

CMA president Laurens P. White loudly protested the fact that the governor was not using Proposition 99's medical service accounts to create, as the initiative specified, new programs expanding the pool of funds available for medical services. He emphasized the CMA's commitment to seeing that the politicians honored the will of the voters: "We are fearful that the administration's budget planners are using the proceeds from the cigarette tax increase approved last November to offset cuts made in the state's health programs. The CMA will work with members of the Prop. 99 Coalition to make sure that does not happen. *When they approved the tax, voters believed they were increasing the amount of money available. We must keep faith with them*" (emphasis added).[41] Although the governor had honored the terms of the initiative by fully funding the Health Education and Research Accounts (the top-priority activities for the voluntary health agencies), the agencies were willing to expend political capital over the supplanting issue—a priority for the CMA—because of the importance of protecting the integrity of the initiative. Nethery, chair of the Coalition, announced, "The voters will be very disappointed that the bureaucrats are trying to raid the revenues from Proposition 99. *In approving Proposition 99, the voters clearly sent a message to Sacramento that they wanted new money for new programs to mitigate the effects of tobacco and teach children about the dangers of smoking.* The Coalition will work to educate the Governor and the Legislature to make sure that the funds are spent consistent with the voter mandate to protect public health and the environment" (emphasis added).[40] Nethery threatened legal action if the governor persisted in violating Proposition 99's stricture against supplanting existing programs because the "proposed budget did not comply with the letter or the spirit of Proposition 99" and the budget would "use the new revenues created by Proposition 99 to replace existing county health services funding eliminated in another portion of the budget."[40]

Assembly Member Lloyd Connelly, who had played a major role in creating Proposition 99, immediately requested a formal opinion from the Legislative Counsel (the Legislature's legal expert). He asked, "May revenues derived from taxes imposed pursuant to Proposition 99 be used to fund existing levels of service for these purposes authorized by Proposition 99 with a four-fifths vote of the Legislature?" The Legislative Counsel's February 24 opinion concluded that the Legislature could not legally fund existing services from these revenues and said that only the voters could change Proposition 99: "Unless an initiative statute grants the Legislature the power to amend or repeal the statute, the Legislature may amend or repeal the statute only by another statute that becomes effective when approved by the electors."[43] Unified opposition forced the governor to back down.

In the end, the governor's initial proposal may not have been a significant threat to the program because Deukmejian, unlike his successor, fellow Republican Pete Wilson, felt bound to implement laws passed by the voters, even if he did not personally agree with them. According to Steve Scott, political editor of the *California Journal,* a widely respected nonpartisan monthly on California politics, "Deukmejian had an interesting attitude about initiatives. He got involved a lot in initiative campaigns. In fact, his staff would sort of get on him for getting involved . . . but by and large, his attitude was if the voters passed it, then the obligation of his administration was to implement it to the best extent possible. And so basically what I've been told recently is that Deukmejian pretty much let Kizer [director of DHS] do it his way."[44]

The first challenge to the integrity of Proposition 99 was thwarted, protecting an important principle for the CMA and other medical service providers. Unfortunately, the CMA would not reciprocate and work with equal vigor to protect the Health Education and Research Accounts.

THE TOBACCO INDUSTRY'S LEGISLATIVE STRATEGIES

On January 17, 1989, the tobacco industry and its consultants met to discuss their short- and long-term strategies for dealing with Proposition 99. For the short term, they hired Sacramento lobbyist Kathleen Snodgrass as the lead "offensive" lobbyist and Paul Kinney from A-K Associates as the lead "defensive" lobbyist. They hired Nielsen, Merksamer, the law firm that had done the industry's political legal work in California at least since Proposition 5, to analyze the budget for the industry and to serve as political consultants.[45] Steve Merksamer was a former chief of staff to Governor Deukmejian and helped put together the Napkin Deal.[19] Jack Kelly, the Tobacco Institute's regional vice president in Sacramento, was to coordinate these efforts, working with the company representatives.

For the tobacco industry, the "major trouble spots" of the governor's budget were the anti-smoking health education program of $175.5 million and the University of California research grants of $43.9 million.[45] The strategy for the Research Account was to limit it: "We believe that appropriate language confining the $43.9 million to hard research would make this item acceptable."[45] The Health Education Account was a greater concern: "Our efforts will have to be very concentrated in this area. The defensive lobbying program will concentrate on the defeat of the dozens of bills that have been or will be introduced to reallocate the Proposition 99 monies to areas unacceptable to our interests."[45]

The long-term strategy was to gut Proposition 99 entirely by putting the revenue into the General Fund and eliminating Proposition 99's requirements that money be spent on anti-tobacco activities. This strategy would be implemented by participation in the Gann Coalition, which was forming to consider modifying some of the state spending rules:

> The long term strategy was developed by our political consultants for two purposes. One purpose was to make the industry "players" in a coalition created to restructure the method of state government finances through an initiative. The discussion motivating such a coalition involves possible repeal or modification of the Gann spending limit, the constraints on the budget process imposed by Proposition 98 [which required that a specified fraction of

state revenues be spent on education], and other constraints such as entitlement programs and automatic cost of living adjustments.

The second purpose was to develop possible goals to mitigate the impact of Proposition 99 on the industry and to strengthen the industry against future excise tax increases.

Our consultant [Nielsen, Merksamer] believes it is possible to fashion a strategy and an implementation plan designed to abolish Proposition 99 earmarking by placing the monies in the general fund instead of the six special funds. . . .

In order for the tobacco industry to be part of this process, which is essential if we are to capitalize on this opportunity, we must be able to offer to the other leaders of the coalition our resources, namely leadership, strategy, and money.

In turn we would want from the coalition a change in the law to abolish earmarking of excise taxes and to direct all revenues into the general fund.

We would also strive to change the law making it more difficult to raise excise taxes by the initiative process and/or a commitment from *our coalition partners (doctors and hospitals)* not to sponsor or support any further increase in excise taxes.

Major players in the coalition are the health care industry, the California Chamber of Commerce, the California Taxpayers Association, public employee groups, and Paul Gann. . . .

The coalition will help strengthen our ties with many groups including the health care industry, and it will also remove tobacco from the major target role. . . .

This second strategy of developing a permanent coalition will be much more visible than the first strategy which is aimed at abolishing Proposition 99 earmarking and sending the tobacco tax revenue from Proposition 99 to the general fund. *The first strategy clearly has to remain an invisible one.*[45] [emphasis different from original]

By February 21, 1989, the State Activities Division of the Tobacco Institute had issued its *Project California Proposal,* together with a detailed budget, amounting to $611,000 on top of the institute's existing lobbying budget for California. Of this money, $545,000 was to pay Nielsen, Merksamer to analyze the budget, to work for diversion of antitobacco funds to other purposes, and to strengthen ties with the CMA, CAHHS, and other health care interests in order to build a coalition that would restructure state finances in a way that would eliminate Proposition 99's earmarked money for tobacco control programs.[46]

The report analyzed the governor's budget to determine what were "acceptable" and "unacceptable" uses of the Proposition 99 revenues:

The Anti-Smoking Health Education program ($176 million) is an "unacceptable" program to receive funds. As currently structured, these funds could be distributed to state anti-tobacco groups for their use in anti-smoking advertising and other campaigns. This budget item was recently amended by the Department of Health to award contracts to private firms to conduct smoking prevention education programs (Attachment C). *We must do everything possible to prevent these revenues from being used in a vigorous anti-smoking public relations or media campaign.*[46] [emphasis different from original]

By February 21, 1989, the long-term strategy was on its way to being implemented: the Tobacco Institute's consultants had already started meeting with the Gann Coalition. The *Project California Proposal* was very specific about the industry's goals in participating in the Gann Coalition. Although they were willing to support modifying the Gann Limit and Proposition 98, which required at least 40 percent of the state budget to go to education, they emphasized that "the *industry's key goals are to eliminate earmarking or dedication to Prop 99 revenues,* and, if possible, also to prevent future excise tax increases through the initiative process" (emphasis in original).[46] While the industry was willing to help the Gann Coalition with "leadership, strategy, and money," this help was conditional, as the February 21 plan made explicit: "It is our firm thought at this juncture that the tobacco industry would withdraw from active participation in the Gann coalition should the industry's goal—eliminate earmarking of Prop 99 revenues—not be included in the coalition's ultimate objective."[46] The long-term strategy would eventually be reflected in an effort subsequently known as Project 90, which remained secret until the summer of 1989.

Nielsen, Merksamer had already begun to study "appropriate" budget items for the Proposition 99 funds to supplement. The firm's recommendation was for all the Health Education money to go to the California Department of Education to be put into the "Program elements" category, which includes bilingual programs, adult education, and vocational programs, among others. Nielsen, Merksamer warned, "There may be some pressure to allocate some of the educational money to the Department of Health Services."[47] If DHS was to receive the money, Nielsen, Merksamer recommended that the money be put into either Maternal and Child Health Care or the Child Health and Disability Prevention (CHDP) program. Both schools and CHDP would eventually receive Health Education money in 1989; by 1994, Maternal and Child Health would also be added to the mix. For the Research Account, Nielsen, Merksamer recommended a requirement that research be performed at all nine University of California campuses, presumably to dilute the effect of the program. Nielsen, Merksamer made no recommendations and expressed no concerns about the Hospital, Physicians, or

Public Resources Accounts. The law firm recommended spending the
monies in the Unallocated Account on hospitals and physicians.[47]

CONCLUSION

Until Proposition 99 passed, the voluntary health agencies had been pe-
ripheral players in Sacramento power politics. This situation changed
with the passage of Proposition 99, when they suddenly became key players in a fight over how to allocate $600 million a year in new tobacco
tax money, including $120 million for tobacco use prevention programs
and $30 million for research. Despite the fact that they were designing
the largest tobacco use prevention program in the world at a time when
state resources were declining, they did not expand their lobbying staffs
or enlist the support of outside technical experts. They were entering the
world of hardball politics with a popular mandate but had not committed the resources necessary to protect that mandate.

In contrast, the tobacco industry had already developed a strategic
plan to undo Proposition 99, with specific plans to divert funds into "acceptable" medical services for children and pregnant women. The industry had started to enlist other powerful players interested in changing the
way California government was financed, including the CMA, the Western Center for Law and Poverty, and other medical interests that the voluntary health agencies hoped would work with them.

CHAPTER 6

Proposition 99's First Implementing Legislation

Governor George Deukmejian's proposals for Proposition 99 revenues did not carry much weight with the Legislature. Legislators had their own ideas about how to allocate the money from the Health Education and Research Accounts and what programs should be established with the money. By introducing a bill, a legislator could jockey for a dominant position in the allocation of the Proposition 99 revenues. A total of thirty-eight pieces of legislation were introduced in the Senate or the Assembly to implement Proposition 99's six accounts. The simplicity of the initiative language helped win the support of the voters and minimize political attacks by the tobacco industry during the initiative campaign, but it also encouraged individual legislators to interpret the initiative in ways that belied its original public health roots.

THE VOLUNTARY HEALTH AGENCIES' LEGISLATION

As preparation for working with the Legislature, members of the Coalition for a Healthy California met on February 3, 1989, to discuss their proposals for how the Proposition 99 monies should be spent. They agreed that their first priority was making sure that the Health Education and Research Accounts were spent for the purposes specified in the initiative. The Coalition supported Senate Bill (SB) 1099, sponsored by Senator Diane Watson (D-Los Angeles), chair of the Senate Health Committee; the bill required that the Health Education money be used to fund tobacco use prevention programs through both the Department of Health Services (DHS) and the California Department of Education (CDE), using a grants mechanism rather than an entitlement-based program. Watson and her chief of staff, John Miller, had a close relationship with the voluntary health agencies, particularly the American Lung Association (ALA). They expected opposition to their plan because both the county health departments and CDE wanted all the money.[1] The voluntary health agencies also worried that the Proposition 99 money would not be used for real tobacco control efforts, but would instead disappear into existing generic programs under the assumption that these programs would include a tobacco control component.

By mid-February 1989, Miller, working with the ALA, ACS, and AHA lobbyists, had agreed that an anti-smoking media campaign should be funded from the Health Education Account. They agreed that Superintendent of Schools Bill Honig's "Healthy Kids, Healthy California" proposal should be handled through the grant proposal route and that only the portions of it that dealt with tobacco education would be funded from the Health Education Account. Similarly, proposals for comprehensive health education would be supported only insofar as they dealt with education about tobacco.[2]

Finally, the role and funding of an oversight committee for the health education programs was discussed. An oversight committee would be an independent body that would monitor only the Proposition 99 health education programs, as opposed to a legislative committee that has oversight over an extensive array of programs. While such a committee could both monitor and protect the program, its creation would take resources from direct program services, and the voluntary health agencies wanted to insure that most of the Proposition 99 revenues would go toward funding programs, not administration. (This concern would also manifest itself in fights over the amount of overhead research universities would receive from the Research Account.) In order to deal with ACS concerns about creating a new bureaucracy and the amount of power it would have, they agreed to limit the oversight committee's funding to one-fourth of one percent of the total Health Education Account budget.[2]

The conversations with CDE continued. On March 7, 1989, Coalition chair Jim Nethery and ALA representative Carolyn Martin wrote to Honig, summarizing what they believed to be "the essential areas of agreement" between the Coalition and CDE, based on a February 8 meeting: 70 percent of the money would go to programs focused on people aged eighteen or younger, with an emphasis on school-based programs, a media component, the use of competitive grants for distributing the money, and the appointment of an oversight committee with some financial support. There was also agreement that DHS and CDE would each have half of the available money and that CDE would use Proposition 99 monies to fund only those portions of Healthy Kids, Health California that dealt specifically with tobacco.[3]

In March 1989 Watson introduced SB 1099 to allocate Health Education funds. The bill largely drew upon language contained in SB 2133, the bill she had introduced in the previous session. The language on what constituted tobacco education was specific: "It is the intent of the Legislature, therefore, to require the State Department of Health Services and the State Department of Education to both cooperatively and individually conduct activities directed at the prevention of tobacco use and tobacco related disease."[4] SB 1099 also authorized the oversight committee to appoint an executive director and necessary support staff if it chose to do so. If the oversight committee could appoint an executive director and support staff, then it could indeed serve as an independent oversight commission. If it was forced to rely on staff from DHS or CDE, it would be less independent and potentially more subject to political pressures. By codifying the oversight committee's power to appoint staff in SB 1099, the Coalition was trying to establish the independence of the oversight committee.

The proponents understood that they were venturing into uncharted territory. No one had ever designed and implemented such a large and comprehensive tobacco control program. As a result, they sought to stress the experimental nature of the effort with the goal of refining the program as it developed. The three key elements underlying SB 1099 reflected this philosophy:

The creation of an outside oversight and policy committee to monitor the anti-tobacco program. The committee, which would be appointed by the Legislature and the Governor, would consist of both education and health interests and be responsible for the development and focus of the overall policies and guidelines for the Health Education Account funds.

An initial period of experimentation and evaluation to refine the program. It was decided that the first two years of the expenditure of the Health Education Account funds would support experimental projects and would also be used to evaluate existing programs. Funds would be distributed by a grant approach to public, nonprofit, and for-profit sectors based on guidelines developed by the oversight committee. Both DHS and CDE would be involved in distributing money, but the plan was to have a varied approach to tobacco use prevention which would be better achieved through grants than by an entitlement-based program.

The development of a master implementation plan. After two years, an evaluation of the effectiveness of the programs would be conducted. The oversight committee would then develop a master plan to utilize the most successful programs with the goal of reducing tobacco use in California by 75% by the year 2000.[5]

In addition to a general framework, SB 1099 established several specific priorities for anti-tobacco education: (1) a focus on youth, with a minimum of 70 percent of the funds to be utilized for programs targeted at young people; (2) an emphasis on high-incidence/high-risk groups, recognizing that the tobacco industry was targeting lower-income and minority smokers; (3) a multifaceted approach, with 50 percent of the funds going to programs in schools and the other 50 percent to a variety of community-based programs; (4) cessation activities targeting people who were already smoking; and (5) efforts to protect nonsmokers from the health dangers of secondhand smoke. CDE was responsible for the school-based programs of the Health Education Account while DHS was responsible for the community-based programs. The oversight committee was to coordinate both departments' program implementation.

OTHER SIGNIFICANT
TOBACCO EDUCATION LEGISLATION

Watson's bill was not the only bill dealing with how the Health Education Account money would be spent. By the end of March, two other bills were also being given serious attention—Assembly Bill 1695, introduced by Assembly Member Bruce Bronzan (D-Fresno), and SB 1392, introduced by Senator Barry Keene (D-Benicia). Unlike SB 1099, which concentrated on reducing tobacco use, these two bills represented the interests of forces that sought to use the Health Education Account money for medical service programs with a much less direct connection, if any, to tobacco control.

Assembly Bill (AB) 1695 concentrated on developing a comprehensive health education program instead of one aiming to reduce tobacco use. Although Bronzan authored AB 1695, the bill was chiefly proposed and lobbied by Steve Thompson, director of the Assembly Office of Research, on behalf of Assembly Speaker Willie Brown.[6] The new program, which was called the Comprehensive Maternal and Child Health Program, targeted women, children, and adolescents and resembled the programs suggested to the Tobacco Institute by Nielsen, Merksamer in December 1988 for moving money into "acceptable" areas.[7] Although a tobacco education component was included as a small part of the program, the bill's main purpose was to consolidate several state health programs into one single new program, which would include provisions for health education and dental disease prevention through grade school programs; nutritional supplements to pregnant women, new mothers, and their children; and childhood immunizations, health screening, and hospital and physician services for the target populations. The bill would have appropriated $123.3 million from the Health Education Account to fund the program.

In reaction to AB 1695, Assembly Member Lloyd Connelly (D-Sacramento) again went to the Legislative Counsel, this time asking if the Comprehensive Maternal and Child Health Act could be funded legally from the Health Education Account. On May 4, 1989, the Legislative Counsel issued the opinion that it could not be funded with money from the Health Education Account because the funding of medical services was not the purpose of the account as presented to voters.[8] Despite the fact that it violated Proposition 99, the voluntary health agencies had to give the bill serious attention because comprehensive health issues were popular and Bronzan was chair of the Assembly Health Committee, the program committee that would likely hold hearings on the plans for the Health Education Account funds. In addition, AB 1695 had the support of Assembly Speaker Willie Brown and of the county health departments, which would benefit financially because most of the proposed programs were to be operated at the county level.

SB 1392 was also a major competitor to SB 1099 because Keene, its author, was the Senate majority leader and the former chair of the Assembly Health Committee. In addition to Keene's sponsorship, the bill had other powerful supporters: the Service Employees International Union (SEIU), which represented county-level heath workers, the County Supervisors Association of California (CSAC), and numerous other county medical service providers and their proponents. The County Health Officers Association also supported it. In addition, the administration, acting through the Health and Welfare Agency, had stated that its priority was to channel as much of the tobacco tax revenue as possible to county programs, thereby alleviating the counties' demands on the state's General Fund.

Instead of a centrally organized basis for distributing tobacco tax funds like SB 1099 and AB 1695, SB 1392 proposed a locally based distribution system using policy recommendations from DHS but preserving local autonomy. Targeted recipients included pregnant women, children, and workplace and community services, including smoking cessation and tobacco control programs. No money was set aside for schools. It was more difficult for proponents of SB 1099 to criticize SB 1392 than AB 1695, since it specifically mentioned anti-tobacco efforts. There were still several items of concern, however, because the target groups were narrowly defined, there was little state oversight or direction, and there was enough latitude to make all kinds of health education, such as alcohol or nutrition, legitimate under the bill. DHS was to develop programs for use in local communities, but the money would essentially go to the counties as block grants with some strings attached. Nevertheless, because of Keene's sponsorship and the fact that the bill gave financial assistance to the counties, Proposition 99 advocates recognized that it would be given consideration along with SB 1099. CDE opposed the bill.

Most of the competition for the Health Education Account money took place in late spring and early summer in behind-the-scenes negotiations among the various interests that were pushing their programs. Although it was clear from the opinion polls conducted at the time of Proposition 99 that the public wanted the Proposition 99 funds to go to anti-tobacco education and research more than it wanted the money to go to indigent health care (see table 1), the Legislature was on record through its previous actions as being unsupportive of tobacco control efforts but supportive of health care screening for children. In particular, funding health care for sick children was attractive to liberals and keeping money out of tobacco education was attractive to members across the political spectrum who supported the tobacco industry.

THE CHILD HEALTH AND
DISABILITY PREVENTION PROGRAM

In December 1988 Nielsen, Merksamer had recommended to the Tobacco Institute that the Child Health and Disability Prevention (CHDP) program was an "acceptable" way to spend Health Education Account funds.[7] The program was popular and had very strong political backing from Speaker Brown, who had carried CHDP's initial authorizing legislation. Brown was closely allied with the tobacco industry,[9] so shifting money from anti-tobacco education to CHDP would meet both Brown's and the industry's needs.

CHDP originated in 1973, when the California Children's Lobby approached Assembly Member Willie Brown and his staff member Steve Thompson about creating a program that would offer free health screens to all children, not just poor ones.[10] At the time, children's advocates were dissatisfied with California's implementation of the federal child health screening program, Early and Periodic Screening, Diagnosis, and Prevention. The federal program had been set up in California as a welfare program rather than a health program, and it provided mass screenings by paraprofessionals instead of doctors, which the medical establishment did not like. In addition, the screenings were divorced from the provision of medical care and providers were reimbursed at very low rates, which reduced the incentive to provide services. Brown and Thompson created CHDP to solve these problems.

CHDP was to be administered by the health department, not welfare, and incorporate doctors into program delivery.[10] The CMA and the California chapter of the American Academy of Pediatrics supported this program. Once the costs of implementing the full program were clear, however, the target population was "temporarily" redefined to be children between the ages of four and six whose family incomes were no more than twice the poverty level; only the costs of screening, not treatment, were covered.[10] When Proposition 99 passed in 1988, CHDP was a popular program with strong political backing that needed money to be more fully implemented. Using the Health Education Account to finance CHDP would advance the policy agenda of important legislators, provide money for doctors, and reduce funds for programs that could damage the tobacco industry.

NEGOTIATIONS AND AGREEMENTS

By May, several of the Assembly bills to implement Proposition 99 ended up in the Assembly Health Committee. Bronzan, the committee chair, decided to consolidate all of the Proposition 99 bills into one omnibus bill. The voluntary health agencies convinced him to incorporate the language of Watson's SB 1099 into his bill and to drop AB 1695. No dominant bill emerged in the Senate, so the legislative leadership agreed to have the Senate pass a related bill that had already passed the Assembly, then let a conference committee consisting of members of both houses work out the final implementing legislation for Proposition 99. That bill was Assembly Bill 75. Authored by former Willie Brown staffer, now Assembly Member, Phil Isenberg (D-Sacramento), AB 75 dealt with some of the Proposition 99 medical accounts and could thus be used to resolve issues related to the other accounts as well. Since it was the only bill that was close to being ready for a conference committee and Isenberg was an acceptable chair to all the major parties, including the Deukmejian administration, Speaker Brown, and Bronzan, he became the chair.[11] According to Isenberg, "By the time my little bill doing nothing got over to the Senate, it was the only survivor. And all the giant gorillas of the Legislature had killed each other, because they didn't want anybody else to have control over the issue. . . . Also the interest groups became very interested in doing that because as time passed there was an actual chance the money wouldn't be divided for a while and there's nothing worse if you expect to get some money than the thought that the getting may be delayed."[11] The Conference Committee included Assembly Members Isenberg, Bronzan, and Bill Baker (R-Walnut Creek) and Senators Keene (D-Benicia), Herschel Rosenthal (D-Los Angeles), and Ken Maddy (R-Fresno), some of whom represented significant interests that had been involved in developing the Proposition 99 legislation. Maddy, the Republican Senate minority leader, represented the administration's interests. Watson, the tobacco control forces' strongest advocate, was left off the committee.

Although the tobacco industry stayed out of public view, it was very active behind the scenes. The tobacco industry spent $2.2 million on lobbying in the 1987–1988 election cycle and another $2.2 million in 1989–1990 (compared with only $274,394 in 1985–1986 before Proposition 99 passed).[9] Between the 1985–1986 and 1989–1990 election cycles, tobacco industry campaign contributions to California legislators more than doubled, from $266,488 to $563,366.[9] Assembly Speaker Willie Brown had received $124,900 for the twelve-year period between 1976 and 1988. In 1989–1990 alone, he received $62,250, more than any other member of the Legislature and more than most members of the US Congress. Senator Ken Maddy (R-Fresno), the leading Republican on the AB 75 Conference Committee, received $38,500 in 1989–1990, more than twice the $19,500 he had received between 1976 and 1988.[9]

During the summer, the Conference Committee staff, lobbyists, and other key individuals worked out the specific language for spending the Health Education Account. By the time the committee met, according to John Miller, "We pretty much knew how we wanted to spend the money and had . . . defeated or derailed most of the really ugly [suggestions for spending the money]. What remained of the ugly ones, we had already accepted. . . . The process inside the Conference Committee was to actually put it into words and put dollars beside each agreement."[12] For the most part, the voluntaries had been successful in defending the language originally in Watson's SB 1099, which had also been sent to the committee to consider in its deliberations. However, they also believed that in order to achieve the necessary support for the provisions in Watson's bill, they would need to come to an agreement with the other organizations that had made a pitch for Health Education Account revenues.

According to Miller, the strategy he and Najera settled on was based on their perception that they had little real support inside or outside the Capitol.

> We had unreliable allies (Heart/Cancer); a fearsome opponent (tobacco); various supporters (hospitals, counties, CMA); an indifferent Legislature; and a mildly antagonistic administration (Deukmejian). We also had a completely untested, unproven theory on reducing smoking. We did have popular support, but it was broad, shallow, and skeptical.
>
> In our estimate, the tobacco industry had the political capacity to bury tobacco control. They could do so either by diverting the funding, or by implementing the mandated program so ineffectually that diversion was unnecessary. This could be done by their "insider" methods.
>
> Tony [Najera] and I resolved that we would avoid an absolutely direct confrontation. We were not strong enough to prevail against a united tobacco/Republican/medical provider coalition, and we determined to buy (literally) time to establish an effective, highly visible, and hopefully popular anti-tobacco program. . . . We resolved to make financial and programmatic concessions when we had to (we had more than enough money) and to associate ourselves with powerful friends such as the CMA, the counties, and Western Center. We did not know the full extent of their duplicity during the first few years, but we did know their support of Prop 99 was opportunistic and we were aware they would pursue their own narrow interests if events evolved in such a direction.[13]

They completely discounted their ability to mount an effective public campaign directed at the Legislature, abandoning their most powerful weapon, public opinion.

At the end of June, the Coalition had reached an agreement with Senator Keene and his competing bill, SB 1392.[12] Under this agreement, funding would be evenly divided among local county-based anti-smoking programs, school-based anti-smoking programs, and state-run competitive grants. Money would also be used for an anti-tobacco media campaign. Thus, SB 1099 now included assurances that local jurisdictions would receive a share of the Proposition 99 funds.[14] According to the June 30, 1989, minutes of a meeting held by the Coalition, the negotiations with the SEIU and health officers resulted in the following allocations: 10 percent of the available funds in the Health Education Account ($12 million) for media, 30 percent ($36 million) to schools through CDE on an entitlement basis, 30 percent ($36 million) to state grants through DHS, and 30 percent ($36 million) to local health departments on an entitlement basis. This meant that over half of the money was going to the county level on a noncompetitive basis, which the voluntaries had been trying to avoid because they worried that it would disappear into local school and health department budgets. They believed that a centrally run program conforming to state standards would be stronger and more likely to actually reduce tobacco use. Sending some of the money to the counties was seen as a way to stop SB 1392 and to make the counties happy but not necessarily as a route to strong programming.[12] This ambivalence about the value of the local programs was to continue in subsequent versions of the Proposition 99 implementing legislation.

The pressure was also heavy to include some funding for CHDP from the Health Education Account, along the lines that Nielsen, Merksamer had suggested to the Tobacco Institute seven months earlier, in December 1988.[7] From a political standpoint, CHDP was popular with several legislators, key lobbyists, including SEIU and the Western Center for Law and Poverty, and the administration. Funding for CHDP directed additional funds to the counties, which also pleased them. Steve Thompson was an important player in the decision to move Health Education Account money into CHDP.[15] In return for the Coalition's support of CHDP, the administration agreed to support SB 1099 and to include anti-tobacco education in the CHDP screening interview. According to Carolyn Martin, a volunteer who represented ALA on the Coalition, "DHS was to meet with the voluntaries to develop the anti-tobacco education component of CHDP. That never happened. Instead, they just added three questions about smoking to the screening interview. That was DHS's idea of an 'effective tobacco education program.' Ha!"[16]

Rather than making a strong public argument that spending Health Education Account money on CHDP violated the intent of the voters, as they had done when Governor Deukmejian proposed using the medical service accounts to supplant funding for local medical programs, the Coalition agreed to divert some money from the Health Education Account to CHDP. In a June 26 memo, Miller told Watson, "If the administration wanted to steal some of the Education funds for themselves, and were willing to let us establish good programs in return, we would let them steal a little (say 20 or 25 million). Anything we can do to reduce the block-grant structure of the program is also welcome." [17] On June 30, with the American Heart Association abstaining, the Coalition passed a motion to go along with the diversions: "The Coalition supports funding for CHDP, $20 million for year one and $20 million for year two [of the two years that AB 75 covered], from the reserve account [in the Health Education Account]. These funds are to be used exclusively for anti-tobacco education. The program will be subject to standard accounting and evaluation procedures. There will be a two year sunset." [18] The decision to divert funds from Health Education to medical services through CHDP established a precedent for deviating from the will of the voters as well as for funding medical services from the Health Education Account. As Isenberg observed, "This support would haunt them in years to come." [19] Giving up $39.1 million for CHDP (out of $271.9 million appropriated from the Health Education Account over two years) in exchange for getting a decent bill, viewed from a Sacramento insider's perspective, was a reasonable and appropriate action. From the standpoint of mobilizing public support to protect the anti-tobacco programs, it was not.

To protect the anti-tobacco programs mandated by Proposition 99, public health advocates could have framed the issue for the public simply as "following the will of the voters." By agreeing to diversions, the voluntaries surrendered the "voter mandate" rationale, clearing the way for medical groups and others to frame the fight over Proposition 99 revenues as sick children versus health education or as just another fight over money among Sacramento special-interest groups. The health groups lost the moral high ground. Moreover, the fact that the Coalition agreed to funding medical services from the Health Education Account demonstrated to the CMA, the tobacco industry, and others that they did not have to pass a new initiative to move Health Education Account money from "unacceptable" tobacco control to "acceptable" medical services; they could negotiate it.

The die was cast.

PROJECT 90

While the Coalition spent most of 1989 concentrating on convincing the Legislature to use Proposition 99 funds to establish effective tobacco control programs, the tobacco industry continued to push its long-term strategy of passing a new initiative that would eliminate the Health Education Account. This strategy, articulated in secret plans the previous February as the *Project California Proposal* (discussed in Chapter 5),[20] involved providing financial, legal, and political support for a coalition of medical, labor, and business groups that were seeking to amend the Gann Limit and change the way the state finances were managed. While staying out of the limelight, the tobacco industry had budgeted $330,000 for Nielsen, Merksamer "to represent industry in coalition, lobby coalition members, draft legislation/initiatives, prepare background materials."[20] The original effort, known as the Gann Limit Coalition, had been renamed the Project 90 Coalition. Steve Merksamer, who had helped facilitate the Napkin Deal, was the principal advocate behind the redirection of funds. David Townsend, who ran the campaign against Proposition 99 for the tobacco industry, was hired to conduct the campaign for Project 90. Jeff Raimundo, who worked on the campaign against Proposition 99, was the spokesman for the Project 90 Coalition.[21,22,23] The industry's support was explicitly tied to using the planned initiative "to eliminate earmarking of dedicated Prop 99 revenues."[20]

While Project 90 stayed in the shadows and its tobacco ties remained unknown until mid-June, the Coalition started to get wind of its activities earlier. On May 17, 1989, the ALA's executive director, George Williams, commented, "We were told at a coalition meeting that the CMA is working on an initiative that would divert all Prop 99 money, except research, to a fund to provide health insurance for uninsured workers. As a side note, it's interesting that CMA has the money to do this, but not to support Prop 99—so much for friends."[24] Assembly Member Lloyd Connelly, writing to the California Taxpayers' Association, a participant in Project 90, on behalf of Assembly Member Tom Hayden (D-Santa Monica), ACS, ALA, AHA, and the Planning and Conservation League, reported,

> While we are in agreement with the basic thrust of Propect [*sic*] 90, we view with concern reports that Project 90 is contemplating including amendments to the allocation and purpose sections of Proposition 99. . . . Before taking any irrevocable action impacting the purposes and integrity of Proposition 99, and the prospects of the Project 90 initiative succeeding, we ask that you con-

sult with all the members of the Coalition for a Healthy California.

It would be unfortunate if the Project 90 initiative does not have the broadest possible coalition supporting it. An initiative that amends Proposition 99 inconsistent with its purposes will have the active opposition of the below signatories, including the signing of the opposition ballot argument and conducting a free media campaign.[25]

This letter did not deter the backers of Project 90.

One of the Coalition's members, the CMA, was not a signatory to the Coalition's letter and was part of Project 90 in order to secure additional funding for health care, which the CMA intended to get by revising Proposition 99. The CMA's specific proposal was to give 5 percent to Research, 7.5 percent to Public Resources, 35 percent to Hospital Services, 10 percent to Physician Services, and 42.5 percent to a new account for "uncompensated health care services, preventive health care services, health education, or the state's subsidy of a health insurance program for the medically uninsured."[26] The CMA would have ended the requirement that any money be spent on anti-tobacco education. The CMA knew it was serving the tobacco industry's interests by pursuing the initiative. On June 27, 1989, Jack Light, a CMA staffer, wrote an internal memo reporting that "the tobacco industry initiated this request to eliminate education and they did it because they realize that a massive educational campaign is the most effective deterrent to smoking there is."[27]

On June 15, *Sacramento Bee* political columnist Dan Walters exposed the connections between the CMA, the tobacco industry, and Project 90 in a column entitled "A Lousy Way to Make Policy."

> The Project 90 executive committee is to meet this week to make final decisions on the content of the initiative.
>
> And one of those decisions will be whether to accept a quarter-million dollar commitment of campaign funds from the tobacco industry in return for placing in the initiative a significant change in Proposition 99, the cigarette tax initiative approved by voters last year.
>
> One portion of Proposition 99, which boosted taxes on cigarettes by 25 cents a pack, requires funds, currently $120 million, to be spent on a massive anti-smoking educational program among California school children and the larger public.
>
> The tobacco industry wants that provision to be axed. It wants to trade the quarter-million-dollar commitment (plus a promise of more later) for a provision to remove all funds from the anti-smoking program and shift them to general health care programs. The move has the support of some medical provider groups such as the California Medical Association, but not such public health groups as the American Cancer Society.[22]

On June 29, Walters' next column on Project 90 appeared, entitled "A Smoky Fight over Initiative."

> While Project 90 leaders, most of whom come from business groups, agreed to the tobacco industry deal as a means of obtaining badly needed campaign funds, it created a big split among health groups, pitting the doctors and other professional providers against volunteer anti-smoking organizations. . . .
>
> The matter came to a head this week during what sources described as an acrimonious, two-hour telephonic meeting of CMA's executive board.
>
> The Board was deeply divided over the issue and finally settled on a strangely worded statement that is to be submitted to the CMA's governing council next month.
>
> While the statement says CMA "disassociates itself" from attempts to eliminate anti-smoking education money and reaffirms the organization's commitment to a smoke-free environment, it also implies that it could not be held responsible for what others might do, including the shift of anti-smoking funds into a broader substance-abuse program and/or direct health care. In effect, the CMA seems to be washing its hands of the deal while leaving open the possibility that its members could profit from it.[21]

The column triggered a firestorm of protest from the public health groups, particularly the ALA and ACS.

The initiative proposed by Project 90 would both revise the Gann spending limit and raise the gas tax. The intent of the supporting organizations was to free state revenues for spending on a variety of public programs and to allow gas taxes to be raised for transportation improvements. Although Project 90 was directed toward putting the proposed initiative on the ballot through legislative action, it was deemed unlikely that the Legislature would pass it, meaning that a signature drive would be necessary. This meant that members of the campaign executive committee, known as Taxpayers for Effective Government, each had to contribute $100,000 for the campaign.[28] The tobacco industry had agreed to provide $250,000 to the effort if the initiative also included language stripping the Health Education Account of money.[22]

The CMA initially confirmed its relationship with the tobacco industry. According to a story in the *Santa Maria Times,*

> The Medical Association's spokesman confirmed last week that deals have been made at the Capitol between doctors and the tobacco industry.
>
> "Yeah, it's true, but the world is not black and white," said Chuck McFadden, communications director for the association.
>
> "We would like it to be morally pure and black and white. Unfortunately you have to engage in trade-offs to enact good public policy. That does not, by any stretch of the imagination, put us in bed with the tobacco companies."[23]

With or without Project 90, however, the CMA stood by its intentions to redirect the money from the Health Education Account. In a July 14 letter to a member of the Legislature responding to a news article critical of the CMA's actions, CMA president William Plested III wrote,

> Advocates of developing a stronger publicly operated delivery system (e.g. free clinics, county hospitals, etc.) want all of the tobacco tax revenue committed early and permanently to the support of that system. CMA and other health providers want the short-term commitment to go toward temporary programs so that the long-term uses will go toward reform of the existing employer-based health insurance delivery system. I do not claim that the CMA is motivated by higher moral purposes than any of the other interested parties who are fighting for this money like jackals over a carcass. We have, however, unlike the others, openly presented our priorities and articulated our rationale for those priorities.[29] [emphasis added]

On July 12, the CMA's position on AB 75, the implementing legislation for Proposition 99, was to oppose it unless it was amended to move the funds in the Unallocated Account into a Physician Services Fund to pay for uncompensated physician services.[30] On July 21, the CMA Council adopted its general policy for Proposition 99 implementation, which had three chief features. First, the CMA wanted all health care money from Proposition 99 to go to a health care insurance program for the working uninsured and their dependents. Second, the CMA opposed any legislation that did not make funds available to all physicians for a portion of their uncompensated services. Third, the CMA supported using the Unallocated Account for physicians who treated patients with emergency conditions.[31] While the council reaffirmed its "total dedication for achieving a tobacco free California by year 2000" and emphasized that "CMA will not participate in any activities which might compromise that goal,"[31] CMA's actions regarding the Health Education Account should not have reassured the voluntary agencies and other defenders of the Health Education Account. There was no promise to support the 20 percent allocation for health education.

The voluntaries went back to the public to defeat the Proposition 99 proposal advanced by the Project 90 Coalition. They organized statewide press conferences in Sacramento and Los Angeles.[32] The press conferences, which received widespread media coverage, articulated the voluntaries' point of view, including a threat on their part to sue if the health education programs did not receive full funding. They encouraged their volunteers to drop their CMA memberships.[33,34] On August 21 physicians Lowell Irwin and Donald Beerline, the president and president-elect of ACS, wrote their volunteers urging them to write to Plested with a request to respect the integrity of Proposition 99.[35] Project 90's threat to the Health Education Account dissipated under the glare of public attention, again demonstrating the power of public sentiment and attention in overcoming the power of the vested interests who had controlled tobacco policy making in Sacramento.

On August 29, the CMA's vice president for government affairs, Jay Michael, tried to distance Project 90 from the tobacco industry: "The Tobacco *Institute* never offered to contribute $250,000 or any other amount to a campaign to redirect the anti-smoking revenue from Proposition 99. Various companies associated with or owned by tobacco companies had . . . offered to contribute money to . . . Project 90. . . . Tobacco *owned* companies (not tobacco or cigarette manufacturers, per se) indicated a willingness to contribute $250,000 'or more' to the overall campaign" (emphasis in original).[36] To health groups, this was a distinction without a difference.

When the Legislature and the governor reached an agreement on revising the Gann Limit, the entire Project 90 effort lost momentum.

THE BATTLE OVER THE MEDIA CAMPAIGN

By August 24, the Conference Committee had made its report available. The Coalition seemed satisfied with the result regarding the Health Education Account. An internal ACS memo concluded that the recommendation was "quite close to the agreement reached by the Coalition and other parties in the form of amendments to SB 1099."[37] At this point, the revenue was divided into one-time and ongoing expenditures. One-time expenditures included $15 million in reserves, $30 million in competitive grants, and $14 million in unallocated funds. Ongoing expenditures were broken down into state programs and local programs. State programs included $3 million for oversight and data collection and analysis, $15 million for the media campaign, $20 million for CHDP screening, and $12 million for competitive grants. Local programs included $36 million for school-aged populations and $36 million for high-risk populations.

At Miller's request, the Coalition members reaffirmed their support for SB 1099 as it existed on August 18, 1989. Miller had asked the Conference Committee to incorporate the substance of SB 1099 into the AB 75 package and reported that SB 1099 would not have a separate hearing. At that point the Coalition decided that a single bill should cover appropriations from the Health Education Account and the medical service accounts; tobacco interests and the CMA would presumably have more difficulty killing the anti-tobacco education program if it were part of a larger bill that included the appropriations for the medical services accounts.[38] According to Miller, "We wanted to make it so that they couldn't have all that money for their clinics and their hospitals unless they voted for health education as well." [12]

The media campaign was the main bone of contention; Miller expected the industry to try to kill it. Steve Scott, political editor of the *California Journal*, observed that the media program "was the main issue because . . . it was that component that bothered them [the tobacco industry] the most. I mean the tax was the tax, there was nothing they could do about it, but the notion that Californians would be educated and that there would be a specific media component to it was what terrified them." [39] As Miller and Scott expected, in September, after AB 75 had moved out of the Conference Committee, the tobacco industry emerged from the shadows and launched an all-out lobbying blitz to kill the anti-tobacco media campaign.

During the final days of the Conference Committee, tobacco industry contract lobbyists saturated legislators.[19,40,41] On September 13 Assembly Members Bronzan and Isenberg and Senators Keene and Rosenthal sent an alert to their fellow members warning them that twenty-five lobbyists had been hired by the tobacco industry to try to kill the provisions authorizing the anti-smoking television ads.[42] Miller recalled the dramatic standoff inside the Conference Committee:

> The blitz of lobbying was awesome—the tobacco industry brought in the "first team" from Washington, D.C., and New York. They literally hired every contract lobbyist around. They would hire a lobbyist just to win one vote. Judge Garibaldi, then the preeminent contract lobbyist, told Senator Watson the industry offered him a blank check—he could fill in any amount he wished, just to add his clout to the contest.
>
> *Prior to adoption of the Conference Committee report, the industry had brought high pressure on the six members to target all tobacco education to youth.* They clearly had the Republican members, and were about to win some of the Democrats (and destroy health education). Before a vote could be taken, however, Phil Isenberg and Bruce Bronzan stood up from the table, stepped to the front of the room, and publicly refused to have anything further to do with the conference. *Both men shamed their colleagues, Isenberg described the youth proposal as one of the cheapest tricks he had witnessed. The demonstration by both men effectively killed the "youth only" effort and assured adoption of a legitimate health education proposal.*[13] [emphasis added]

When the bill moved to the Assembly floor, tobacco lobbyists were lined up three and four deep along the public railing outside the Assembly chamber, sending messages in to legislators and talking to them as they went into the chamber.[43] Mary Adams, the ACS lobbyist at the time, noted, "The tobacco industry was handing out $10,000 checks to any and every lobbyist it could find who would work on the issue. It was a hoot to see who was at the railing! They would have hired my cat if she had been a registered lobbyist!"[44] The industry was successful in reaching some legislators, most notably Senator Maddy and Speaker Brown, both of whom questioned the value of using Health Education Account money for a massive and untested media campaign.[19]

Fortunately for public health advocates, the tobacco industry went too far and generated a backlash among many legislators. In Bronzan's words, the lobbying campaign became "so gross and so obvious that it becomes dangerous for [lawmakers] to associate themselves with it."[43] The health advocates alerted the media to the tobacco industry's lobbying tactics. Walters summed up the effort in his *Sacramento Bee* column: "The tobacconists may have made a tactical error. Their heavy-handed push drew attention from news media, which put the politicians on the spot and, in the end, they abandoned the drive and the ad money remained."[45] Walters declared the industry's defeat a public victory over narrower interests.

In 1989 politicians still saw implementing the voter mandate as a priority. The industry had put itself in the limelight with a too-obvious lobbying effort. Once again, outside attention had worked to the advantage of the health groups and to the defeat of the industry.

THE RESEARCH ACCOUNT

While the Health Education Account was widely debated and many proposals were floated for how to use the money, the Research Account attracted far less attention. The Research Account, like the Public Resources Account, was not "on the table" because it was viewed as an earmarked account.[46] Everyone assumed that the 5 percent allocation specified by the initiative would be put into research. Three issues had to be resolved concerning the Research Account: (1) who would administer it, (2) how indirect costs (overhead) would be handled, and (3) what kinds of research would be funded. None of the preferences that the voluntary agencies had initially expressed ended up in the final legislation.

Instead, the preferences of the governor and the University of California (UC) prevailed.

The voluntaries wanted DHS to administer the money and limit the amount of indirect costs that could be charged to research grants funded out of the Proposition 99 Research Account. In their view, indirect costs would involve general support for the universities rather than support for tobacco-related work. By January 20, 1989, the California research universities had drafted their own statement of principles, supporting UC as the lead agency, establishing scientific merit as the basis for awards, and requiring the payment of all research costs, both direct and indirect, consistent with federal guidelines.[47] The private universities opposed limiting overhead. (Stanford's overhead at the time was higher than 80 percent.[1]) On March 7 the UC proposal, supported by Stanford, Cal Tech, the University of Southern California, and the California State University system, was on the table. It proposed UC as the administrator, a system of outside peer review based on the National Institutes of Health model, a policy advisory committee, and full-cost reimbursement of indirect costs "consistent with federal guidelines."[48]

The research program was eventually authorized by Senator John Garamendi's (D-Walnut Grove) SB 1613. It specified that the Research Account was to be managed by the University of California, and the university was directed to appoint a Scientific Advisory Committee to advise it in administering the account to conduct research related to tobacco. The private universities got full indirect costs, but UC did not. The university was given wide latitude in administering the Research Account. Deukmejian approved SB 1613 on October 2, 1989, which authorized the research programs through December 31, 1993.

THE OUTCOME

AB 75 appropriated a total of $272 million from the Health Education Account, which included the money raised from January 1, 1989, through June 30, 1991. The bill appropriated $978 million for indigent health care from the Physician Services Account, Hospital Services Account, and Unallocated Account for medical services. (A separate bill allocated $74 million from the Research Account for tobacco-related disease research; $74 million from the Public Resources Account was distributed through the budget for environmental protection.) The Child Health and Disability Prevention (CHDP) program was funded from the

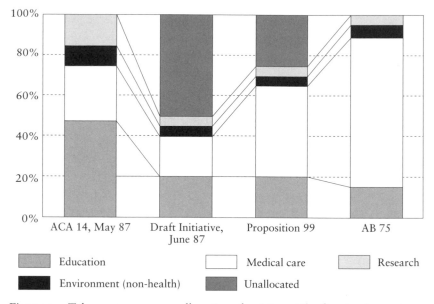

Figure 5.   Tobacco tax revenue allocations for AB 75. The first implementing legislation for Proposition 99 appropriated more money for medical services than the initiative allowed and less for anti-tobacco education than it required.

Health Education Account, even though it was a medical service program. In total, AB 75 appropriated $1,017 million for medical services, or 69 percent of the total revenues available from the tobacco tax increase, including $96 million that the voters had earmarked for anti-tobacco education. AB 75 did not follow Proposition 99's directive that 20 percent of revenues be spent on anti-tobacco education (figure 5). For true anti-tobacco education it appropriated only $229 million, or 15.8 percent of total revenues.

The Health Education Account money was to target "high-risk populations," particularly school-age youth and their families, blacks, Hispanics, Native Americans, pregnant women, and current smokers. The money for local health department programs was allocated to "local lead agencies," California's fifty-eight county health departments and three city health departments. Amounts were included in the 1989–1990 and 1990–1991 budgets to fund the competitive grants for other public and nonprofit agencies. School programs were to be administered by the California Department of Education (CDE), and money to school districts was to be distributed as an entitlement on the basis of average daily attendance. Ninety percent of the money allocated to CDE was to be allocated to school districts and county offices of education. The remaining 10 percent was to be awarded as grants for innovative programs. All other programs were to be administered by the Department of Health Services.

AB 75 also established an eleven-member Tobacco Education Oversight Committee (TEOC), which was charged with advising DHS and CDE on programs funded by AB 75 and developing and updating the Master Plan. Members were to be appointed by the governor, the Senate Rules Committee, the speaker of the Assembly, and the superintendent of public instruction to represent specific constituencies, including voluntary health agencies, health care employees, university faculty, and target population groups. While TEOC was more limited in authority than originally envisioned by tobacco control advocates, they still hoped that TEOC would play an important role in guiding and evaluating the new program.

Throughout the development of AB 75, extending as far back as Watson's first proposal a year earlier (SB 2133), tobacco control advocates had recognized explicitly the experimental nature of the tobacco control program they sought to develop. In order to ensure accountability, they had included a sunset clause, requiring a return to the Legislature after two years to obtain new spending authorization. The idea behind this decision was to provide adequate oversight and adjustment for the new program during its developmental period. The sunset provision was incorporated into AB 75, requiring a new bill authorizing the Proposition 99 programs to be enacted by July 1, 1991. While this two-year period of initial experimentation seemed reasonable at the time, in fact only twenty-one months elapsed between the signing of AB 75 and the date when new legislation was required. Far from providing a more rational approach to developing the new program, the sunset provision was to create a new opportunity for the tobacco industry and its allies among the medical service providers to continue their efforts to divert Proposition 99 funds into "acceptable" programs.

AB 75 passed the Assembly by a 72-2 vote and the Senate by a 38-0 vote, and the governor signed it on October 2, 1989.

CONCLUSION

The primary source of protection for Proposition 99 during the initial implementation phase was public pressure. With the election less than a year in the past, the Legislature was conscious of what the public wanted. As the *California Journal* noted, "Their [the tobacco industry's] most important ally at the time was Speaker Brown, but with the election still fresh in memory, even Brown's muscle couldn't pull enough votes for the industry to get its way in this battle. It was one of the first major losses suffered by the industry in the Legislature until that time." [49] But as the election faded from memory, the public health groups had to find other ways to keep public interest activated and the media involved.

The need to keep the public involved reflected the different dynamic faced by the voluntaries in their legislative fight compared to that of the initiative campaign. In drafting Proposition 99, the voluntary health agencies were able to control most of the critical policy decisions, and they succeeded in the election by presenting a broad and generalized concept that allowed for minimal attack. Once Proposition 99 arrived in the Legislature, however, many more players got involved in policy decisions. Another key to the voluntaries' success in the initiative campaign was that their only major opponent in the fight over the initiative was the tobacco industry. Within the Legislature the industry could find allies. While not succeeding in diverting all the money away from "unacceptable" anti-tobacco programs to "acceptable" medical services, the tobacco industry was able to exploit its common interests with medical service providers during the legislative battle. The conservative CMA and the liberal Western Center on Law and Poverty had used CHDP funding as a wedge that would expand diversions away from genuine anti-tobacco education in future years.

The insider forum of the Legislature was not an environment where the voluntaries were generally successful in creating tobacco policy. According to Cliff Allenby, Deukmejian's secretary of health and welfare in 1989, the voluntary health agencies were not well positioned for the insider game. When asked about the voluntaries and their power relative to the other groups who sought money from AB 75, he said, "They had a lot going for them. They had this whole education thing, and they really believed that that was their initiative." [50] He commented that they probably did not realize their potential strength but went on to say,

> Nobody ever realizes their potential. . . . My theory is the assertion theory . . . you just say you're right. And if you know where you're going to go, then you really are in a stronger position than the opponent who is kind of defensive. Because they had to defend in discussions why the money shouldn't go to provide screening for kids to determine whether they had problems with their teeth. . . . We knew how the education money should be spent. . . . They didn't really have a clue of what they wanted to do or how they wanted to carry it out, and we did. I mean, we knew what we wanted to do. And that's a hell of an edge. [50]

When asked if the voluntaries would have done better by going on the offensive, he remarked, "To go on the offensive, they would have had to have been better prepared than they were. So, if they had gotten their act together, maybe. They had no act." [50] The voluntaries were relying on the election victory to create an "entitlement" for them to the Health Education monies, but the other legislative players were likely to give this mandate only minimal respect unless the voluntaries kept public attention on the negotiations. As Allenby noted, the administration was working to establish the issue as "health care for children" versus "tobacco education," a framing that the voluntary health agencies had to avoid.

From Miller's perspective, the diversion of money into CHDP was in the best long-term interest of the Proposition 99 programs: "The tens of millions we 'gave away' bought time for us to establish a real program. We gave our opponents no opportunity or justification to eliminate health education and no justification for CMA or the counties to abandon us. Yes, we surrendered a moral position, but we won three years to prove Prop 99's promise." [13] But for those who had to protect Proposition 99 in the long run, the surrender of the moral high ground in pursuit of a workable insider political strategy was problematic. By compromising, the health groups lost the ability to make a compelling argument: that the Legislature had to follow the will of the voters. They themselves had agreed to compromise the voters' will; why should the politicians flinch at doing the same thing?

AB 75 established the basic structure of how the health education program would operate in California. It created the largest tobacco control program in the world and featured several types of interventions: a media campaign; state-level programming; and local, community-based programs in the schools and county and city health departments. [51] Although AB 75 was close to what the voters had specified in Proposition 99, the health groups had made compromises with medical service providers that would seriously undermine the anti-tobacco education and research programs that had led the public to vote for Proposition 99 in the first place.

More important, by compromising on the money, the health groups lost the moral high ground by abandoning the demand that the politicians respect the will of the voters.

CHAPTER 7

Implementing the Tobacco Control Program

Despite the budgetary compromises that tobacco control advocates had made in AB 75, they still emerged with the largest budget ever allocated to a tobacco control program. The field of play shifted to the state bureaucracy, which had to implement California's Tobacco Control Program. While the Department of Health Services (DHS) ran the anti-tobacco media campaign and some competitive grants, the vast majority of the money flowed through DHS and the California Department of Education (CDE) to the county health departments, county offices of education, and local school districts. This program design meant that two state-level agencies, sixty-one local health departments, fifty-eight county offices of education, and over 1,000 school districts went overnight from having virtually no money dedicated to tobacco control to having over $100 million annually. The challenge for these organizations was to put into place immediately, with virtually no existing infrastructure, an unprecedented tobacco control program. Throughout the development and passage of Proposition 99 and the subsequent battle over the implementing legislation, there was a constant tension between those who wanted the money to go to programs specifically designed to reduce tobacco consumption and those who wanted to see the money go into health promotion generally, with the promise that there would be a tobacco control component.

In addition to active efforts by the tobacco industry to undermine the program (discussed in chapter 8), there were five significant operational barriers to successful implementation of a well-coordinated tobacco control program. First, the administration of the program was split between two state agencies that reported to different, and competing, elected officials. The director of DHS reports to the governor (who in 1989 was Republican George Deukmejian) while CDE reports to the independently elected superintendent of public instruction (in 1989 this was Democrat Bill Honig, who, to complicate matters, was thinking of running for governor). This partisan division between DHS and CDE persisted through the first ten years of the Tobacco Control Program. Honig was succeeded by Democrat Delaine Eastin, and Deukmejian was succeeded by Republican Pete Wilson. There was no authority available to mediate disputes between the two departments. Second, in the absence of a sure model for tobacco use prevention, each agency could define its approach to tobacco control as it saw fit, and very different models emerged. DHS dealt with tobacco specifically, and CDE subsumed tobacco control within a larger health promotion model. Third, with so many independent agencies participating in the program, a scheme for monitoring and oversight had to be developed that combined program accountability with creativity in achieving goals. Program administrators found these two goals—accountability and creativity—difficult to achieve simultaneously. Fourth, lacking experience in tobacco control, health and education agencies had little capacity to mount a massive tobacco control program. Fifth, AB 75 gave these agencies only a short time to produce results; as noted in the previous chapter, AB 75's sunset provision took effect just twenty-one months after the bill was signed.

TWO DIFFERENT MODELS

Although the voluntary health agencies had insisted that health education programs focus specifically on tobacco issues, the final legislation was permissive about what could be done with Proposition 99's Health Education Account money. According to the final language of AB 75, the agencies were to provide "preventative health education against tobacco use." The bill broadly defined what such education might be. It included "programs of instruction intended to dissuade individuals from beginning to smoke, to encourage smoking cessation, or to provide information on the health effects of tobacco on the user, children, and nonsmokers. These programs may include a focus on health promotion, disease

prevention, and risk reduction, utilizing a 'wellness perspective' that en-
courages self-esteem and positive decision-making techniques."[1] The
tobacco-specific model, which the voluntary health agencies had advocated, and the blended model, which the legislation allowed, were both
implemented, the former by DHS and the latter by CDE. Because these
differing models became the basis for programming in health departments and schools, they complicated the relationship between health
and education agencies.

DHS chose to develop a tobacco-specific program based on a model
for tobacco control developed at the National Cancer Institute (NCI).[2]
According to this model, tobacco use, especially the adolescent progres-
sion to adult smoking, was the result of a specific and identifiable set of
influences—including the tobacco industry's promotional activities (figure 6). The program sought to break the chain of events which led people
to smoke or continue smoking. The NCI model guided program planners
in designing tobacco interventions for delivery through four channels—
health care settings, schools, community groups, and worksites—using
one of three types of programs: mass media, policy, or direct program
services. The first comprehensive plans from local health departments
used a slightly modified version of this model.

In contrast, CDE simply incorporated the tobacco money into existing school-based programs designed to deal with the factors that put children "at risk" for using illegal drugs and alcohol.[3,4] In the "risk factor"
approach, children who have problems in their own lives or with family,
school, peers, or the community are considered at risk (figure 7). This
approach seeks to enhance protective factors for these youth through the
following specific activities:

1. Promoting bonds to family, school, and positive peer groups
through opportunities for active participation.

2. Defining a clear set of tactics against drug use.

3. Teaching the skills needed to learn the tactics.

4. Providing recognition, rewards, and reinforcement for newly
learned skills and behaviors.[5]

With the advent of Proposition 99, tobacco was added to this model because it was considered a "gateway" drug to the use of other drugs. CDE,
citing data showing that youth tend to use drugs such as tobacco, al-

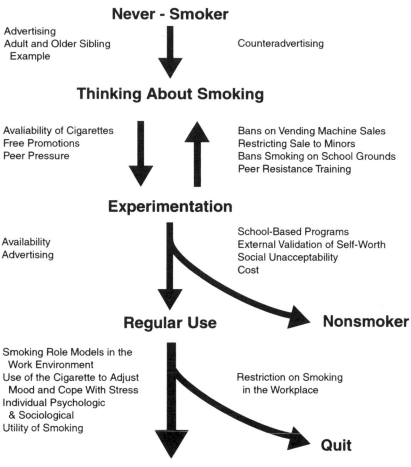

Never - Smoker

Advertising
Adult and Older Sibling   Counteradvertising
  Example

Thinking About Smoking

Avaliability of Cigarettes   Bans on Vending Machine Sales
Free Promotions   Restricting Sale to Minors
Peer Pressure   Bans Smoking on School Grounds
                                    Peer Resistance Training

Experimentation

                                    School-Based Programs
Availability   External Validation of Self-Worth
Advertising   Social Unacceptability
                                    Cost

Regular Use   **Nonsmoker**

Smoking Role Models in the
  Work Environment
Use of the Cigarette to Adjust   Restriction on Smoking
  Mood and Cope With Stress   in the Workplace
Individual Psychologic
  & Sociological
Utility of Smoking

                                    Quit

Dependent Smoker

Figure 6.   The National Cancer Institute's model of the factors influencing to-
bacco use. The model of tobacco uptake is linear and offers specific points of
intervention. The DHS tobacco control program is based on this model.
Source: National Institutes of Health, *Strategies to control tobacco use in the
United States: A blueprint for public health action in the 1990s* (Bethesda,
MD: National Institutes of Health, 1991), 23.

cohol, marijuana, and other drugs in a predictable sequence, concluded
that "the nature of multi-drug use indicates that preventive efforts should
not be targeted to any single drug."[5] To curb the use of tobacco, along
with other substance use, schools were urged to concentrate on alleviating the factors that put a child "at risk."

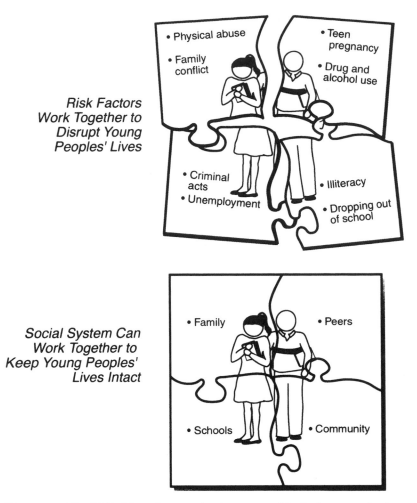

Risk Factors Work Together to Disrupt Young Peoples' Lives

Social System Can Work Together to Keep Young Peoples' Lives Intact

Figure 7.   The CDE risk and protective factors model of tobacco and substance abuse. The model is diffuse and does not offer specific intervention points that can be coordinated with community-based tobacco prevention programs. *Source:* California Department of Education, *Not schools alone* (Sacramento: California Department of Education, 1991), 2-3.

LEADERSHIP AT DHS

The Department of Health Services is part of the State Health and Welfare Agency, which reports to the governor. At the time Proposition 99 passed, DHS was headed by Dr. Kenneth Kizer, who was personally committed to the success of the Proposition 99 programs and recognized that Proposition 99 created a unique opportunity to create a whole new approach to public health, especially tobacco control. He took a strong personal interest in seeing that an effective and innovative tobacco control program was put in place and was willing to stand up to the tobacco industry and its allies inside the state government in order to do so. Jennie Cook, an American Cancer Society (ACS) volunteer, a national chair of ACS, and a member of the Tobacco Education Oversight Committee (TEOC) since its inception, observed, "Kizer was probably the most honest person I've ever run across where tobacco was concerned. . . . You knew up front he was an advocate for tobacco control. He felt strongly that he was going to make this program really work."[6] In a 1995 interview, Kizer himself expressed his strong commitment to the program:

> I can tell you in all candor that basically the approach that we took was one that we were going to try to do it right. . . . The Health Department took the position early on . . . that the Health Education Account should be used for health education, for media and local education campaigns, etc. That was not supported, or at least it didn't appear to be supported, strongly at the agency level. And it was absolutely not supported at the Governor's Office. . . . I think they [the Health and Welfare Agency] felt that was a huge amount of money . . . and there was no way that we could reasonably spend that in the time period.[7]

Kizer created a separate Tobacco Control Section (TCS) within DHS and ordered the administrative support units within DHS to give priority to staffing, issuing its requests for proposals, and adding other services needed to get the fledgling program up and running as quickly as possible.

TCS was to develop the state's anti-smoking media campaign and run a series of statewide projects and technical support activities as well as develop, fund, and oversee local tobacco control activities. The local activities were to be delivered and coordinated by local lead agencies (LLAs) in each of the California's sixty-one local health departments. Each LLA was designed to be an identifiable, tobacco-specific organization. This local structure, which was to emerge as one of the California Tobacco Control Program's greatest strengths, however, was relatively long in coming. TCS had to write guidelines for the local programs, the LLAs had to develop and submit plans, the plans had to be reviewed and approved, and the money distributed. And, of course, hundreds of people had to be recruited and trained to complete all these tasks, a process that took nearly a year.

THE MEDIA CAMPAIGN

In contrast to the complexities of getting the local programs off the ground, it was a relatively simple bureaucratic task to launch the antismoking media campaign that AB 75 had established. It merely required writing one request for proposals and issuing one contract to one advertising agency. It was the one way that DHS could show the public and politicians that it was doing something with Proposition 99 money in a hurry.

DHS moved quickly to implement the media campaign. The request for proposals was released on December 1, 1989, fifty-nine days after Governor Deukmejian had signed AB 75; responses from advertising agencies were due just six weeks later, on January 10, 1990. On January 26, DHS selected the Los Angeles advertising agency keye/donna/ perlstein to run the campaign.[8] The first anti-tobacco advertisements reached California's television viewers on April 10, 1990, sixty-five days after the contract was signed.[9]

The campaign was like nothing the world had ever seen. Rather than talking about the dangers of smoking, or even secondhand smoke, the campaign directly and explicitly attacked the tobacco industry.

The first television advertisement, "Industry Spokesmen," showed a group of actors portraying tobacco industry executives sitting around a smoke-filled room (figure 8). Their leader says:

> Gentlemen, gentlemen. The tobacco industry has a very serious multi-billion-dollar problem. We need more cigarette smokers. Pure and simple. Every day, 2,000 Americans stop smoking and another 1,178 also quit. Actually, technically, they die.
>   That means that this business needs 3,000 fresh, new volunteers every day. So, forget all that cancer, heart disease, stroke stuff.
>   Gentlemen, we're not in this for our health.

At the end, he laughs, joined by the other executives.

This radical new approach grew out of discussions between Kizer, Dileep Bal, head of the Cancer Control Branch (which includes TCS), and ad agency principal Paul Keye, who brought a new perspective to the question of how to reduce tobacco consumption. As Keye later explained,

> The cigarette companies were never in any of the advertising agency's original thoughts or conversations with the Department of Health Services. You can't find the topic in our first work. . . . What happened was that—as we dug into each topic—there, right in the middle of everything were the Smokefolk, mak-

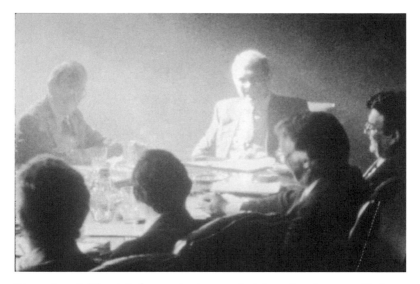

Figure 8. California's first anti-tobacco television advertisement, "Industry Spokesmen," was a frontal attack on the tobacco industry. This advertisement set the tone for the California Tobacco Control Program when it was first aired in April 1990. (Courtesy California Department of Health Services)

> ing their quaint, nonsensical arguments and—by sheer weight of wealth and power and privilege—getting away with it. . . . Frankly, the tobacco industry pissed us off. They insulted our intelligence.[10]

Instead of falling back on the traditional public health messages ("tobacco is bad for you"), Keye urged that the campaign directly attack the tobacco industry. The first reaction to the campaign within TCS was surprise, with some wondering aloud, "Can we say that?" But TCS soon agreed that it could and should, and the anti-industry emphasis became an integral part of the campaign.[10,11] TCS was out to raise the temperature around tobacco as an issue, convincing people that smoking was not normal, ordinary behavior and the tobacco industry was not just another legal business.

To reinforce this message and to announce the new aggressive campaign against the tobacco industry, TCS ran full-page advertisements in all the major newspaper in California on April 11, 1990, with the headline "First, the Smoke. Now, the Mirrors" (figure 9). The text began:

> In less than a generation, the bad news about cigarettes has become no news. Most Americans—even the very young—know the unavoidable connection

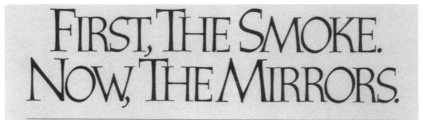

Figure 9. California's first anti-tobacco newspaper advertisement. The Department of Health Services announced the new California Tobacco Control Program with this full-page advertisement in newspapers throughout the state on April 11, 1990. (Courtesy California Department of Health Services)

between smoking and cancer, smoking and heart disease, smoking and emphysema and strokes.

Today a surprising number of us can tell you that cigarettes are our #1 preventable cause of death and disability.

So, we seem to know about the smoke. But what about the really dangerous stuff—all those carefully polished, fatal illusions the tobacco industry has crafted to mess with our minds so they can mess with our lives?[12]

Smoking was not just a health problem; it was also a social and political one.

The tobacco industry and its allies in the advertising industry went wild. Walker Merryman, vice president for communications at the Tobacco Institute in Washington, protested that "the ads themselves have broken faith with the voters. . . . They are an unsavory assault on tobacco companies." He claimed that they were not educational advertisements.[13] Tom Lauria, a spokesman for the Tobacco Institute, agreed: "They pitched Prop 99 as: 'We want to reach underaged children. We want to educate children to the purported health effects of smoking.' . . . anything beyond that is not educational, it's political."[14] Bob Garfield, a columnist in *Advertising Age,* an advertising industry trade newspaper, accused TCS of inciting racial paranoia by trading on "a vile stereotype: the wealthy, white embodiment of evil. . . . This 'public service' message is inflammatory and racist and it will feed paranoia. . . . Californians should indeed be careful of what they breathe. There is something foul on their air."[15]

Governor Deukmejian was cool toward the advertisements. One of his spokesmen explained: "It's not in the nature of the governor to go on an attack like this. He's always been genteel and civilized in his approach to public affairs."[16] Deukmejian, however, took a hands-off approach to the campaign and allowed Kizer and DHS to proceed according to their professional judgment. Indeed, the Tobacco Institute lamented the way Governor Deukmejian was giving Kizer free rein over the campaign: "As a 'lame duck,' the Governor is not likely to get into a public sparring match with Dr. Kizer, even though he disagrees with the Department of Health Services' attack approach with the anti-tobacco advertisements."[17] Rather than submitting the detailed, multilayer political review of the media campaign that came to be required when Pete Wilson succeeded Deukmejian as governor, TCS simply made a "brown bag run" to the Governor's Office the night before new ads were aired so that the governor would know what was about to hit.

The other first-wave advertisements in 1990 were just as strong. One featured black rappers attacking the tobacco industry for targeting African Americans with mentholated cigarettes, using the tag line "We used to pick it; now they want us to smoke it." [13] Another showed a husband and his pregnant wife sitting together. When the man lights up and inhales deeply, the smoke comes out the woman's mouth. The tag line was "Smokers aren't the only ones who smoke." [15]

The advertisements attracted international attention. Indeed, in 1997, seven years after it had originally run and over a year after Governor Pete Wilson's administration had ordered it off the air permanently, "Industry Spokesmen" still had the highest recall rate—96 percent of adults and 93 percent of teens—of any advertisement that DHS produced.[18] The advertisements stimulated strong public interest in the Tobacco Control Program. They also set the overall tone for the program as one that considered tobacco a social and political problem well beyond the bounds of traditional public health thinking at the time.

THE LOCAL LEAD AGENCIES

While the media campaign was jump-starting the Tobacco Control Program, the LLAs were still getting organized. In addition to the efforts within each local health department, each LLA was required to encourage the formation of a "local coalition" made up of players from the private and nonprofit sectors, including local units of the voluntary health agencies as well as new players in tobacco control. These local coalitions would play an increasingly important role in the evolution of California's Tobacco Control Program. The counties were required to submit preliminary plans in December 1989, before the media campaign had reached the public.

For most counties the tobacco revenue represented a substantial amount of new money, especially since Proposition 13 had hit the counties so hard. Each county received at least $150,000 a year, with the larger counties receiving considerably more: Los Angeles ($12.2 million), San Diego ($1.8 million), San Francisco ($1.6 million), and Santa Clara ($1.6 million). Even medium-sized counties like Ventura and Sonoma received over $460,000.[19]

TCS recognized that, in addition to guidelines, the LLAs needed a state infrastructure that would provide them with ongoing training and technical assistance. TCS hired a contractor to establish the Tobacco Education Clearinghouse of California, which kept existing tobacco resource materials on file and added to its collection all materials developed by Proposition 99–funded health programs. TCS also created the California Tobacco Survey, a large statewide telephone survey of tobacco use in California, to provide information on how well the tobacco control program was working. Dr. John Pierce of the University of California at San Diego won the contract to run the survey. The survey was to provide feedback throughout the program on the overall effectiveness of the California Tobacco Education Program and some of the reasons for the program's success or failure. To provide technical assistance to the LLAs and competitive grantees, TCS contracted with the American Nonsmokers' Rights Foundation (ANRF), Stanford University, and the Western Consortium for Public Health to create the California Tobacco Control Resource Partnership, which was to provide ongoing training, conferences, and other forms of technical assistance to DHS-funded programs. Over time, the California Tobacco Control Resource Partnership, particularly through a series of regular teleconferences, became the "central nervous system" for the local programs. The teleconferences were hosted by ANRF and designed to give the LLAs (and other Proposition 99 participants) help in countering pro-tobacco strategies as well as other technical assistance. The rapid sharing of information—especially about tobacco industry tactics and how to respond to them—increased reaction times of the local programs and thus their effectiveness.

Getting the LLAs off the ground, however, was a cumbersome process. Although Kizer had forced DHS to help TCS get up to speed quickly, most county tobacco control operations got no such special treatment. The slowness of county paper processing and the complex nature of county procedures impeded rapid program development. Part of the problem faced by one LLA director had to do with the unusual nature of her program design. She said, "The reality is no one had really had money like that to do anything innovative in the health department. So I think people had to get used to the idea of something different, including purchasing. I mean, you never had people buying some of the things we were buying before all this. Now they're used to it but it was unusual. . . . it took a lot of work, we had to go back two, three times sometimes."[20] Eventually some LLAs cut back the number of grants to local groups for tobacco control work simply because of the time it took. On the other hand, some county administrators and politicians were important program advocates. Another LLA director described her health officer as "a very strong tobacco [control] advocate [who] . . . was willing to fight battles and take the heat." She emphasized that the health officer was "one of the reasons we had these successes . . . and it wouldn't have happened without him."[21]

In contrast to the state level, the earliest local program designs reflected a traditional view of public health, focused on promoting smoking cessation, even though "policy" and "media" were part of the NCI model. But smoking cessation programs were comfortable. Most people who had trained in public health were familiar with providing direct services, especially cessation. The tobacco industry generally sits quietly when people run smoking cessation programs because such programs are expensive and not very effective. Generally only about 10 percent of those enrolled in cessation programs are still abstinent a year later, and cessation programs, because they approach smokers one person at a time, simply cannot reach a significant portion of the smoking population. Cessation programs do nothing to keep people from starting to smoke.

The media campaign was launched in the midst of the LLAs' efforts to get their programs up and running. Cynthia Hallett, then with the Los Angeles LLA, thought the advertisements were "great" but that they hit the streets almost too fast: "In trying to launch our education campaign, it was really difficult, given that media was out there and talking about how bad the tobacco industry was. And here we were just trying to start our program. People were calling us saying, 'Those ads. Well, what are you guys doing? And can I get some service?' And we were still training staff."[22] Whether intentional or not, the anti-industry focus of the media campaign began to shift the emphasis of the other programs toward policy interventions. In addition, Americans for Nonsmokers' Rights was continuing to support communities in developing and passing local tobacco control ordinances. ANR's policy-oriented approach already permeated the state and the LLAs felt its influence. Even so, it took a year or so to move beyond cessation programs to activities that would change the social environment enough to reduce tobacco consumption.

One LLA director commented that she moved into other programmatic areas almost immediately because she had done cessation before and did not want to do it again. But for most LLAs the transition to community-based strategies took longer. One LLA director described the process:

> We ended up funding Stop Smoking and Smoking Prevention Programs for every ethnic group and every age group. We even had a preschool program. It was very much a cessation model, helping individuals quit smoking. People

thought that was the logical way to spend the money. . . . We had a Stop Smoking Program for the Vietnamese, another one for the Spanish-speaking. We had another one for African Americans. We had another one for senior citizens. We had one for teenagers. (laughter) I remember thinking, driving around one year later, "Is my program having any effect on this community?" Because everywhere I looked people were smoking inside and outside. I just had the sense that I was wasting public dollars.

And meanwhile, people were calling me with bad secondhand smoke prob-lems at their workplace. Totally bombarded. I would look up their [local clean indoor air] ordinance and say, "There is nothing I can do for you. Your em-ployer can smoke at your workplace." So the laws were very bad at that point. . . . So I remember driving down the street one day, thinking maybe we could just make everything smoke free.

So I talked to one of the higher-ups in the county, and said, "Why don't we just get a good county ordinance going here?" And she leaned over and she patted my hand and she said, "Oh no, dear, you don't know what you are talking about. This person on the Board [of Supervisors, the county legisla-tive body] smokes, that person on the Board smokes. Their secretary smokes. Don't do it, don't even consider this." So I said, "Well, OK, what if the cities passed ordinances and that would like peer-pressure the county into it?" And she kind of smiled. So I just hung in and got started, changed the whole pro-gram orientation to policy and ordinances.[23] [emphasis added]

This interest in doing policy work was not, however, universal. People worried about getting involved in local controversies and wanted to avoid confrontation with the tobacco industry and its political allies. People in public health departments who had trained as traditional health educa-tors were not used to being confrontational or political. Their lack of ex-perience was exacerbated by the ambivalence of coalitions consisting of other public health professionals or representatives of local units of the voluntary health agencies who were reluctant to get involved in politics.

Over time, however, the values and approaches of the Tobacco Con-trol Program changed, and most program participants became more policy-oriented. In 1998, when asked what she would do differently if she had it to do over again, one of the reticent directors responded, "I would be more pro-active with local leaders. I would probably get into it, and say, 'Oh well, if we're going to have a conflict, let's just go for it.'"[24]

ENCOURAGING DIVERSITY

Beginning with AB 75, tobacco control programs were required to fo-cus on certain target populations, especially pregnant women, minori-ties, and youth. Public health groups viewed these subpopulations as im-

portant targets because pregnant women who stop smoking early nearly
eliminate the excess risk of delivering a low-birth-weight infant and because the tobacco industry was targeting minorities and youth in its advertising. In agreeing to focus on youth and pregnant women, tobacco
control groups may have played into the hands of tobacco interests. After all, Nielsen, Merksamer had recommended the Child Health and Disability Prevention (CHDP) and Maternal and Child Health programs as
good candidates for the diversion of Health Education Account funds.[25]
The industry appears to accept tobacco prevention programs focused
on pregnant women and youth because they have limited impact on cigarette consumption. At any given time, there are not many pregnant
women, so messages directed at this group will not be relevant to most
of the population. And primary prevention programs directed solely at
youth are of limited effectiveness because they may inadvertently reinforce the belief that smoking is an acceptable adult behavior.[26]

Fortunately, TCS never interpreted this focus narrowly, and the result
was a campaign that addressed the general population while including
these groups. The effort to create an inclusive program brought a wide
range of community-based organizations into the program, such as the
Asian American Health Forum, the Watts Health Foundation, the California Healthy Cities Project, the East Los Angeles Health Task Force,
and KCET Public Television.

For public health professionals working at the state and local level, it
was a challenge to reach minority populations because health departments tended to be made up primarily of white, middle-class people.
The LLAs addressed this problem by encouraging groups that were already working in the target communities to apply for LLA grants to
fund tobacco control activities in those same communities. While this
approach often worked, it ignored the need for capacity building around
the tobacco issue. As a result, as the program evolved, the LLAs developed more directed strategies to involve these community groups. One
county eventually created a "Tobacco 101" orientation that a group had
to complete before they were eligible to receive grants from the health
department. Eventually TCS also funded Ethnic Networks, which provided resources and networking capacity to community-based programs
funded either directly by TCS or by the LLA to serve African Americans,
Native Americans, Asian Americans, and Latinos on a statewide basis.[27]

As the thrust of the LLA programs began to shift away from cessation
to community-based, policy-oriented work, the reliance on community-

based organizations (CBOs) also meant that these groups had to be educated in the new paradigm and away from cessation classes. According
to one LLA director, leaders of these community organizations often reacted skeptically: " 'Why the hell should I be interested in this? I know
that tobacco's bad, so what?' *Moving them more toward looking at this
issue globally, how does it impact them, what can they do about it.* And
again giving them the skills then to say, 'Okay, now that I know that this
is bad, what do I do?' *Trying to get the CBOs to understand that they
had to have an ongoing relationship with the community, to get them to
understand why it's important to have smoke-free environments"* (emphasis added).[28] While there were difficulties in involving the new constituencies in tobacco control in California, community activities were
to emerge as one of the strongest and most innovative aspects of the California Tobacco Control Program.

Peter Hanauer, a veteran of the Proposition 5, 10, and P campaigns,
was impressed with the difference that this outreach made in the tobacco
control movement:

> Things had changed. I walked into a meeting in San Francisco, . . . this was
> sometime in the late eighties or early nineties, and I had been used to going
> to meetings with almost all white males, a few women occasionally, a token
> black occasionally. I walked into this meeting and it was like every spectrum
> of San Francisco society was represented there. . . . And I was overwhelmed
> when I walked in there and saw all of these people from all the different mi-
> nority communities, who were up in arms because they had come to realize
> that the industry was preying on them, that the industry was not the good Sa-
> maritan that it pretended to be.[29]

While the original goal of involving community organizations had simply
been to reach their constituencies with tobacco control messages, this
effort was having much deeper effects. In particular, it was beginning to
undermine the acceptance that the tobacco industry had built up over
the years in these communities by providing financial support for community groups.

The effort to create diversity through grants, however, was more successful than creating diversity through volunteers. The LLAs were required by TCS to create a diverse coalition to help with their programs.
But there were almost universal problems in trying to keep a coalition
active and involved. In two of the fifteen counties where interviews were
conducted, the coalition was an active body, involved in program design
and local politics. Dynamic chairs from outside the LLA provided a great

deal of leadership. In the other counties, the coalition was more reactive, made up of paid staff from other public agencies, the voluntary health agencies, and grantees.

TCS's push for coalitions brought mixed reactions from the LLAs, as did some of TCS's other actions. In the early days, life for the LLAs was chaotic, and people at the county level had mixed feelings about the TCS. In general, the directors of the larger, urban LLAs seemed to be happier with TCS than the smaller, rural ones. One LLA director from a large county made this comment:

> They [TCS] were very, very supportive. And TCS has always been profoundly advanced in terms of policy, Carol Russell [who headed the local programs unit] especially. They could not have been better. They funded teleconferences through ANR [ANRF, American Nonsmokers' Rights Foundation]. They had workshops directly. I mean, they just did everything they could; they understood early on how important this was. *And they began to encourage us to move away from changing individual behavior more into the community norm and changing the environment.*[23] [emphasis added]

Those working in the rural areas, however, felt from the beginning that the TCS program was not designed with them in mind. One blunt LLA director said,

> They [the staff at TCS] are very controlling, very, very strong. . . . TCS has a very strong hand in what we do and what we don't do and how we do it. They want it on the paper in a certain way. They want us to do X, Y, Z and only X, Y, Z. And don't be interjecting any of your own creative problems into it. You do what you are told, you accept our money, and you play with our money within our realms. . . . They have no sense or feel [of] what is going to happen in a rural environment. We've never been asked by TCS, not to my knowledge have we ever been asked for input on what our areas of priority should be.[24]

A number of the rural LLA directors, when they were interviewed in 1998, were still stung by early accusations that they were racist when they protested that the targeted groups excluded the vast majority of their population, which was white.

The other major complaint from the rural areas had to do with the concentration of the media campaign in the major media markets. According to one LLA director, "When the media campaign was all over the state, that really was good, that was just so helpful and so beneficial. And then they started cutting down on . . . media coming up into this area, based on . . . population. . . . California does extend 300 miles north of Sacramento, and I was really indignant about [it] when they cut the media. And I still think it's a big loss to us." [30] In another rural county, the LLA director wished that the advertisements at least existed in a format that could be shown in the local movie theater.[24] In general, there was a feeling that not a lot of creative thinking had gone into reaching the rural markets. This problem was aggravated by the dominance in some rural areas of out-of-state satellite television and other media.

Some of these tensions between the field and TCS would remain throughout the program, reflecting the struggle between local-level program autonomy and state-level control. On March 12, 1993, TCS hosted a Statewide Projects Meeting in San Francisco, where the LLAs again expressed a desire for TCS to provide more leadership and less project supervision.[31] Despite these problems, the local programs funded by Proposition 99 emerged as a key element in its success. They quickly evolved away from traditional smoking cessation efforts to a variety of approaches designed to change the social environment—through passage of local clean indoor air ordinances and other efforts to counter directly the influence of the tobacco industry in their communities. In addition, TCS directly funded some service delivery projects whose scope was multicounty and sometimes statewide. In one innovative project, a tobacco-free race car brought a tobacco-free message to racetracks, a venue where pro-tobacco messages, both on the cars themselves and around the track, had gone unchallenged. The involvement of minority groups and other new players deepened and strengthened the statewide constituency that was working actively to reduce tobacco consumption in California. In California's war against tobacco, the media campaign provided the air cover and the local groups provided the ground troops.

THE SCHOOLS: A DIFFERENT APPROACH

If it was a challenge for local health departments to build a mechanism for delivering tobacco control programs quickly, the schools faced an even greater problem. Every county had a health department, and those health departments had a tradition and mandate to do prevention-oriented activities directed at specific diseases or risks. Within schools, the situation was different. Health was not a central part of their mandate, and schools varied in their capacity to provide any kind of health education, much less something as specialized as tobacco use prevention. Moreover, teaching health issues of any kind in schools can expose the local elected board of education to controversy, which it may not be willing to tackle. This approach, avoiding controversy, contrasted sharply with DHS's approach: using controversy in the media campaign to engage the public in the debate over tobacco.

From the beginning, the schools viewed the tobacco money as just another categorical program. Educators tend to resent categorical programs because they believe that such programs limit their authority to do what is best for their students and because the programs require excessive paperwork. Thus, while the Proposition 99 dollars were welcome, the mandate that the schools provide tobacco-specific prevention activities was not. In addition to these problems, AB 75's rapid sunset also caused difficulties. No one knew what would happen when AB 75's twenty-one months ran out, and this uncertain future made the schools even less interested in developing a long-term commitment to tobacco education.

When Proposition 99 passed, California schools were under financial siege. Proposition 13, which had limited the ability of local governments to raise local revenues, had hit the schools particularly hard. Bill Honig, who served as superintendent of public instruction when Proposition 99 passed and when AB 75 was being implemented, explained the situation this way:

> There are four things that were going on in California that would make anything hard. Number one is this huge growth. Many places are just trying to accommodate new kids. . . . They're just coming out of the woodwork and we are not building the buildings. . . . Secondly, there has been this demographic shift of poverty. The explosive growth of poverty conditions makes schooling much tougher. More kids are coming with deep problems. Then the third one was this whole language demographic shift where you've got now, one out of three kids in that early elementary school level doesn't speak English. So we've got that problem. And then you have the funding crisis on top of that, we're trying to do it with less and less and less dollars.[32]

In this difficult climate, Proposition 99's new money was viewed by the schools as a way to solve some of their pressing problems.

At approximately the same time that Proposition 99 was passed, the California school superintendents were working to establish a regional structure to provide the school districts with health expertise. At the state level, CDE had already established a program and an administrative unit called Healthy Kids, Healthy California, which was responsible for carrying out health and drug-related programs. CDE decided to use the Healthy Kids Regional Centers to implement Proposition 99. CDE pooled the Proposition 99 monies with two other funding sources to create the Drug, Alcohol, and Tobacco Education (DATE) program. CDE required each county office to have a Tobacco Use Prevention Education (TUPE) coordinator, and generally this person was also responsible for the drug and alcohol programs and, in smaller counties, other categorical programs as well, including some that were not health programs.

According to Kathy Yeates, who was the acting director of the Office of Healthy Kids, Healthy California in 1994, schools were not really committed to doing much about tobacco for a variety of reasons:

> There was no commitment to it. It was like one more thing, given reading programs and bilingual and all the pressing problems—the obvious problems. "Yeah, some kids smoke, but who cares. You know, smoking. Big deal. . . . It's the least of our discipline problems right now. We've got kids fighting with guns; tobacco, that's just a passive problem. It's not as active as fighting or something like that." A lot of school folks smoke and it was just too controversial with unions and whatever. So schools really didn't want to take it on. In addition to everybody having someone that's an alcoholic, everybody's got somebody in their families that smokes. And people on staff. . . . So they kind of tiptoed around it and didn't want to take it on. Didn't see it as a problem . . . as long as they weren't smoking in their classrooms, who cares what they do? . . . I mean like "Oh yeah, bad drugs," but you know that's not the biggest problem.[33]

This attitude, coupled with the risk and protective factors model, provided schools with an opportunity to spend their Proposition 99 monies creatively. For schools, a program that addresses the problems that educators consider most pressing was much more appealing than taking on tobacco directly. From this perspective, if school failure is an underlying cause of tobacco use, then tobacco money could be spent on just about anything that would improve the schools.

The method used to distribute funds added to the problem. In contrast to the critical mass of funding created in the health departments, money went to the county offices of education and the school districts based on average daily student attendance. Once the money was spread over 1,003 districts, fifty-eight county offices, and ten regional centers, the amounts could be quite small. Some of the small districts received under $500, hardly enough to create an identifiable presence for tobacco control. By contrast, even the smallest county health department received $150,000. With a lack of commitment to Proposition 99 at the top, inadequate programming, and sometimes small amounts of money, it is not surprising that schools saw themselves as the recipients of a categorical funding stream, driven by entitlements, which they could try to use for the dominant priorities of the schools. And tobacco, especially at first, was not a particularly high priority for schools.

The poor condition of health education generally in California, due to years of Proposition 13–inspired budget cuts, created further problems for implementing meaningful tobacco prevention programs in the schools. (Increasing numbers of districts were cutting back or eliminating their school nurses at that time.) As one TUPE coordinator said, "All of this money has been flowing to schools with the assumption that there was an infrastructure in place for health education." [34] The infrastructure to absorb this money and use it effectively simply did not exist. There is no high school graduation requirement for health education in California, and there is a very minimal requirement for health education in teacher credentialing. One of the county TUPE coordinators explained how the lack of infrastructure in schools set them up for failure, not just in tobacco programs but other health programs as well:

> There wasn't an infrastructure there to accept the money. A lot of us were afraid that all this money was coming down and it was going to be misused because there wasn't anybody in place. This is kind of a Catch-22, it's a chicken-egg thing. We've got the money but nobody in place, so then we put the money in, we say, "Look, it's failing, it isn't working. . . ." This is the typical thing that's happened in health education in many instances where the person who ends up teaching it at the high school is the person who's on their last leg. "We don't know what to do with Charlie so we'll have him teach health." [35]

The $36 million that schools were given each year during the two years of AB 75 would have been a substantial increment to an existing backbone for the delivery of health messages in the schools had it existed.

A coherent approach to tobacco education in the schools was further undermined by the absence of training, materials, or expertise in tobacco use prevention. This lack of materials reinforced the tendency of the schools to teach health as "body systems." There was little in the way of good age-appropriate material that focused on tobacco as a social and political issue.

For early program implementers, CDE's lack of commitment to the program was reflected in the nature of its tobacco-free mandate. Schools were not required to have tobacco-free policies in order to qualify for Proposition 99 funds, and they were given until 1996 to become tobacco free. CDE promulgated a definition of "tobacco free" that was more rigorous than the definition used by other organizations—schools could not allow any smoking in the buildings, on the grounds (including service yards), or in vehicles. But with the long deadline, schools could receive Proposition 99 funding without having to do anything at all about tobacco use on the school site. For those believing in policy-based health interventions, this long deadline was not a good start to the program.

EARLY LEADERSHIP PROBLEMS

It might have been possible to overcome the financial and structural problems that the schools faced in delivering anti-tobacco education if there had been strong and committed leadership at high levels within CDE, as Kizer had provided for DHS, but such leadership never materialized. Robert Ryan, who was the head of the Healthy Kids, Healthy California office and responsible for the anti-tobacco education efforts until he left in 1994, brought the right credentials to the job. With a background that combined training and education in both health and prevention, he had vision for the program, but his own drug and alcohol problems got the better of him and he quit coming to work.

Kathy Yeates, who worked with Ryan and his assistant Bill White (who headed CDE's tobacco program) and who was eventually named to succeed him, described the leadership problem:

> Robert was already in big trouble with his own using of drugs, alcohol, and tobacco. He was in big trouble. . . . I had told Robert that if he messed up one more time that I would have to do something about it, which I followed through and went . . . [to an] associate superintendent who went to the deputy and they just called him in and chewed him out. Nothing happened . . . so I watched Robert go downhill. . . . He hated confrontation of the mildest kind. And he just didn't come to work. . . . And it was too big of a task for the two of them to do without more competent staff. And they just didn't have additional competent staff that understood prevention. . . . And he didn't have the support of the agency, because he had jeopardized that. So he was taking all this flack—deserved, a lot of it deserved—but it was doing him in more than supporting him. So I think that he had the potential but he lost it. And the field was disenchanted. The CDE staff was disenchanted. And so because of that the program did suffer.[33]

At a conference in Millbrae, held in the spring of 1990, White told educators to put enough tobacco material in their drug programs so that if any parent was an executive at a local voluntary health agency, he or she would see something for the Proposition 99 dollars. Rather than encouraging schools to become a partner in the larger California Tobacco Control Program, the leadership appeared to be offering cash-strapped school districts a wink and a nod to use the money however they wanted.

MONITORING AND ACCOUNTABILITY

CDE's initial program simply involved distributing the money based on average daily attendance (ADA), with few program or fiscal guidelines. ADA-based funding is easier to distribute and is politically less volatile than a contract or grants program because it avoids the need to apply what some may consider subjective criteria. Distributing the money according to such a formula also means that no one has to consider the minimum amount of money that a small district needs to mount a credible program or the maximum that a large district can responsibly use.[36] (Severe understaffing at CDE—three people were charged with monitoring 1,003 school districts—aggravated this problem.) In addition, when funds are distributed on an ADA basis, monitoring the expenditures presents difficulties because districts receive an entitlement regardless of their interest in participating in the program.

Carolyn Martin, the first TEOC chair, was asked whether the accountability problems were the result of incompetence or a lack of interest in keeping track of the money. She replied, "I think it was both. I think that they were incompetent or they could have written much tighter guidelines for the schools. They full well knew that schools were in desperate shape for money, and, man, if they didn't ride herd on every penny, it was going to disappear. I mean you don't have to be a genius to figure this out. Nonetheless, the message that was sent out was 'Do the best you can, guys.' Well, if you tell the schools to do the best you can, . . . believe me, the money will disappear. And indeed it did just go down a hole."[37] Assembly Member Phil Isenberg (D-Sacramento), who chaired the Conference Committee that wrote AB 75, also became cynical about how schools were spending their money. He was invited to a celebration of Red Ribbon Week, an anti-drug program, during the 1989–1990 school year and was not happy to discover that the ribbons and balloons for the anti-drug week were purchased with tobacco funds. According to Isenberg, this incident inspired him to keep after the schools about their tobacco program:

> They had this elaborate anti-drug program that was funded by the tobacco funds. And sure, did I mention that? Yes, I did. They were so pained because I probably mentioned it in at least three or four speeches. But nobody tried to take that money from them. On the other hand, it's pretty clear that health people don't control where the money goes once it reaches the schools. I mean it's just out there. It may be wonderfully spent, it may be well intentioned, but if the smoking rate of kids is any indication, it's not having . . . much im-

pact. . . . Once the money reaches the school site, nobody has much of an idea how it's spent or whether it does any good. And as we got into the latter years, and began to fumble around with performance information and outcome tests and so on, it reinforced again, the schools don't comfortably deal with that conceptually whether it's the cigarette tax money or anything else.[38]

Adding to the accountability problem of the blended model was the lack of a plan to evaluate program effectiveness. When asked about evaluation and reporting requirements at the first tobacco orientation conference held by CDE in San Diego in 1990, White simply told one TUPE coordinator, "Do the best you can."[34]

CDE did not attempt to account for how the schools were spending the Proposition 99 Health Education Account until 1993, when it included use of these funds in its biennial Coordinated Compliance Review, whereby CDE evaluated how local districts were implementing state education mandates. The effort to put TUPE into the Coordinated Compliance Review reflects the effort under Yeates to give the program more accountability. By 1998, the inclusion of tobacco in the Coordinated Compliance Review was regarded as a help by virtually all of the county-level TUPE coordinators. According to one, "It took me a long time to come to this. I used to think if you just gave education the money and leave them alone, they will do the right thing. But I have learned that is not always the case."[39]

FORMALIZING NONCOOPERATION BETWEEN DHS AND THE SCHOOLS

Even though it was theoretically desirable to have a close relationship between the DHS-funded community programs and the programs in the schools, there were many political and bureaucratic impediments to effective collaboration. The increasingly specific tobacco control programs of DHS, the LLAs, and their coalitions diverged over time from the schools' diffuse efforts. Tobacco control advocates increasingly viewed the schools as black holes into which money would disappear with little or no effect on tobacco consumption. TCS decided to limit LLA involvement in the classroom because of concern that the schools would coopt LLA funding to serve needs that CDE was supposed to be financing. TCS was also worried that, as with the early focus on cessation, LLAs would spend their time doing one-shot presentations in the schools rather than moving into policy-based activities for community change.

In September 1990 TCS was sufficiently concerned about the way that CDE was spending its money that it drew up the following guidelines:

> 1. DHS funds cannot be used for the development or implementation of in-classroom curriculum in public schools without prior state contract approval.
>
> 2. DHS-funded programs in school settings must be non-curricular programs that supplement ongoing Department of Education (DOE) funded curriculum programs in the classroom or are extra-curricular activities for which DOE funding is not available to support.[40]

In 1993, in a study of eight counties, the three LLAs that were trying to collaborate with the schools voiced strong objections to the guidelines because the guidelines second-guessed and impeded their efforts.[41] By 1998, when fifteen of the sixty-one LLA directors were interviewed, no one mentioned them because most were no longer trying to work in schools very much.

Carolyn Martin, who headed TEOC at the time the classroom guidelines were established, was angry about them:

> We found out later that, as the money became tighter, Dileep Bal had told his friends at DHS, "Under no circumstances are you to do anything whatsoever in the schools. They have their own money and we don't need to help them out." Well, on the community level this is a source of great anger and resentment because it's stupid . . . and the local yokels know it. So we have absolutely given Dileep marching orders that they are to cooperate and spend time and money in the schools. Now whether or not that will happen, I don't know.[37]

The LLA directors had mixed reactions about the Proposition 99 program in the schools, generally more negative than positive. Of the fifteen LLA directors interviewed in 1998 for this book, seven thought that their schools had done very little on the tobacco issue. Five thought some tobacco programming had occurred, although they had hoped for better. Only three of the fifteen were supportive of the effort in their schools.

CONCLUSION

Thanks to the strong leadership that Ken Kizer showed at the Department of Health Services, the Proposition 99 program got up and running quickly. The media campaign was developed rapidly—so rapidly that it was on the air before the tobacco industry and its political allies could stop it. Rather than offering traditional anti-smoking messages, the media campaign set an aggressive tone that confronted the tobacco industry directly. While DHS's local programs started as traditional smoking cessation programs, they rapidly evolved into ones that concentrated on public policy interventions, particularly encouraging passage of local clean indoor air and other tobacco control ordinances. The DHS was on its way to redefining tobacco as a social and political problem (as opposed to a medical one) and undermining the whole social network that supports tobacco use and the tobacco industry.

In contrast, the schools failed to make effective use of the money to develop and implement specific programs for reducing tobacco use. The justification was based on a broader desire to reduce high-risk behavior among students, but the schools never produced convincing evidence that this program worked. This failure to develop effective tobacco control programs stemmed partly from the unique financial and political problems that the schools faced in post–Proposition 13 California and partly from a lack of leadership or even interest in tobacco control within CDE.

These two different approaches to spending the money that Proposition 99 made available were reflected in how these two communities reacted to potential controversy. The DHS programs often sought to create controversy as a way of engaging the public and increasing the visibility of the tobacco issue. The schools sought to avoid controversy. DHS sought to build a local network of people and institutions seeking to confront the tobacco industry and stimulate social change; the schools were trying to survive.

All the pressure was amplified by the size of the amount of money that Proposition 99 had suddenly made available and the knowledge that AB 75 would last only twenty-one months before the Legislature would have to pass a new law to continue authorizing the Proposition 99 programs. Joel Moskowitz, the project director for one of DHS's early evaluation contracts, observed, "The Legislature basically had set this whole thing up for failure anyway with the short enabling legislation. . . . When they passed AB 75, the word had gone out that this program was going to end with the demise of AB 75. The Legislature was going to rip off the money. I think that many people believed that, on the health side as well as the education side, the Legislature wasn't real serious about this program, just because of the short period of the enabling legislation."[42]

Nearly two years before AB 75 passed, the health groups had originated the idea for a sunset provision in Senator Diane Watson's SB 2133 to ensure experimentation, evaluation, and accountability in the new programs that Proposition 99 created. But instead the sunset provision impaired program development.

At the same time that tobacco control advocates were struggling to get the programs up and running and develop some idea of what worked and what did not work, the tobacco industry was already developing a sophisticated understanding of the damage that the media campaign and the local programs were doing and could do. The industry also recognized that the schools would not be a problem.

The fact that AB 75 would end only twenty-one months after it passed created unanticipated political problems for the people implementing the programs. It would take the Legislature several months to pass new authorizing legislation and additional time to launch the new Proposition 99 programs, which meant that proponents would be back in the Legislature debating the future of Proposition 99. This situation would create tremendous political problems for tobacco control advocates interested in defending the fledgling programs.

No one understood this reality better than the tobacco industry and its allies who wanted to see Health Education money diverted to medical services.

CHAPTER 8

The Tobacco Industry's Response

The organizational and program design barriers faced by Proposition 99's Tobacco Control Program would have been hard for any new program to overcome. But, unlike traditional public health programs that involve attacking bacteria or viruses, tobacco control advocates were dealing with an intelligent and rapidly evolving adversary—the tobacco industry. Far from sitting quietly while the new program was put in place, the tobacco industry undertook a major effort to dissect the program, to identify its strengths and weaknesses, and to shift money away from its strengths. The tobacco companies appreciated the importance and effectiveness of two parts of the California program—the media campaign and the local health department programs—well before the health groups had convincing evidence that these programs worked. The industry was not worried about how the schools were spending their Proposition 99 money.

THE INDUSTRY AND THE MEDIA CAMPAIGN

In the first authorizing legislation (AB 75), the tobacco industry tried to prevent any of the education money from being spent on an anti-tobacco media campaign. They hired dozens of lobbyists to kill off the media campaign, but failed because their effort was so obvious and heavy-handed. They would not make this mistake again; future efforts against the media campaign would be conducted through intermediaries.

After the media campaign hit the airwaves on April 10, 1990, the tobacco companies complained loudly in the press that the advertisements
were tasteless and a waste of money and that they were "political" rather
than "educational." According to the *Los Angeles Times*,

> "They pitched Prop. 99 as: 'We want to reach under-aged children. We want
> to educate children to the purported health effects of smoking,'" said Thomas
> Lauria, a spokesman for the Tobacco Institute, a Washington-based industry
> group. . . .
>
> He said he had not seen the state's anti-smoking ads and that industry lead-
> ers would view the ads before deciding whether to respond further.
>
> But, he said: "These ads sound like they are trying to lay the ground-
> work for a next phase of a political agenda, which is to ban advertising from
> cigarette companies. These people are on a long march toward prohibition of
> tobacco." [1]

The Tobacco Institute briefly considered a lawsuit to stop the media
campaign and consulted with both Covington and Burling (its law firm
in Washington, DC) and California legal counsel. But the institute decided that a lawsuit against the media campaign would be a tactical error and that "there is no basis for a suit which would have a realistic
chance of success." [2] Within RJ Reynolds, H. E. Osmon put it more
bluntly: "I believe that we should take no overt legal action. It increases
the rhetoric, sustains the story, and, if we lose, it would be a major embarrassment." [3] The institute had also considered a counteradvertising
campaign but rejected it: "If the industry attempts to meet the Department of Health Services head on in the media, the controversy is likely
to shift from the advertisements to the industry." [3]

On April 11, 1990, the day after the media campaign started in California, Samuel D. Chilcote, Jr., president of the Tobacco Institute in
Washington, DC, sent a memo to his executive committee, with copies
of the "Industry Spokesmen" ad and the other broadcast and print advertisements attached, describing the Tobacco Institute's three-pronged
approach for dealing with the California campaign: "(1) Encourage California legislative leaders to intervene, (2) *Through third party allies,* attempt to convince Health Services head [Ken] Kizer to either pull or modify the current advertisements, (3) Encourage the Governor to intervene
against the current advertisements" (emphasis added). [4] Using sympathetic legislators to attack the funding and content of the media campaign while pressuring the administration to channel the campaign into
messages acceptable to the industry would remain the industry's strategy
against the media campaign throughout the history of Proposition 99.

Chilcote went on to describe the tobacco industry's legislative efforts to eliminate the media campaign by putting the Proposition 99 funds to other "acceptable" uses. While acknowledging the loss on AB 75, he was clearly anticipating the next battle over authorization as another opportunity to shut down the media campaign, working with the industry's allies who wanted to see the money going to medical services:

> Despite Herculean efforts [on AB 75], our goal of completely eliminating the media dedication was not met. But through our work, the media component was sliced to $14.3 million for fiscal year 1989–90. Another $14.3 million is allocated for fiscal year 1990–91, for a total to date of $28.6 million.
>
> *The industry has been approached by representatives of county governments, as well as physician groups, expressing an interest in working with us so that they may receive monies that are currently earmarked to the media "education" campaign. These avenues continue to be explored with the California State Association of Counties and the California Medical Association.*[4] [emphasis added]

Chilcote described the tobacco industry's efforts to line up opposition to the advertisements in the minority community: "The black and Hispanic communities also are upset because very few Prop 99 dollars have found their way to the poor in the form of new health services. A substantial amount of the Prop 99 revenues are being use [*sic*] to 'replace' previous state funding from other sources."[4]

The industry was also planning to conduct its own focus group research "in order to support our position that the advertisements are more propaganda than information."[4] There was, in fact, a chance that people would not consider the advertising as "education." The innovative nature of the California media campaign was based on the recognition that merely providing information about health-compromising behaviors did little to reduce smoking. Heavily promoted by the industry as attractive, glamorous, and necessary for social acceptance, smoking had to be shown instead as a deadly, addictive habit foisted on people by a cynical industry with seemingly endless amounts of money to spend on lying about its product. The campaign was thus designed to "unmarket" smoking rather than inform people about the health effects of smoking, which traditional health educators thought an "education" campaign was supposed to do. If the industry could demonstrate that the public did not see the advertisements as "educational," then it might have additional ammunition to take to the Legislature.

On April 18, 1990, Chilcote sent another, more detailed memo to members of his Executive Committee providing a "further update on our efforts to deal with the anti-smoking advertising campaign in California."[4] By this time, Kurt L. Malmgren, the Tobacco Institute's senior vice president for state activities, had added a fourth part to its earlier strategy for dealing with the media campaign: "Cooperate with minority, business and other groups in developing their opposition to the advertising program."[2] On the Tobacco Institute's list of options, this tactic became second only to working with the legislative leadership.

In the week between these two memos, the Tobacco Institute realized that Kizer of DHS would fight to protect the campaign and that Governor George Deukmejian, while not agreeing with the specifics of the campaign, would back him up:

> After analysis from our California team, it is clear that our efforts should center on the first two strategies [the Legislature and other groups], with the hope that these efforts can have some effect on the other two strategies.
>
> The reasons for this approach are (1) Dr. Kizer is not likely to pull or modify the advertisements without strong pressure from the Administration; (2) as a "lame duck," the Governor is not likely to get into a public sparring match with Dr. Kizer, even though he disagrees with the Department of Health Services' attack approach with the anti-tobacco advertisement.[2]

Seeing little chance of success with the Deukmejian administration, the industry decided to concentrate its efforts on getting the Legislature to eliminate funding for the media campaign.

By April 18, the industry had made more than one hundred contacts about diverting money away from the media campaign and was already working to create a "focused coalition willing to take the lead in an effort to end funding for media from Prop 99 taxes and redirect it elsewhere."[2] In addition to the county supervisors and the California Medical Association (CMA), this coalition was to include the black and Hispanic communities, the Western Center for Law and Poverty, the Asian community, hospital groups, and business groups. According to Malmgren,

> Intelligence to date shows a range of reasons why these groups are ill at ease and concerned with the advertising campaign. Black concerns, for example, vary from resentment at the denigrating nature of the advertisements, to concern that Prop 99 dollars are not being channeled to pressing health care needs for minority groups, to the fact that Prop 99 media dollars are not being funneled to black-owned media. . . .
>
> *The doctor and hospital segment appears to believe the media funds would be better spent to pay medical costs.*[2] [emphasis added]

On May 3, New York–based KRC Research delivered a public opinion survey regarding the media campaign to Covington and Burling, followed on May 18 by a qualitative study of the advertisements.[5,6] The survey was based on a questionnaire administered between April 26 and 29, just two weeks after the advertisements started. By then, 66 percent of California respondents were already aware of the campaign, and 46 percent were aware of discussions about the campaign. The Tobacco Control Section's plan to create some noise was clearly working. Forty-five percent of respondents thought the campaign would help smokers stop and 70 percent thought it would be effective in stopping nonsmokers from starting. However, an even larger share of respondents (83 percent) thought school-based smoking education programs would be more effective than the ads. In addition, 74 percent said they would rather see the money spent on health care for the poor than on the media campaign. There was an even split, 43 percent to 43 percent, between those who thought the advertisements were an appropriate use of state money and those who did not. KRC concluded,

> To engage in a public debate over this advertising campaign (i.e., whether it is an appropriate use of state funds, and whether it will actually be an effective deterrent to smoking) will most likely serve only to escalate the controversy.
> We believe it will be more effective for the Tobacco Institute not to engage in this battle, but rather to attempt to focus attention on the ways that people would prefer to see state money spent in the pursuit of improved public health.
> To this end, we believe that the questions we develop for use in Field's California Poll should be designed to identify the types of health care and educational programs that people believe will be more effective and that they would prefer to see funded.[5]

The Field California Poll is a widely regarded survey whose results are always made public, regardless of who commissions the survey. The fact that the industry did not pursue a Field California Poll suggests that it was uncertain of getting the answers it wanted.

The qualitative analysis of the advertisements was based on a series of eight focus groups. The report concluded,

> The atmosphere in California appears to be rapidly evolving into an anti-smoking environment. This "reality" is *accepted* by smokers and *advocated* by non-smokers. Smokers believed that smoking is potentially harmful, yet they cannot quit and cannot be forced to do so. However, they want their children to be smoke free.
> Neither smokers nor non-smokers voiced strong opposition to Proposition 99. They all empathized with people who could not afford healthcare, and supported making it more accessible to the poor. There was general support for the $221 million education campaign, and a mixed reaction (though

only one or two respondents were strongly opposed) to $28 million being spent on an anti-smoking media campaign.

As for the five commercials, they were perceived to have slight to no impact on the marketplace. These ads will not change smokers' behavior. The ads do, however, add to the general anti-smoking environment.

It is important to understand that the commercials' lack of appeal was not based on the idea that government infringed on the rights of smokers. Rather, opposition was based on the perception that these ads were not strong enough.

Respondents generally agreed that an effective non-smoking ad campaign should be more "medically" informative and visually explicit.[6] [emphasis in original]

The report was not encouraging to the tobacco industry, since it suggested that the public wanted an even stronger anti-tobacco campaign.[4]

On May 14 Walter N. Woodson, the Tobacco Institute's vice president of state activities, wrote to Chilcote advising him that the industry was moving ahead with efforts to shift the media money to specific service providers:

We are working with several groups who share our interest in having the funds targeted to *real* health care concerns. Among them:

California Health Foundation

Black Health Network

California Rural Counties Association

California Hospital Association

California Medical Association

A just-formed, and as yet unnamed, confederation of most state minority health organizations[7]

By November, the Tobacco Institute seemed to be making some progress in this strategy. A report noted that "prompted by minority health groups such as the Watts Health Foundation and the Black Health Network," two Democratic legislators "attempted to reopen the funding of the media program and dedicate the funds to other programs benefitting their communities."[8] The effort was stopped in a conference committee by Republicans who would not support the effort without a promise of support to amend Proposition 98, which required that 40 percent of the state budget go to education. The Democrats refused to reopen Proposition 98, so this effort to divert the media campaign money died.[8]

The industry strategy then focused on the 1991–1992 legislative session, when a new piece of implementing legislation would be needed for the Proposition 99 programs.[8] The tobacco industry and its allies would be working with Governor Pete Wilson and his new administration, which would prove more sympathetic to the industry's positions.

"IT'S THE LAW"

While most local ordinance activity in California was concentrated on clean indoor air at this time, there was also growing interest in passing local ordinances that would make it harder to sell cigarettes and other tobacco products to children. In response to this development, which was matched by a similar climate in other states for reducing youth access to tobacco products, the Tobacco Institute developed "It's the Law." This program provided stickers that merchants could post to warn consumers that it was illegal to sell cigarettes to children. It was designed to head off laws that could impose meaningful enforcement provisions or penalties on retailers or tobacco companies.

By 1991, the tobacco industry was actively planning ways to use its "youth initiative" to undermine Proposition 99. Philip Morris intended to introduce legislation in several states to address sales penalties and vending machine restrictions in terms that were acceptable to the company.[9] Despite its ostensible goal, however, the program had nothing to do with decreasing the youth smoking rate: "The ultimate means for determining the success of this program will be: (1) A reduction in legislation introduced and passed restricting or banning our sales and marketing activities; (2) Passage of legislation favorable to the industry; (3) Greater support from business, parent and teacher groups."[9] Although the tobacco industry claimed to have designed the program "to promote our objectives in preventing youth smoking while protecting our sales and marketing practices,"[10] its main purpose was clearly the latter.

The youth strategy was an important aspect of undermining Proposition 99. In a December 21 memo, T. C. Harris of RJ Reynolds wrote, "I believe that a concentrated implementation of the Youth Non-Smoking Program is a critical component, as it gives us a *credible* way to show that the Proposition is unnecessary, whether we do it via advertisements or in negotiations" (emphasis in original).[11] By 1991, the Tobacco Institute was also interested in how it could use the youth issue to gain the ear of elected officials. In May, Walter Woodson of the Tobacco Institute, was preparing a mailing to 6,000 California elected officials containing a press release on the Tobacco Institute's youth smoking initiative and a press kit on "It's the Law." According to Woodson,

The industry is being hit hard at the local level in California this year. We currently are facing more than forty local ordinances, many of which address more than one issue. As might be expected, a number of these bills have been introduced under the premise that youth have easy access to tobacco products. . . . Sending the youth materials to all elected officials in the state may help to alleviate the surge of introductions for the time being, and provide us with a vehicle to go in and meet with some of the representatives there. Additionally, such a mailing could assist with efforts to achieve broad distribution of the youth program throughout the state.[12]

In other words, the purpose of the program was to head off legislation restricting tobacco marketing.

THE INDUSTRY AND THE SCHOOLS

In contrast to its reaction to the anti-tobacco media campaign, the tobacco industry seemed satisfied with the school-based programs that the California Department of Education (CDE) was running. Indeed, some schools were actually using "educational" materials produced by the tobacco industry, even though these materials were widely viewed by tobacco control advocates as subtly encouraging smoking. CDE, unlike DHS, did not understand that the tobacco industry had to be treated as an adversary.

RJ Reynolds hired the consulting firm of Stratton, Reiter, Dupree & Durante from Denver to provide a thorough analysis of the structure of TCS, CDE, and the Proposition 99 anti-tobacco program.[13] By April 1991, the firm had concluded that the program in the schools did not threaten the industry and perhaps represented an opportunity. In a memorandum summarizing his conversations with the firm's Rick Reiter, Tim Hyde of RJ Reynolds wrote,

$72,000,000 [of the Health Education Account money] goes to the Department of Education for K–12 classroom uses. The specific allocation of this money is fairly straightforward. It is primarily being used for training and materials to be included as a tobacco supplement to drug and AIDS curriculum. There are also a few odds and ends, such as numerous "tobacco-free" contests and the like. Rick's preliminary suggestion is for us to take advantage of the review-committee opportunity to get industry personnel involved in the overall DOE decision-making process because *the goals of this program are consistent with our own views on youth smoking.*[14] [emphasis added]

The industry's consultants recognized the schools' lack of commitment to doing something about tobacco with the new Proposition 99 money. The report comments,

> Coincidently [*sic*], it wasn't until after passage of Prop 99 that CDE suddenly discovered tobacco prevention as being tantamount to promotion of healthy lifestyles for children. In reviewing HKHC [Health Kids, Healthy California] workshop materials developed *prior to 1990, seemingly every health-related issue at the school level was emphasized except tobacco*. . . . *With the recent discovery of tobacco as a health threat came the discovery of a funding mechanism to supplement the newly introduced HKHC comprehensive health program*. This co-mingling effort of shared resources suggests that CDE tobacco excise revenues are being used to supplement activities related to drug and alcohol prevention and cessation. These two areas are the priority health and safety concerns in the public schools.[13] [emphasis added]

The report was uncertain about the degree to which tobacco had, in fact, become part of the schools' program and suggested that the cutbacks could "be of some relief to the industry; funds are being shifted to areas outside of the Health Education Account, and CDE will continue spreading [the reduced allocation] among drug and alcohol programs rather than tobacco exclusively."[13] The chief threat posed by the schools, according to the report, was that schools had helped frame the smoking issue as a health issue, which the tobacco industry had consistently tried to avoid in California. When smoking was framed as a health issue, not one of individual choice or taxation, the industry generally lost its political battles.

The tobacco industry had its own strategy for schools. It produced curricula designed to "educate" kids about tobacco without clearly discussing the health dangers of smoking or the fact that it killed adult smokers. RJ Reynolds produced "Right Decisions, Right Now"; the Tobacco Institute produced "Tobacco: Helping Youth Say No," originally entitled "Helping Youth Decide." Both packages were slickly produced and were free to schools. Rather than presenting tobacco as a dangerous product that should be avoided by everyone, these materials emphasized "the choice to smoke" and that "smoking was for adults." The industry justified their materials with the objective of ensuring that "minors receive support and education in regard to smoking being an adult practice."[9] These messages are consistent with traditional tobacco industry advertising themes—that smoking makes kids look grown up—and even convey the notion that smoking is a desirable "forbidden fruit" for youth.[15–17] The curriculum materials also seemed to serve an important political purpose for the industry: they supported the argument that there was no need for government to spend tax dollars to reduce smoking; the industry would take care of everything.

In the early years of Proposition 99's Tobacco Control Program, educators who should have known better contacted the tobacco companies and ordered some of the industry's materials for use in the schools. In April 1992, two and a half years after CDE began receiving Proposition 99 monies, Bill White (head of CDE's Tobacco Use Prevention Education program) telephoned RJ Reynolds to ask about the "Right Decisions, Right Now" program. H. E. Osman, to whom White had spoken, ran his response by his superiors, "given the sensitivity of sending anything to the Prop 99 people." Osman's paranoia about White, however, was ill founded. A year later, some of the "Right Decisions, Right Now" posters were decorating the walls in the Healthy Kids, Healthy California office.

White was not the only person from the schools requesting these materials. Schools all over the state requested copies of the tobacco industry's "educational" materials, including one director of a Healthy Kids regional center.[18]

CONCLUSION

The DHS anti-smoking advertising campaign clearly identified the tobacco industry as a threat to the public health, and the industry reacted quickly and vigorously to develop a political strategy to fight the media program. The industry learned from its defeat in the AB 75 battle that it would have to stay in the shadows and work through surrogates to fight the media campaign in the Legislature.

The schools did not threaten the industry. While some efforts to place tobacco industry materials were rebuffed in schools, the CDE leadership showed little commitment to anti-tobacco efforts. Many were even willing to cooperate with the industry in distributing its curricula, despite the fact that this material was widely criticized in the public health community. For the industry, the Proposition 99 programs in the schools posed no threat and even presented an opportunity to advance its own legislative strategy. Industry documents contained no strategy to kill off the schools program.

The media campaign and the local government programs were not so fortunate. The fight against anti-tobacco efforts at the local level, in fact, became a central piece of the industry strategy, one in which the industry would invest substantial time and money.

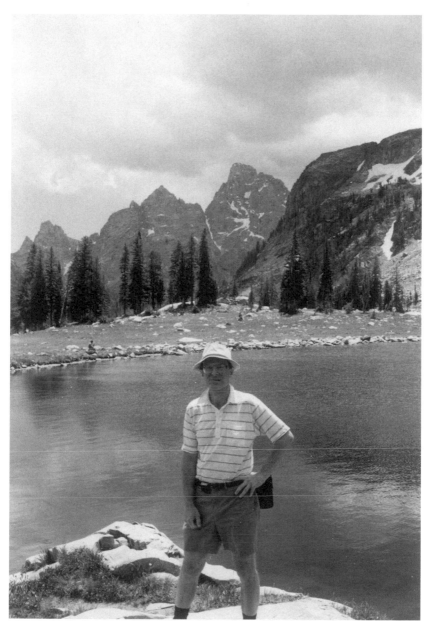

Peter Hanauer, one of the early leaders of the nonsmokers' rights movement in California, viewed secondhand smoke as an environmental problem, as opposed to a medical one. (Photo courtesy of P. Hanauer)

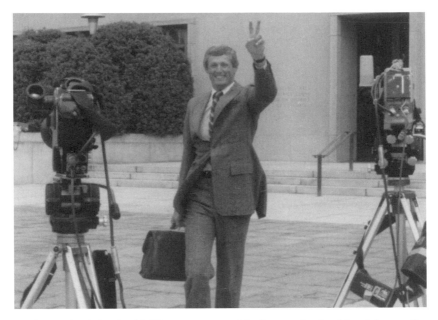

Paul Loveday joined with Hanauer to provide the core leadership of the 1978 and 1980 efforts to enact clean indoor air laws in California through the initiative process. While the tobacco industry defeated these initiatives, non-smokers' rights advocates developed the political skills and strategies to defeat the tobacco industry at the local level. The photo shows Loveday leaving the US Court of Appeals in Washington after arguing that the Federal Communications Commission should require disclosure of tobacco industry sponsorship of advertisements in political campaigns. (Photo courtesy of P. Loveday)

Tony Najera, the American Lung Association's lobbyist, joined Mekemson and others in developing and passing Proposition 99. Najera, a continuous presence in the Capitol, led insider efforts within the Legislature to implement tobacco control programs. (Photo courtesy of Tony Najera)

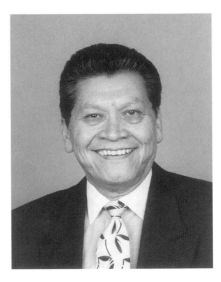

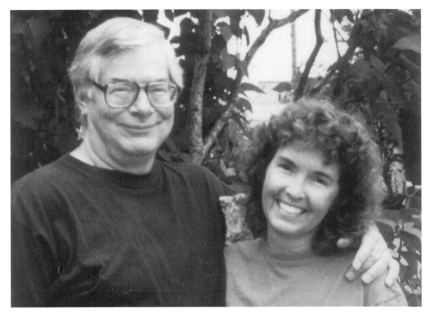

Curt Mekemson (shown here with his wife Peggy), working with environmentalist Gerald Meral, originated the idea of raising the tobacco tax and allocating a portion of the revenues to tobacco control. This idea was realized in Proposition 99. (Photo courtesy of C. Mekemson)

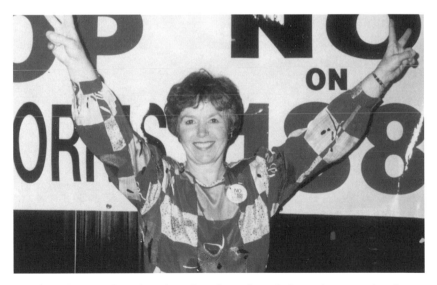

Carolyn Martin, a longtime American Lung Association volunteer, played a leading role in passing Proposition 99 and organizing the early opposition to the Philip Morris initiative, Proposition 188. She also served as the first chair of the Tobacco Education Oversight Committee. (Photo courtesy of C. Martin)

Julia Carol rose from secretary of Americans for Nonsmokers' Rights to become its executive director and the champion of local grassroots efforts to protect nonsmokers. She also played a leading role in the 1996 public campaign to rescue Proposition 99 by moving from insider to outsider strategies. (Photo courtesy of J. Carol)

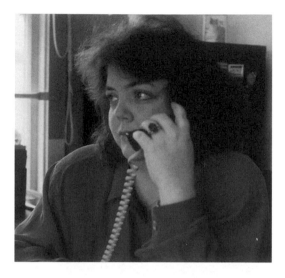

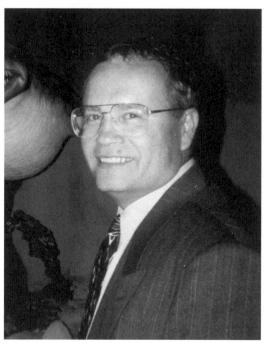

John Miller, chief of staff to Senator Diane Watson and the Senate Committee on Health and Human Services, was the primary inside player within the legislative staff who worked to support tobacco control efforts. (Photo courtesy of J. Miller)

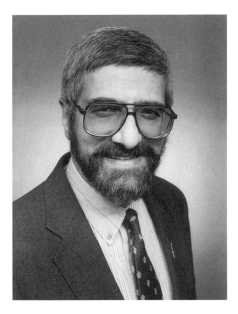

Dileep Bal, the head of the Department of Health Services Cancer Control Branch, which includes the Tobacco Control Section, provided the vision and bureaucratic savvy that helped California develop the most aggressive tobacco control program in the nation. (Photo courtesy of D. Bal)

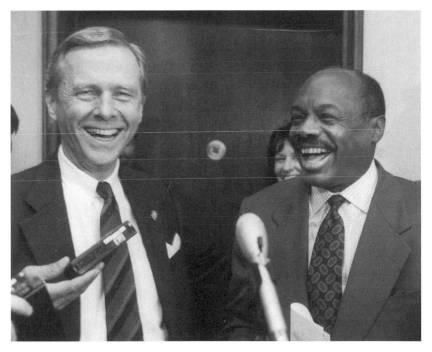

Republican Governor Pete Wilson (left) and Democrat Assembly Speaker Willie Brown (right) clashed on many issues but worked together to gut California's tobacco control program. (Photo by Rich Pedroncelli)

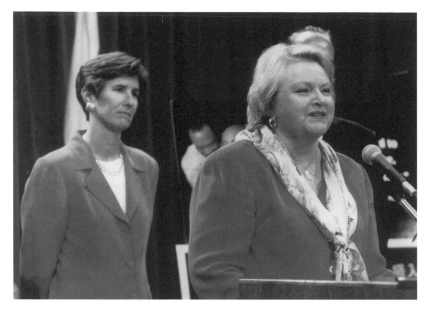

Sandra Smoley (right), secretary of health and welfare in the Wilson administration, voted against the Sacramento clean indoor air ordinance when she was
a member of the Sacramento Board of Supervisors. She took the lead in forcing
the California Tobacco Control Program to tone down attacks on the tobacco
industry. Kimberly Belshé (left), director of the Department of Health Services,
campaigned against Proposition 99 for the tobacco industry in 1988, then
occasionally advocated for the Tobacco Control Program behind the scenes,
but ultimately implemented administration policies to tone down the campaign. (Photo courtesy of California Department of Health Services)

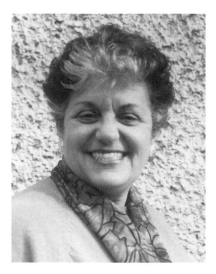

Jennie Cook, an active volunteer with
the American Cancer Society who
rose to become the national chair of
the board, worked on tobacco control
activities in California and became the
second chair of the Tobacco Education
and Research Oversight Committee.
Cook generally avoided confrontation
with the administration, but eventually
took the lead in using TEROC as a
platform to pressure the Wilson
administration to strengthen the
anti-tobacco media campaign.
(Photo courtesy of J. Cook)

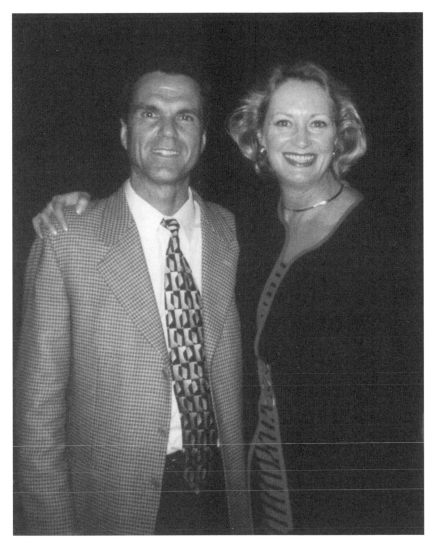

American Heart Association lobbyist Mary Adams (right) convinced Executive Vice President Roman Bowser (left) to join in an aggressive public campaign to force the California Medical Association away from the tobacco industry and hold Governor Pete Wilson accountable in the successful drive to restore funding for Proposition 99. (Photo courtesy of M. Adams)

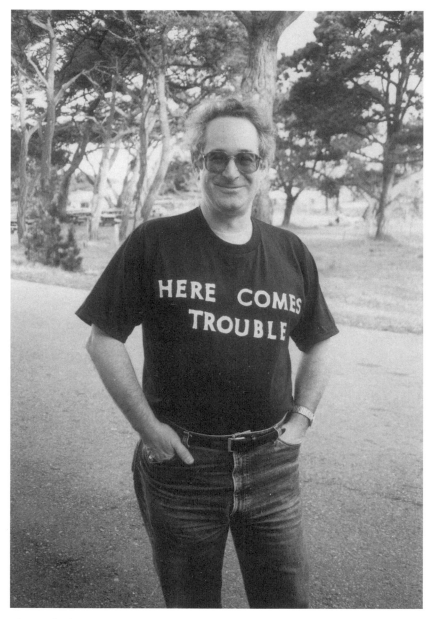

The staff of the Department of Health Services Tobacco Control Section gave UCSF Professor Stanton Glantz a t-shirt labeled "Here Comes Trouble" in honor of his role—both in public and behind the scenes—in pressuring the administration to strengthen the tobacco control program.

CHAPTER 9

The Battle over Local Tobacco Control Ordinances

Unlike the media campaign and school programs, which started from scratch after the voters passed Proposition 99, the effort to pass local tobacco control ordinances was already well under way by the time that the Department of Health Services (DHS) set up its tobacco control program. By the time DHS started to implement Proposition 99 in 1990, 213 California communities, working with Americans for Nonsmokers' Rights (ANR), had passed local clean indoor air ordinances. After Proposition 99 passed, this effort received a substantial boost. DHS, the local lead agencies (LLAs), and the local coalitions rapidly adopted the local ordinance strategy that had grown out of Propositions 5, 10, and P a decade earlier and that ANR had been pursuing since. The media campaign raised public awareness of secondhand smoke issues, and DHS provided resources and technical assistance with which the LLAs and other groups could engage the public in developing and implementing local tobacco control policies.

The tobacco industry also recognized the power of local action. It worked in the shadows to undermine local efforts, because it lacked credibility with the public. In a 1989 opinion poll conducted by the Gallup Organization, the Tobacco Institute received the most unfavorable rating among nine nationally recognized interest groups.[1] This poll confirmed the results of a secret poll done for the Tobacco Institute by Tarrance and Associates in 1982, which found that overt industry opposition *increased*

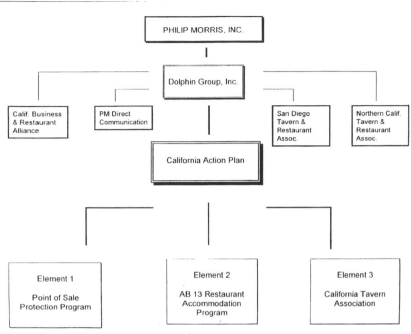

Figure 10. Philip Morris's secret California Action Plan network. Philip Morris hired the Dolphin Group to create this coalition of "business and restaurant associations" to obscure the industry's role in orchestrating opposition to local clean indoor air laws. *Source:* Philip Morris (?), *1994 California Plan,* 1994 (Bates No. 2022816070/6080).

popular support for proposed clean indoor air legislation.[2] As a result, lobbyists for the Tobacco Institute tried to stay out of public view. For example, the institute's West Coast lobbyist, Ron Saldana, attended hearings on local smoking control ordinances but rarely testified; when asked why, he said, "I've learned from experience that as soon as I'm identified as a representative of the Tobacco Institute, I lose all credibility. They just sneer us away. . . . So I try to work behind the scenes whenever I can."[3] Over time, the tobacco industry would use public relations firms to create a network of front groups—"restaurant and business associations"—to fight clean indoor air ordinances (figure 10).

While hundreds of California communities would enact local tobacco control ordinances, a few of these battles with the tobacco industry will capture the flavor of all the fights. The first such battle occurred in Beverly Hills in 1987, the year before Proposition 99 passed.

BEVERLY HILLS

In 1987 the Beverly Hills City Council proposed a 100 percent smoke-free requirement for the city's restaurants. This ordinance would have been only the second such ordinance in the country and the first in California. For the proposal to become law, the council had to approve it on two separate readings. The ordinance passed its first reading without public opposition.

Between the first and second readings, the Tobacco Institute hired political consultant Rudy Cole to create the Beverly Hills Restaurant Association (BHRA) to oppose the ordinance.[4] To drum up membership for BHRA, Ron Saldana, the Tobacco Institute's regional director, spoke to the local restaurant owners and the Chamber of Commerce to "make them aware of the potential impact the ordinance will have on the community."[5] The Tobacco Institute's role in creating the BHRA was not disclosed. At the second reading, Cole appeared as spokesperson of the newly formed Beverly Hills Restaurant Association to protest the ordinance. Nonetheless, the city council unanimously passed it in March 1987, making Beverly Hills approximately the 130th community in California to pass a clean indoor air ordinance and the state's first to make restaurants entirely smoke free.

Mickey Kantor, a prominent attorney in the well-connected law firm of Manatt, Phelps, Rothenberg and Phillips, was hired to represent the BHRA. (Kantor, a power in California Democratic politics, went on to become President Bill Clinton's foreign trade representative, secretary of commerce, and a key personal advisor in the Monica Lewinsky controversy.) The BHRA attempted to get a temporary court order to stop the implementation of the ordinance, but the effort failed.[6] Kantor then filed a lawsuit against the city claiming that the ordinance was unconstitutional, discriminatory, and disastrous for business. This action also failed.[7] The Tobacco Institute paid BHRA's legal bills.[8]

Having failed to void the law in court, the BHRA complained that restaurants had suffered a 30 percent drop in business after the ordinance took effect.[9-11] While being touted widely in tobacco industry publications, this claim was not challenged or investigated by the health community at the time. As a result, the claim of a serious impact on business was widely accepted. In July, four months after the ordinance went into effect, the city council voted 5-0 to allow restaurants to establish smoking sections of up to 40 percent of their seating.

Six years later, Barry Fogel, BHRA's nominal president, wrote to the New York City Council to endorse its planned ordinance making restaurants smoke free. He recounted the history of BHRA:

> There was no Beverly Hills Restaurant Association before the smokefree ordinance. We were organized by the tobacco industry. The industry helped pay our legal bills in a suit against Beverly Hills. The industry even flew some of our members by Lear Jet to Rancho Mirage, another California city considering smokefree restaurant legislation, to testify before their City Council against a similar smokefree ordinance. Tobacco Institute representatives attended some of our meetings.
>
> The tobacco industry repeatedly claimed that Beverly Hills restaurants suffered a 30% decline in revenues during the 5 months that the smokefree ordinance was in effect. Figures from the State Board of Equalization using sales tax data, however, showed a slight increase in restaurant sales.
>
> I regret my participation with the tobacco industry. In 1991 when I learned that secondhand smoke caused cancer, I made all Jacopo's restaurants 100% smokefree, including bar and outdoor patio areas. Even in this difficult economic climate, our sales have risen.[12]

The tobacco industry could claim a victory in Beverly Hills because this was the first time a nonsmokers' rights ordinance had been weakened after it was enacted. Even so, while Beverly Hills represented a setback for clean indoor air advocates, the 60 percent minimum nonsmoking requirement still left Beverly Hills with the strongest ordinance in the state at that time.

LODI

The movement toward a smoke-free society took a big step forward in the small farming community of Lodi (population 50,000) in California's Central Valley. Armed with the recent US Environmental Protection Agency report that identified secondhand smoke as a Class A carcinogen,[13] the San Joaquin County Smoking Action Coalition, a group of residents formed to promote smoking ordinances, approached the Lodi City Council in December 1989 to request consideration of a smoking control ordinance. Sandy Stoddard, a coalition member and American Cancer Society (ACS) staff member, had grown up in Lodi and knew three of the five council members personally.[14]

During the spring of 1990, the Lodi City Council formally considered a smoking ordinance. After promoting the ordinance, the community health activists took a back seat as elected officials, particularly Mayor Randy Snider, molded the proposal. On May 16, the city council voted 4-1 in favor of an ordinance prohibiting smoking in almost all indoor public places. (Bars, motel and hotel rooms, retail tobacco stores, private offices, and residences were excluded.) Before the proposal became law, the council was to vote on it again, within one month after the initial vote.

During the intervening three weeks, RJ Reynolds learned of the proposal and sent an Action Alert letter to residents of Lodi, urging them to call their council members and attend the council meeting to voice opposition to the proposal. The names and telephone numbers of council members were included in the letter, as well as a toll-free RJ Reynolds telephone number for anyone with questions.

Meanwhile, in June 1990, a group called Taxpayers United for Freedom (TUFF) was formed in Lodi to oppose the ordinance. TUFF claimed to be a grassroots organization that did not receive support from the tobacco industry. Adam Dados, a spokesperson for the group, said, "We've only received some ashtrays and lighters from the tobacco companies." [15]

In contrast to the first city council meeting, where little opposition was evident, the June 6, 1990, meeting was a raucous affair with 400 people attending, some hissing and booing during testimony by the ordinance's supporters. Local physicians, ANR, and the local chapters of the ACS and AHA spoke in favor of the ordinance. ANR's executive director, Julia Carol, said after the meeting that she had been to many similar hearings but "none so hostile." [16] Those who spoke in opposition to the proposal were all local residents. Dados presented petitions with over 3,000 signatures to the council.

Despite efforts by RJ Reynolds and TUFF to organize opposition to the ordinance, the Lodi City Council passed it on second reading by a 4-1 vote. Lodi became the first 100 percent smoke-free city in the United States.

After the vote, Bill Stamos, a Lodi resident, armchair legal scholar, nonsmoker, and opponent of the ordinance, drafted a referendum for TUFF to force a popular vote on the ordinance.[17] Supporters of the referendum had thirty days to gather 2,369 signatures for it; they turned in petitions with 5,051 signatures. The council had two choices: repeal the ordinance or put it on the ballot. They voted to let the people of Lodi decide.

Soon after TUFF submitted the petitions, ordinance supporters formed the Lodi Indoor Clean Air Coalition (LICAC). This group, led by a physician and a retired waitress, was formed without the assistance of any established health organization. On July 10 LICAC held a public meeting; about 175 local residents attended, $2,000 was raised, and volunteers were identified for the campaign. Assuming that TUFF would mount a well-organized campaign, LICAC decided to hire a professional campaign coordinator.

During the initial weeks LICAC mobilized support and asked for contributions from concerned citizens through advertisements in the local newspaper. Most of the larger contributions came from medical professionals. Of the $6,250 in contributions amounting to $100 or more, $3,200 came from individual doctors and medical companies, groups usually hesitant to become involved in local political campaigns.[18] LICAC raised a total of $12,025, almost half of which was in contributions of less than $100.[19]

Independently of LICAC, the local ACS sent out approximately 1,250 letters to patients and volunteers in Lodi urging them to support the referendum on the smoking ordinance.[14] No effort was made by the other local voluntary health agencies (ALA or AHA) to mobilize support for the referendum. The California Medical Association was asked to support LICAC but did not contribute to the campaign.[20]

LILAC's campaign strategy was to discredit the opposition, not by attacking TUFF directly but by indirectly labeling the group as a tobacco industry front.[21] LICAC used newspaper advertisements borrowed from health activists in Fort Collins, Colorado, who had faced a similar campaign in 1984. These advertisements included one portraying a tobacco spokesman waving his cigar, saying, "So long Lodi, it's been good to know you," as he hopped into his limousine to leave town after the election, his briefcase full of tobacco industry money.

TUFF's advertisements focused on smoking as an issue of rights and freedoms, embedded in the U.S. Constitution. One ad, framed with the American flag, proclaimed, "The smoking ban . . . is ANTI-AMERICAN and in violation of the very precepts of our inalienable rights as Americans."[15] TUFF also used the specter of severe punishments for ordinance offenders. One cartoon showed two prisoners in a jail cell, one saying, "I'm in here for murder, extortion and grand theft! What did you do?" The other replied, "I lit up a cigarette in Lodi!"[15]

TUFF collected more than $11,439 in monetary contributions from local individuals, businesses, and fund-raising events.[22] The vast majority of donations were less than $100; the source of these donations was not subject to disclosure, but presumably they came from concerned local residents. Responding to the charge that TUFF was a front for the cigarette companies, Dados said that Philip Morris had contacted him in the early weeks of the campaign to offer support but that nothing ever came of the offer. According to Dados, tobacco industry support would gladly be accepted.[23] In fact, the tobacco industry supported TUFF. TBP Political Consulting in San Francisco, the firm of RJ Reynolds consultant Tim Pueyo, loaned TUFF $1,200.[22] When asked about the San Francisco connection, Dados said Pueyo was just a friend. Rudy Cole of the tobacco industry's BHRA appeared in Lodi in October, where he was the keynote speaker at a major TUFF fund-raiser. On August 29, 1990, RJ Reynolds hired a firm in Winston-Salem, North Carolina, to send letters to Lodi residents encouraging them to vote against the ordinance.[24]

In November, despite the efforts of TUFF and the tobacco industry, the voters in Lodi approved the ordinance by an overwhelming 60 percent (1,986 to 1,470).

Even after they lost the election, TUFF did not give up.[25] They threatened a recall of the council members who voted for the ordinance and targeted Mayor Randy Snider when he ran for reelection; Snider won. They filed a legal challenge against the ordinance, which failed. They attempted to organize noncompliance. In the end, however, the ordinance went into effect and was enforced, making Lodi the first city in California to enact and maintain a law requiring 100 percent smoke-free restaurants.

Other cities began to follow suit. In August 1990 the coastal college town of San Luis Obispo implemented the nation's first law creating smoke-free bars.

SACRAMENTO

While the battle in Lodi was taking place, both Sacramento and Sacramento County enacted strong ordinances ending smoking in all public and private workplaces and in all public places, including restaurants.

The most significant factor in Sacramento's success was the strong connection between the American Lung Association of Sacramento–Emigrant Trails and community leaders. The Sacramento ALA had recruited influential civic leaders from various backgrounds to serve on its thirty-five-member board of directors. It was no coincidence that a county supervisor, a city council member, and the chair of the Environmental Commission—individuals who were instrumental in passing the ordinance—had served as volunteers or staff members of Sacramento ALA. Commission chairman Rob McCray, an attorney and former ALA volunteer, appointed a task force that included the local chapters of the three voluntary health agencies (ALA, AHA, and ACS), the Sacramento Restaurant Association (a bona fide organization of restaurants), the Chamber of Commerce (one representative from a small business and one from a large business), Arco Arena (the indoor sports arena), Pacific Gas & Electric (a major employer), and the airport.

The health advocates on the task force successfully pushed to recommend a total smoke-free policy in the workplace. They also wanted to increase the percentage of nonsmoking seats in restaurants from a minimum of 10 percent (under the previous ordinance) to 50 percent. The task force recommendations went to the Environmental Commission, which held public hearings on the recommendations. Significantly, the Chamber of Commerce, an organization representing 2,600 local businesses, endorsed the recommendations.

At the hearing before the County Board of Supervisors, the tobacco industry flew in its "expert witnesses" who frequently testify before legislative bodies. Among those out-of-towners testifying against the ordinance were Gray Robertson of Fairfax, Virginia, a tobacco industry "consultant" who had been set up in a series of businesses by Philip Morris to play down secondhand tobacco smoke as a significant cause of indoor air pollution;[26,27] David Weeks, a physician from Boise, Idaho; Malinda Sidak, an attorney from Covington and Burling in Washington, sent to represent the Tobacco Institute; and John C. Fox, an attorney from San Francisco.

County Supervisor Sandra Smoley, a registered nurse and ACS volunteer, voted against the ordinance. (Smoley had accepted a $250 contribution from the tobacco industry in 1988.[28]) Echoing the tobacco industry, Smoley said that if the county approved such stringent measures against smoking, then it should also "outlaw alcohol and fatty foods and mandate that everyone ride their bikes."[29] On October 2, 1990, despite the industry's efforts, the Sacramento County Board of Supervisors passed the ordinance on a 3-2 vote, making all workplaces and most public places smoke free. Restaurants were to become smoke free with a three-year phase-in period; bars were exempted. A week later, on October 9, the Sacramento City Council passed a nearly identical ordinance by a vote of 8-1. The only difference was the phase-in time for restaurants to become smoke free. For the county, the period was three years, for the city, eighteen months.

The tobacco industry did not give up.

On October 3, the same day that the County Board of Supervisors passed the ordinance, the Tobacco Institute loaned $20,000 to a referendum campaign committee that had not yet formed.[30] On October 5, three days after the county vote and prior to the city council vote, Sacramentans for Fair Business Policy (SFBP) filed a statement of organization to force a referendum on the smoking ordinances. Tim Pueyo, the San Francisco political consultant for RJ Reynolds, was hired to run the campaign for SFBP. The same day, the company contributed almost half of its total contribution of $134,000. The other four major domestic cigarette manufacturers at the time, American Brands, Philip Morris, Lorillard, and Brown and Williamson, had all contributed thousands of dollars by the end of October. As of December 31, 1990, SFBP had received $375,971 in cash, loans, and services, only $9,150 (2.4 percent) of which came from nontobacco interests, mostly restaurants. As in past campaigns, the tobacco companies' contributions to the referendum effort were in proportion to their market shares.[31]

In Sacramento SFBP hired Nielsen, Merksamer, the tobacco industry's usual law firm in California, to fulfill legal obligations. Within two weeks, SFBP was using the tobacco money to distribute referendum petitions through the mail. Despite being organized and funded by out-of-state tobacco companies, throughout the campaign SFBP posed as a local independent organization. On November 1 Pueyo told the *Sacramento Bee* that his organization "is a grassroots coalition of business operators and individuals who oppose government sticking its nose in our business." [32]

The county required 30,433 signatures and the city required 19,334 to force referenda. Most of the tobacco money went to a Sacramento company specializing in petition drives. Of the approximately 60,000 signatures submitted to the county, enough were valid to force a referendum. Of the 31,135 signatures submitted to the city, not enough were valid to meet the minimum requirement. Therefore, the county ordinance was delayed until the next countywide election in 1992, which gave the tobacco industry another chance to overturn it. The city's ordinance went into effect on December 14, 1990.

THE ESCALATING FIGHT OVER LOCAL ORDINANCES

Things were not going well for the tobacco industry. In particular, its efforts to organize grassroots smokers and encourage them to fight against local tobacco control ordinances on their own was not proving successful, probably because these ordinances enjoyed general support among smokers. As a result, the industry moved to a more sophisticated strategy that involved using public relations firms to fight local ordinances directly, with the local "smoker's rights" groups playing only a cosmetic role.

By September 1990, the tobacco industry was worried about what was going on at the local level. Things were already getting out of control. In a Tobacco Institute memo from Terry Eagan to George Mimshaw, Eagan commented,

> *Frankly the gravest threat we face comes not from the Legislature but from local government.* At present there are disastrous proposed ordinances at work in such major metropolitan areas as the City of Los Angeles, the City of Sacramento and the County of Sacramento. . . . This new wave of action on local ordinances is being financed by revenues from Proposition 99 as disbursed to local entities by AB 75 of 1989. . . . Using state allocated Prop 99 funds earmarked for anti-smoking purposes, local governments create citizens committees designed to further the stated goal of a smoke-free society by the turn of the century. More often than not these committees come back to their city councils or boards of supervisors with a proposed smoking ordinance. These ordinances run the gamut from total bans in all public places, including restaurants, bars, and the workplace, to bans on vending machines in areas accessible to minors. . . .
>
> Given the tremendous amount of money dedicated to anti-smoking purposes it is more than a safe assumption that we will be facing dozens of local actions each year from here on out, either new ordinances or proposals to strengthen old ordinances. Health groups have admitted that they have been unsuccessful in obtaining state-level legislation banning or restricting smoking. *They will oppose to the death any attempt on our part to obtain preemption of local authorities. They have shifted the battleground to the local level where they are confident they will be more successful. The evidence more than indicates that success will be more readily available to them than in the Legislature. San Luis Obispo, San Francisco, Lodi, and Sacramento testify to their presumption.* . . .
>
> *The Tobacco Industry does not have the resources in place to fight local ordinances at a multitude of locations at the same time.* We were able to stop the Richmond billboard ordinance with an intense effort by our industry, its consultants, the distributors, the billboard companies and the minority business community.

In Vista and Riverside we were able to convince city attorneys, supervisors and council members that they were pre-empted by state law from regulating vending machines.

In Los Angeles we formed a new restaurant/business organization which is leading the fight against the Braude [clean indoor air] ordinance. But the industry's resources are stretched so thin that things will begin to happen by default.[33] [emphasis added]

By April 17, 1991, the Tobacco Institute had reorganized and added staff to fight local ordinances. Bob McAdam was brought in to replace Ron Saldana as the Tobacco Institute's regional director. The industry was also expanding its California effort by bringing in major political and public relations firms, including the Dolphin Group and Ray McNally and Associates. According to a memo written by Mark Smith to Tom Ogburn of RJ Reynolds,

The days of having to hope for return phone calls from Ron Saldana are fast becoming a bad memory. McAdam is reachable and open about what is going on. And McAdam's weekly conference call not only enhances communication by all parties, but increases the sense of accountability. The Dolphin Group and Ray McNally, both paid for by PM [Philip Morris], but reportable to TI [Tobacco Institute], appear at this early stage to be competent and hard working. The addition of John Hoy to the RJR team has been a big plus that will pay dividends down the road, especially as the L.A. Basin heats up.[34]

The reason for this intense effort was simple: as more ordinances restricted smoking, people stopped smoking or reduced their cigarette consumption, costing the tobacco industry hundreds of millions of dollars in annual sales.[35,36]

The industry's front groups continued to deny or downplay their connections with the tobacco industry. The tobacco companies understood that their role in the effort to stop local clean indoor air ordinances would be controversial and that they had to keep a low profile; they had to rely on other groups to do their bidding. As McAdam explained,

While the industry has coordinated the process, we have effectively used surrogates throughout this effort, and we have several organizations started which serve to facilitate the organization of local interests. These entities provide us with the negotiation necessary to limit our referenda exposure. First, *we have created Californians for Fair Business Policy,* which is the name given to our operation that has conducted the various referenda, and it is clearly identified as a "tobacco organization." *Then there is the California Business and Restaurant Alliance (CBRA). This organization has a tax exempt status and is operated by The Dolphin Group with assistance from our consultant,*

Joe Justin. Finally there is Restaurants for a Sound Voluntary Policy (RSVP) operated by Rudy Cole. While this organization was active in the Los Angeles battle, and to some extent in Bellflower and Culver City, it has not grown since then and does not have a presence outside the Southern California region. A variety of RJR-sponsored *local smokers' rights organizations have been created for specific battles* to assist in the grassroots effort.[37] [emphasis added]

McAdam observed that the tobacco industry's "strongest weapon" was its mobilization of local businesses: "This has been accomplished through CBRA and our full-time consultant, Joe Justin, and a great deal of work by The Dolphin Group. If our battle is to continue on this level, this part of the operation is essential. If PM [Philip Morris] will continue to fund this group, which again can be triggered by both circumstances and our Regional Vice President, it will fit into our defensive strategy."[37] McAdam went on to say that "as the opposition gets more aggressive (and they will)," the Tobacco Institute would have to be prepared to respond. He proposed that two new consultants be hired with institute funds but added, "These consultants will be retained by one of our surrogate organizations."[37]

McAdam also realized that the tobacco industry needed one final piece of the puzzle, evidence that smoke-free ordinances had a negative economic impact: "We need to produce some hard information about the economic impact of the smoking bans. . . . Now that the bans have had one or two quarters to take effect, we can look at tax data that will be available this fall and create a study that can be used across the state. A Price-Waterhouse study with some credibility in this area would cost $25,000."[37] The proposed study of California ordinances using tax data never materialized; either it was never conducted or the data, when obtained, showed no adverse effect from the smoke-free restaurant laws.

The tobacco industry's efforts to use the argument that smoke-free restaurant ordinances hurt the restaurant business was eventually discredited as a result of a chance meeting of Lisa Smith and Professor Stanton Glantz of the University of California, San Francisco, in the ornate lobby outside the Los Angeles City Council chambers in 1990, just after the tobacco industry defeated a proposed clean indoor air ordinance. Smith was working on local ordinances in the Sacramento area and had attended the hearing to see the industry in action; Glantz was at the hearing to testify about the dangers of secondhand tobacco smoke. After the hearing, Glantz expressed his doubt over the now-familiar industry claim that smoke-free ordinances reduced restaurant sales by 30 percent. The

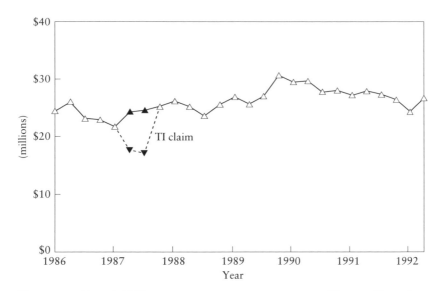

Figure 11.   Beverly Hills restaurant revenues, 1986–1992. The 100% smoke-free restaurant ordinance did not reduce revenues by 30% when it was in force in Beverly Hills, as the tobacco industry had claimed. The ordinance (solid triangles) actually had no significant effect on sales. *Source:* S. A. Glantz and L. R. A. Smith, The effect of ordinances requiring smoke-free restaurants on restaurant sales, *Am J Pub Health* 1994;84:1081–1085. Reproduced with permission of the *American Journal of Public Health* (copyright 1994 by American Public Health Association).

number seemed illogical to Glantz since only about 25 percent of Californians smoked at the time. He mentioned that analyzing the sales tax data would be an objective way to test the effect, if any, on sales. Smith overheard the comment and responded that such information was publicly available and that she knew where to get it. This chance meeting led to a collaboration that lasted several years and produced a series of reports documenting that smoke-free restaurant ordinances—and, later, smoke-free bar ordinances—did not affect revenues, contrary to industry claims at the time. The reports were based on an analysis of restaurant sales tax receipts from many cities, including Beverly Hills (figure 11).[38–43]

This research would cause the industry problems. According to a 1993 internal Philip Morris e-mail, "The economic arguments which only a year ago prevented a ban in Los Angeles and San Francisco, are losing the ability to pursuade [*sic*], as more and more communities, small and

large, have banned smoking without apparent economic effect (Glantz'
'studies' are still more credible to the media and elected officials than
restaurateurs' anecdotal accounts of lost business)." [42] Price Waterhouse,
sponsored by the San Diego Tavern and Restaurant Association, produced a study for the tobacco industry claiming that smoke-free restaurant ordinances adversely affected business,[44] as did other firms. These
"studies," however, were based on opinion surveys and failed to carry
much weight in the face of studies based on sales tax data, which were
more complete and objective.

To support the industry's local referenda effort in the coming year,
1992, McAdam wanted $750,000 in ready reserve with Californians
for Fair Business Policy. This money would be used to fund signature-
gathering if it became necessary in Los Angeles. He also wanted $40,000
to fund efforts in each of four elections: Paradise, El Dorado County,
Oroville, and Visalia, where the industry had forced local clean indoor air laws onto the ballot, and $1,500,000 for the renewed effort in
Sacramento County. In total, the California Local Referendum Project
required $2,060,000 for its first year of operation.[37] In the end, the in-
dustry spent $1.71 million attempting to overturn ordinances in Sacra-
mento County, Oroville, Paradise, El Dorado County, and Visalia. Each
company's contribution was based on its share of the prior year's production of cigarettes and manufactured tobacco.[45]

With a more organized and sophisticated strategy, the tobacco industry was prepared to continue its fights against local ordinances all over
the state. When confronted with an ordinance, the industry would first
attempt to force the local government to drop or weaken it; if this ploy
failed, the industry would then start a referendum petition drive to pressure elected officials to modify the ordinance rather than incur the cost
of an election. If these two steps failed, the industry would mount a well-
funded campaign to defeat the ordinance at the polls.

LONG BEACH

The industry's stepped-up efforts were evident in the later local ordinance
campaigns, such as the one in Long Beach, a major urban center. The initiation and development of Long Beach's ordinance came from the Long
Beach Tobacco Control Coalition, a broad-based advisory group of civic,
academic, and health leaders and staff from the Long Beach Department
of Health and Human Services.

In January 1991 the coalition and the health department asked the Long Beach City Council's Quality of Life Committee to strengthen the city's existing ordinance, and the committee went on to recommend that the council adopt an ordinance that would have ended smoking in public places and the workplace, made at least two-thirds of restaurant seating nonsmoking, and restricted vending machines and billboard advertising.

The ordinance was publicly opposed by local restaurant and business owners, the Long Beach Chamber of Commerce, and Rudy Cole of RSVP. (At the time, Cole denied that he was or ever had been paid by the tobacco industry.) Fred Karger of CBRA never testified publicly but attended several city council meetings with the vice president of governmental affairs for the Chamber of Commerce. Karger, at a later Quality of Life Committee meeting, even refused to answer questions from Councilman Evan Braude. Karger's dual role as chief executive officer of CBRA and executive vice president of the Dolphin Group was not widely known, nor was his association with the tobacco industry.

Despite the tobacco industry's efforts, the council exceeded the Quality of Life Committee's recommendations, stipulating that smoking would be completely ended in restaurants by 1994. After lobbying efforts failed to stop the ordinance, the tobacco industry, acting through Californians for Fair Business Policy (CFBP), initiated a referendum petition drive to suspend the ordinance. CFBP spent $87,410 on the petition drive, virtually all of which came from tobacco companies, but the level of industry involvement was not known at the time.

Controversy surrounded the petition drive and the signature gatherers. CFBP hired Kimball Petition Management to collect the necessary signatures. Complaints were reported to city officials of signature gatherers misrepresenting the content and nature of the petition drive. According to CFBP's disclosure statement, the petitioning firm employed at least eighteen signature gatherers who did not live in Long Beach. Despite the objections of health advocates to the tobacco industry's questionable tactics, enough signatures were validated to suspend the ordinance. No investigation of the allegations of misrepresentation or the use of out-of-town signature gatherers was conducted.

Validating the signatures cost Long Beach $1,861.[46] At the time, an election to decide the issue was estimated to cost Long Beach approximately $500,000; this figure was later lowered to $170,000. Rather than incur the cost, the city council rescinded the ordinance and drafted one acceptable to the tobacco industry. This strategy—raising the possibility of an expensive election and then withdrawing the threat when a compromise suitable to the industry was reached—was to reappear in other local ordinance campaigns. It was also one of the experiences that led Philip Morris to produce a statewide initiative, Proposition 188, in 1994.

PLACER COUNTY

Placer County is located in the foothills of the Sierra Nevada range northeast of Sacramento. The Placer County Tobacco Control Coalition (PCTCC), similar to the one in Long Beach, played a key role in developing and passing tobacco control ordinances in the county and several of its cities. During 1991 the PCTCC initiated ordinances in meetings with city managers, arranged study sessions for city councils in the municipalities of Auburn and Roseville, and provided model ordinances as well as written support and public testimony.

The tobacco industry recognized that it could not stop all legislative activity, so it settled on a fall-back position of supporting weak, ineffectual ordinances in the hope that they would forestall tough local tobacco control regulations. By April 25, 1991, the tobacco industry had identified an opportunity to get its "model" ordinance adopted in Placer County.[47] The model ordinance provided for 50 percent of a restaurant's space to be designated as a nonsmoking area as well as for workplace smoking policies to be established by the individual employer. Although the industry proposal was denounced by health groups, it indicated how far and how fast the issue of clean indoor air had advanced in California: the industry's proposed law was stronger than either Proposition 5 or Proposition 10, which the industry had spent over $10 million defeating just a decade earlier.

In Placerville the industry worked through its California Business and Restaurant Alliance (CBRA). In an April 25 memo, Randy Morris, regional director of the Tobacco Institute, wrote to Kent Rhodes, the local CBRA counsel, to specify procedure: "Naturally, this proposal [the industry's model ordinance] is not set in concrete, however, significant changes to the ordinance's provisions, i.e. increasing penalties, further smoking restrictions, etc., must be cleared with appropriate institute staff: the undersigned and Bob McAdam, Vice President for Special Projects. T.I. Staff will then review proposed changes with appropriate member-company personnel, to wit: Sandy Timpson of Philip Morris

and Jim O'Mally of R. J. Reynolds." [47] Incidentally, the Tobacco Institute
wanted to be sure that all memo recipients understood that this "model"
was the standard for California only: "A caveat is in order. While the
Placer County Omnibus Tobacco Control Act of 1991 is a guideline
which will allow Placer County to definitively handle the tobacco issue
by setting a standard for other California counties and municipalities, *it
must be acknowledged that industry policy on California local issues
reflect[s] a distinct and separate environment of tobacco politics unique
to this state*" (emphasis added).[47] In short, a similar ordinance in another state would not be acceptable. California's Tobacco Control Program was succeeding.

In early summer the PCTCC began to develop an ordinance for the
county similar to those being passed in the cities. (The city of Colfax
also passed an ordinance in mid-August with the help of the PCTCC.)
By this time, the tobacco industry had started to intervene aggressively
with its new strategy. On November 1, 1991, the Sacramento Restaurant
and Merchant Association (SRMA), which was a vehicle for Ray Mc-
Nally, cosponsored a meeting to organize opposition and select individuals to speak at the Board of Supervisors' November 6 hearing. Diann
Rogers and Rosabel Tao of SRMA (employees of Ray McNally) conducted the meeting and stated that SRMA was assisting other communities against similar tobacco control ordinances. They distributed detailed
information explaining exactly what local individuals should do to oppose the county ordinance. Rogers asserted that the ordinance would
adversely affect the local economy, impose too much government regulation, and infringe on individual rights. The meeting also presented strategies to counter health advocates' efforts. Rogers stressed that health
advocates would claim that the tobacco industry was assisting the opposition but that it was important to deny such involvement—such
claims would damage the opposition's credibility and the allegations of
industry involvement were not true.

The tobacco industry's new strategy succeeded in mobilizing local opposition. The issues brought up at the November 1 meeting were raised,
and the tactics applied, by opponents at the Board of Supervisors' hearing later that week. Rogers and Tao attended but did not testify. Although
the ordinance had strong support from two supervisors, it was defeated
by a 3-2 vote. A compromise ordinance—one weaker than those adopted
in the nearby Sierra Nevada foothill communities of Auburn, Roseville,
and Colfax—was passed.

The tobacco industry continued to develop an aggressive local strategy to combat the efforts of local health professionals who were aided by resources and education programs funded by Proposition 99. By November 27, 1991, McAdam was formalizing the Tobacco Institute's "California Local Referenda Program." According to McAdam,

> *In the absence of a preemptive state law governing smoking restrictions, we have confronted—and will continue to confront—an unprecedented threat of workplace and restaurant smoking ban actions at the local level in California.* Either through the ballot box by referenda or through reasonable compromise forged with local officials, this increasing threat of local smoking bans must be challenged. . . .
>
> The past eight months of operating at the local level have given us some substantial insight into what organization and resources have been most effective in waging this particular battle to stop these prospective bans.[37] [emphasis added]

The industry mounted a multi-million-dollar campaign using professional public relations and political campaign firms to directly lobby for and organize opposition against local tobacco control ordinances.

THE SACRAMENTO BATTLE OVER MEASURE G

While the 1990 petition drive against the Sacramento city ordinance did not collect enough valid signatures, the county petition drive did yield enough signatures to suspend the ordinance. The Board of Supervisors decided to place the issue on the June 1992 ballot, where it appeared as Measure G.

In Sacramento Ray McNally worked through the SRMA, and the Dolphin Group worked through the CBRA, to conceal the tobacco industry's role in mobilizing opposition to the ordinance.

In December 1991 representatives from the ALA, ACS, AHA, the Sacramento/El Dorado Medical Society, and the Sacramento Sierra Hospital Conference formed Citizens for Healthier Sacramento/Yes on Measure G (CHS). Early in 1992, CHS commissioned a poll to plan its campaign to defend the ordinance. Seventy-two percent of those surveyed supported the county's tobacco control ordinance. The survey also showed that if people knew that Sacramentans for Fair Business Practices was actually a "front" for the tobacco industry, 48 percent would be more likely to vote for the ordinance, and 69 percent felt that such use of a front organization was "dishonest."[48]

The tobacco industry, through CFBP, spent $1,775,379 on its campaign to defeat Measure G, using mailers, radio advertisements, television spots, personalized absentee ballot registration forms, and a Kentucky-based telephone bank. The industry's strategy again emphasized that the ordinance would lead to unneeded bureaucracy, waste taxpayer dollars, and create "cigarette police."

CHS anticipated a major tobacco industry campaign against the ordinance, but realized it could not match the tobacco industry's spending. Instead, it concentrated on raising an adequate budget to run an aggressive grassroots campaign with two key strategies: using the media to constantly inform voters of the tobacco industry's involvement against Measure G and educating organizations in Sacramento County about Measure G and the industry's misleading campaign advertisements.

CHS cultivated substantial media coverage and publicity for Measure G, which yielded nearly 100 newspaper, television, and radio stories. This media attention educated the public about how much the tobacco companies were spending and reported the false claims and controversy surrounding CFBP's campaign commercials and advertisements. This effort led three local newspapers to publish editorials supporting Measure G and criticizing the industry's involvement in Sacramento. *The Business Journal* warned, "They'll [tobacco companies] masquerade as smart, smooth-talking yuppies, complaining in savvy tones on your TV and radio about how Big Brother is at it again. But don't forget who they really are—tobacco companies that don't give a damn about small business or civil liberties, let alone public health."[49]

In addition to its media campaign, CHS used two other key tactics. In April and May, CHS community outreach volunteers visited approximately sixty-five groups to neutralize the tobacco industry's misleading campaign messages and draw key support for the ordinance. Since CHS could not hope to match the industry's television or professional mailer campaigns, CHS got its campaign messages out by spending most of its money ($35,000) on radio advertisements attacking the tobacco industry during the final three weeks of the election.

A turning point in the election was a mailer sent out by CFBP one week before voting took place. Aiming to show that Measure G would create unnecessary "cigarette patrols," the mailer listed several fake emergency telephone numbers, including a number for the "cigarette patrol." Residents were encouraged to place these numbers near their telephones. The back of the mailer featured a copy of a memo from the Sacramento

County Sheriff's Department regarding budget cuts, implying that the sheriff opposed Measure G. In reality, the memo had nothing to do with the ordinance. CHS capitalized on such a media event and joined with police, fire, health, and even telephone company officials who publicly criticized the industry mailer because of its misrepresentation and the potential danger associated with the fake numbers.

CHS's aggressive media strategy, its active community outreach program, and other local grassroots efforts led to a 56 percent to 44 percent victory for Measure G.

THE TOBACCO INDUSTRY'S PLAN: "CALIFORNIA'S NEGATIVE ENVIRONMENT"

By January 11, 1991, the Tobacco Institute's State Activities Division had prepared a secret report entitled "California: A Multifaceted Plan to Address a Negative Environment."[4] The report documented how successful the tobacco control advocates had been:

> With the passage of Proposition 99—the $500 million annual tobacco tax increase measure adopted in November, 1988—the industry faces statewide funding of local anti-tobacco activity, including local measures to ban smoking in workplaces, restaurants and most other public places.
> Ten years ago, the assumption was that most law makers and members of the public who thought about the issue viewed smoking as an occasional nuisance. Today, it seems that many view tobacco smoke as dangerous to the health of nonsmokers.[4]

The report listed three long-term strategies: to "adopt a reasonable statewide smoking law, with preemption"; to "redirect Proposition 99 funding away from direct anti-tobacco lobbying and other activities"; and to "reduce or eliminate Proposition 99 funding." In the interim, the industry was to "assemble a legislative team to monitor and defeat local smoking restriction ordinances in California." The team working on local strategies had a budget of $520,000 in 1991 and $2,085,000 in 1992, with the understanding that "as it becomes necessary to exercise our referenda option in various communities, this amount could increase greatly."[4]

In 1992 Kurt L. Malmgren, the Tobacco Institute's senior vice president for state activities, prepared a report for Samuel Chilcote, president of the Tobacco Institute, in which he generalized from the tobacco industry's experiences in California, Massachusetts, and Washington State to design an "Expanded Local Program" for the tobacco industry to use nationwide. Among the needs identified in California, Malmgren listed the following as "primary":

Sophisticated monitoring of local ordinance introductions

Ability to respond quickly with locally-based advocates

Local consultants who can go door-to-door to educate restaurateurs, business leaders, minority group leaders, representatives from organized labor, and other potential allies

The ability to rightfully project a *local* concern about a given anti-tobacco ordinance, making it more difficult for anti-tobacco leaders to say, "The only people who oppose this ordinance are the out-of-state tobacco companies"

Reasonably coordinated and effective means to trigger direct mail campaigns, phone bank operations and other contacts[50] [emphasis in original]

Malmgren also cited one of the Tobacco Institute's strengths in California: "The industry team quickly employs coalition coordinators who can —quickly and effectively—do the necessary legwork to develop support for individual restaurateurs, retailers, hoteliers, local labor leaders and others."[50] Significant local opposition to local ordinances was unlikely to exist without an employed coalition coordinator. While the industry was able to slow passage of local ordinances using these strategies, in the end the tobacco control community—through a combination of Proposition 99–funded educational programs and privately funded political action—was routinely defeating the tobacco industry at the local level.

An undated Philip Morris memorandum on various state tobacco control programs observed,

In California our biggest challenge has not been the anti-smoking advertising campaign created with cigarette excise tax dollars.

Rather, *it has been the creation of an anti-smoking infrastructure,* right down to the local level. It is an infrastructure that for the first time has the resources to tap into the anti-smoking network at the national level.[51] [emphasis added]

Much as it disliked the anti-tobacco media campaign, the industry recognized that, contrary to its early expectations, there were other potent forces at work that would cause serious problems.

THE TOBACCO INDUSTRY AND THE CALIFORNIA PUBLIC RECORDS ACT

One final tactic strategically used by the tobacco industry to impede state and local tobacco control operations involved freedom of information

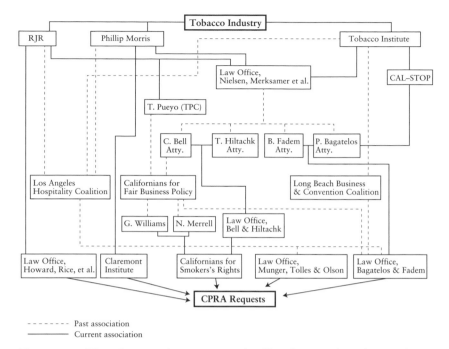

Figure 12.   The tobacco industry's network of law firms and smokers' rights groups, which submitted requests to tobacco control organizations under the California Public Records Act. *Source:* S. Aguinaga S and S. A. Glantz, The use of public records acts to interfere with tobacco control, *Tobacco Control* 1995;1995(4):222–230. Reproduced with permission of *Tobacco Control* (copyright BMJ Publishing Group).

acts. These laws, created to insure that citizenry had access to information collected by their governments, were used as a tool to slow the work of tobacco control offices. The tobacco industry set up a complex web of law firms and smokers' rights groups to submit requests for information under the California Public Records Act (figure 12).

DHS's Tobacco Control Section (TCS) received many more requests for public information than other seemingly controversial state-level health programs, such as AIDS and alcohol and drug programs or the HIV prevention program at the California Department of Education. In fact, TCS was the only health program receiving any requests; between 1991 and 1993, there were fifty-nine requests for 371 documents.[52] For example, on April 4, 1991, Mark Helm of the Los Angeles law firm Munger, Tolles & Olson wrote to the Tobacco Control Section to request "all public records (including all correspondence, memoranda, and other documents) dated on or after November 1, 1988" related to the baseline survey, innovative programs, the independent evaluation, the information campaign, the master plan, and the activities of TEOC. The request appears to have simply replicated the language of Assembly Bill 75.[53] The firm was working in 1990 as Philip Morris's California counsel.[54] From April to June 1991, the freedom of information requests came from the Nielsen, Merksamer law firm, which handled much of the tobacco industry's legal work in California.

This tactic of using the freedom of information act as a form of harassment was to continue throughout the life of the program and eventually included requests to the health departments in the larger counties and the California Department of Education.[52] Program advocates, however, eventually understood how to handle such requests with minimal disruption to their operations: by requiring requests in writing and by assessing reasonable photocopying charges on the requesting parties.

Some of the LLAs responded to the requests by using them to call attention to the tobacco industry. In 1993, for example, the Contra Costa County LLA received a public records act request from a Marietta Stuart. The director replied by saying that complying with the request would disrupt the LLA's work and suggested that Stuart come in personally to inspect the documents and make photocopies. In response, the LLA received a call from the law firm Bell and Hiltachk, representing Californians for Smokers' Rights; the firm scheduled a time for someone to come with a copy machine to photocopy the documents. When Glenn Williams, a Californians for Smokers' Rights employee, arrived with a copier, the LLA director was waiting with the media to denounce what she perceived as harassment by pro-tobacco groups. The incident received wide coverage in the press, and requests to the LLA stopped.

The tobacco industry recognized that the public health community was getting more sophisticated in dealing with its tactics. For example, when Stratton, Reiter, Dupree & Durante was preparing its report for RJ Reynolds, one of the complaints in the report was the effectiveness with which TCS had dealt with records act requests: "TCS's heightened concern over the status of its '91–'92 Fiscal Budget, plus a profound screening process to ward off tobacco industry access to public documents, presented significant barriers to reviewing individual grants and county tobacco control plans. Thus a significant element of this research project involved creating access points to interviews and publications among TCS staff, state government leads, and unsuspecting program contractors."[55] In addition to seeking to disrupt policy making by state and local health departments working for tobacco control, the industry used much of the information obtained through the California Public Records Act in its propaganda. In the upcoming legislative battles over Proposition 99 reauthorization, the information was to emerge in the industry's attacks on innovative tobacco control projects as a waste of money.

CONCLUSION

The local battles of the late 1980s and early 1990s taught tobacco control advocates several lessons.[31,46] First, they could expect the tobacco industry to intervene, although indirectly, through groups like CBRA, SRMA, CFBP, and RSVP, to fight local tobacco control ordinances. Even these groups, however, tried to stay out of the public view by providing behind-the-scenes assistance and information to mobilize local opposition. Second, as the health dangers of secondhand smoke became more widely known and believed, the only way the industry could counter the health message was to generate claims of adverse economic impact. Since these claims were not sound, the tobacco industry had to create "facts" in order to make their arguments. Such facts were often generated and circulated by public affairs firms, particularly the claim that smoke-free ordinances had reduced restaurant sales by 30 percent. Local proponents learned to counter these "facts" with peer-reviewed scientific studies proving the industry charges of adverse economic consequences were not true. Third, while health professionals gained expertise in avoiding the time and expense of defending the ordinance at the polls, tobacco control advocates still had a chance to win if forced to the polls, in spite of the industry's money. In most cases, when tobacco control advocates and elected officials remained active and committed and raised adequate money, the industry's efforts failed. Effective campaigns took advantage of both the tobacco industry's lack of credibility and the voters' understanding of the dangers of secondhand smoke.

Proposition 99–funded education, through the media campaign, on the dangers of secondhand smoke, as well as the messages designed to discredit the tobacco industry, created an environment where it was easier to mobilize public and political support for policies to protect nonsmokers from secondhand smoke. The DHS also gave the Americans for

Nonsmokers' Rights Foundation a contract to provide technical assistance to the LLAs and other organizations involved in the Proposition 99 Health Education program. This assistance helped local tobacco control advocates better anticipate and fight the tobacco industry's tactics. The local programs reinforced these messages, and the local coalitions, the voluntary health agencies, and ANR leveraged this environment to increase the effectiveness with which they fought the tobacco industry in the political arena. Overall, the local ordinance effort was to prove remarkably successful. Between 1989 and January 1, 1995, when a statewide smoke-free workplace law went in to effect, 195 local clean indoor air ordinances were passed or strengthened in California. As the tobacco industry had feared, this new environment contributed to the marked decline in smoking in California.[56–58]

The tobacco industry recognized that its historical ability to control tobacco policy in California was no longer as effective because tobacco control advocates moved successfully to the local level and away from the Legislature. While they were willing to fight local ordinances as an interim measure, the industry was still counting on the California Legislature to rescue it, which it could do in two ways. First, the Legislature could increasingly "de-fund" the LLAs and the media campaign, both of which were supporting local efforts. Second, the Legislature could pass statewide legislation that would preempt the ability of local level governments, either city or county, to pass legislation.[59] With a single, weak state-level law, the local ordinance campaigns would disappear.

CHAPTER 10

Continued Erosion of the Health Education Account

1990–1994

Proposition 99's anti-tobacco programs were off to a good start. The media campaign had achieved high visibility within California and attracted international acclaim. The local programs were up and running, and local clean indoor air ordinances and tobacco control measures were passing at a faster rate. On October 30, 1990, the Department of Health Services (DHS), which was implementing all the Proposition 99 anti-tobacco education programs except the school-based programs, estimated that California had 750,000 fewer smokers than it would have had if Proposition 99 had not passed, that the percentage of smokers over the age of twenty had dropped from 24.6 percent to 21.2 percent, that tobacco consumption was down 14 percent, and that between 62 percent and 85 percent of the target groups were aware of the media campaign.[1,2] With such a strong early-performance record, public health advocates should have been in a position to protect the Health Education Account from the tobacco industry and its allies who wanted to see more money go to medical services.

AB 75's sunset provision took effect on June 30, 1991, only twenty-one months after passage, so the Legislature had to enact new implementing legislation for Proposition 99 in 1991. This situation created a new opportunity for the tobacco industry and its allies to dismantle the anti-tobacco programs. The health groups believed that their earlier compromise with the California Medical Association (CMA) and other medical interests—allowing a relatively small amount of money to be taken from the Health Education Account to fund medical services like the Child Health and Disability Prevention program (CHDP)—would protect the anti-tobacco programs from further incursions. They were wrong.

The state was facing a budget shortfall, which further motivated groups interested in funding medical services to raid the Proposition 99 Health Education Account. Ironically, the very success of the Tobacco Control Program in reducing tobacco consumption magnified this problem: less smoking meant fewer cigarettes sold, which meant lower Proposition 99 tobacco tax revenues. Public health groups recognized from the beginning that the Health Education revenues would decline naturally as smoking did and that, as the program succeeded in reducing tobacco consumption, it would become less necessary. But they did not anticipate that medical service providers would work to cut health education funds faster than the natural rate of decline. For medical service providers, who faced escalating costs and a growing population demanding services, a drop in revenue due to less smoking motivated them to fight for a bigger piece of the shrinking financial pie.

In addition, the tobacco industry was continuing to make substantial campaign contributions to most members of the Legislature, with especially heavy donations going to the leadership. In the 1991–1992 election cycle, the industry spent $5.8 million on campaign contributions and lobbying in California. Because of the importance of Proposition 99, the tobacco industry spent $3,772 per member in the California Legislature in 1989–1990, compared with only $2,451 per member in the US Congress.[3,4] In particular, the industry increased contributions to Assembly Speaker Willie Brown, who was uniquely positioned to defend the industry's interests.

California also had a new governor. In November 1990 Pete Wilson was elected to succeed George Deukmejian. While both were Republicans, their attitudes toward initiatives differed. Deukmejian might oppose an initiative during an election (as he had Proposition 99), but he would then respect the will of the voters and make an honest effort to implement any initiative that passed, including Proposition 99.[5] By contrast, Wilson believed that it was his prerogative to "massage" initiatives.[6]

EARLY POSTURES

Legislative activity surrounding Proposition 99 began in the fall of 1990 with the formation of a steering committee of the organizations that had been most interested in AB 75, including the voluntaries, the CMA, California Association of Hospitals and Health Systems (CAHHS), Service Employees International Union (SEIU), Western Center for Law and Poverty, and others. The committee was to provide a forum for the groups to communicate with each other about new legislation. According to American Lung Association (ALA) lobbyist Tony Najera and Senator Watson's chief of staff, John Miller, the steering committee and Assembly Member Phil Isenberg (D-Sacramento), who had chaired the Conference Committee that wrote AB 75, agreed to extend the existing programs and distribution formulas without substantive changes, to share pro rata in the 14–18 percent reduction in revenues, and to minimize conflicts and press for fast-track passage of legislation authorizing the Proposition 99 programs by March 1991.[7] In light of the political deal that the public health advocates had made to ensure AB 75's passage as well as the newness of the programs, this was not an unreasonable position. The debate was becoming simply how to divide up another pie in Sacramento.

On January 7, 1991, the three voluntaries, the CMA, CAHHS, SEIU, Western Center for Law and Poverty, and other interested parties wrote to Isenberg and the other members of the Conference Committee, urging them to extend the provisions of AB 75:

> Our organizations have worked together through-out the implementation phases of AB 75 to assure that legislative policy objectives are being achieved. We now join in urging your support for a three year extension of the provisions of AB 75, as contained in AB 99 (Legislative Session 1991–92), in order to assure the continuation of the programs and services that are funded with these tobacco tax proceeds. In order to secure a stable and efficient administration at both the state and local level, it is critical to obtain an extension of the provisions of AB 75 well in advance of the sunset date.[8]

This reauthorization strategy meant that if everyone played by the rules, then programmatic issues related to the allocation of money would not be raised, including the issue of using the Health Education Account to fund CHDP. The health groups felt that this was the best strategy to avoid further erosion in funding of anti-tobacco education because it would not force them to defend the efficacy of the Tobacco Control Program, which was just building steam. They did not want to appropriate

Health Education Account money in a bill separate from the medical service accounts because doing so would isolate funding for the anti-tobacco program and make it a better target for the tobacco industry and its allies.[9]

The public health groups honored their side of the agreement, although it meant accepting the continued diversion of funds from the Health Education Account into medical services. The Tobacco Education Oversight Committee (TEOC), the committee created by the Legislature to provide advice about Proposition 99 implementation, supported using Health Education Account money for CHDP. TEOC's position was articulated through statements by its chair, Carolyn Martin, a volunteer with ALA, and Jennie Cook, a volunteer with ACS. At a January 23 press conference, Martin described the activities funded by the Health Education Account, including CHDP: "The prevention message is reaching every group targeted by the enabling legislation (AB 75) in settings as diverse as fast food restaurants, clinic waiting rooms and half time at the Chargers-49ers exhibition game."[10] Jennie Cook explicitly justified the use of Health Education Account funds for medical services: "Pregnant women who smoke become parents who smoke around their young children causing increased respiratory illness, ear infections, and reduced growth. Education efforts have begun in many prenatal care settings and maternal and child health programs."[10] No one was willing to question whether CHDP should continue to receive funding from the Health Education Account.

THE CMA POSITION

In contrast to the voluntary health agencies, which demonstrated commitment to all programs, the CMA was soft on the issue of funding programs other than medical services. Although the CMA signed the January 1991 letter to Isenberg, on November 10, 1990, the CMA Council had adopted a recommendation that the existing Proposition 99 expenditure patterns be extended "until CMA's affordable basic care proposal or a similar proposal is implemented."[11] AB 75 distributions were acceptable only until the money was needed to pay for indigent health care. According to CMA Resolution 9021-90,

> (1) CMA supports funding of tobacco education programs through the years 1990 and 1991, as approved by the voters of California in Prop. 99. (2) CMA will monitor the progress of the State's evaluation of the effectiveness of the

Prop. 99 health education account. (3) CMA will work in conjunction with the legislature and with other groups interested in tobacco education and access to care, toward *the goal of utilizing tobacco tax revenues for access to care as soon as feasible,* while maintaining adequate funding for tobacco education.[12] [emphasis added]

The council had reiterated its basic position that using Health Education dollars for public health programs was an interim measure, that funding health care was the preferred policy, and that anti-tobacco education was entitled only to "adequate" funding, not "full" funding.

In 1990, when chief CMA lobbyist Jay Michael was questioned about CMA policy by Lester Breslow, a member of the TEOC and former dean of the UCLA School of Public Health, Michael responded, "The CMA's policy relating to the distribution of Prop 99 monies until June 30, 1990, was consistent with our long-range policy relating to the ultimate use of Prop 99 funds in the future. . . . CMA's general policy for the short term was to ensure that physicians received their fair share of the health care funding provided by Prop 99, which was intended to temporarily patch up our health care delivery system until such time as an overall solution can be achieved to address our most serious health care problems." [13] He went on to reiterate the CMA position emphasizing that $30 million is enough to mount a massive campaign in the schools and that a public media campaign is not likely to be effective.[13-15]

The CMA was also prepared to contest the evaluation data that showed the programs' effectiveness. When interviewed in 1993, Michael expressed his attitude about the evaluation:

Did you read the study that was done by the Department of Health Services or commissioned by the Department of Health Services? I think that's a sloppy study; it's undocumented; the conclusions, or the data do not support the conclusions. . . . Why? Because the money was vulnerable to being diverted to other purposes in a tight state budget year. And they were desperate and it was a survival response. And I don't fault them for that. I've been in this business for a long time, and that's the way people behave. It's very hard to be judgmental about things like that. . . . But to cloak their biased stacked study in objectivity is offensive to me. . . . The issue is: is that the most cost-effective way to use that money to improve health and to reduce the amount of tobacco addiction? And I don't think that study has ever been made. As an advocate of the point of view that it ought to be given to health care providers and health care providers should be educated, trained to get people to stop smoking, I'm advocating that. I don't have a clue as to whether that's the most cost-effective way to use the money. I'm saying it ought to be evaluated along with every other kind of use of that money by someone who really does an objective job. And the money shouldn't be split up on the basis of these hokey trumped-up biased advocates for a particular interest group.[16]

For the public health groups, or the "dread disease organizations," as Michael called them, these comments were not those of someone who wanted to maintain the status quo.

The CMA's most immediate concern was to prevent any drop in money for health services. The "maintenance of effort" clause in Proposition 99, which required that the new tobacco tax money be used to supplement rather than replace existing state funding, was an issue in the fall of 1990. The 1990–1991 state budget had reduced funding for county Medically Indigent Service Programs and for Medical Services Programs. According to the CMA Council minutes, most counties believed that they could not maintain existing levels of service and thus would not be able to qualify for Proposition 99 funds, so they had asked to have the maintenance of effort requirement waived for fiscal year 1990–1991. The CMA went on record as opposing any waiver of maintenance of effort requirements.[17]

At the same time, on November 1, 1990, the Tobacco Institute was also planning its 1991 legislative strategy for neutralizing Proposition 99. The main goal was to "divert the media funds," and the institute saw a chance to achieve this diversion:

> The decrease in revenues will increase the competition for funding in the 91–92 budget among the various program elements. Additionally, California is expecting a shortfall of as much as $2 billion, possibly more, in the next fiscal year. *That will tempt the new administration and the Legislature to supplant existing general fund revenues with Proposition 99 revenues where appropriate programs exist. The women, infants and children and the health screening programs are appropriate programs since they contain anti-tobacco education elements and would satisfy the dictates of Proposition 99.* . . .
>
> Proposition 99 revenues are down which will pit the sponsors of the initiative against one another as they seek funding for their favorite programs. Confusion and animosity will result. . . . *A coalition of interests could be built to chase the media money. The nucleus of such a coalition could be the minority health communities which feel not enough of the Proposition 99 money is getting to the streets. Other coalition members would be the rural counties, a few of which are facing bankruptcy. Public hospitals desperately need money to fund trauma centers.* Other interest groups would join the chase if they thought the money were in play.[18] [emphasis added]

Rather than battling Proposition 99 in the open, the tobacco industry would help orchestrate other interests who wanted the money. The industry would remain in the shadows, making campaign contributions and lobbying the administration and the Legislature out of the public eye.

GOVERNOR WILSON'S BUDGET CUTS

The hope among health groups for a fast-track reauthorization of the Proposition 99 anti-tobacco programs was shattered when Republican governor Pete Wilson released his first budget on January 10, 1991. Although the Health Education Account contained $161 million ($38 million carried over from previous years, $7 million in interest, and $116 million in new tax revenues),[19] the governor appeared to accept the CMA's plan to spend just $30 million on the DHS anti-tobacco programs.

The governor's budget represented a huge cutback for the Tobacco Control Program. The local lead agencies (LLAs) and the media campaign were each to receive $15 million. The LLAs had previously been receiving $36 million annually, and the media campaign, $14 million annually. The competitive grants program would be ended entirely, after receiving over $50 million during the life of AB 75 and as much as $11 million in 1990–1991. (The Tobacco Control Section of DHS was also budgeted to receive $2 million for state administration.) Wilson proposed cutting the California Department of Education (CDE) to $16 million annually for local programs and state administration, down from $36 million. In total, Wilson proposed that the overall Tobacco Control Program was to receive only 30 percent of the available Health Education Account revenues,[19] or only about 6 percent of tobacco tax revenues (as opposed to the 20 percent specified in Proposition 99). He also proposed cutting the research program in half, to less than 3 percent of tobacco tax revenues (as opposed to the 5 percent specified in Proposition 99).[20]

The major beneficiaries of the governor's cuts in the anti-tobacco programs were a new perinatal insurance program called Access for Infants and Mothers (AIM), which would get $90 million, $50 million of which would come from the Health Education Account, and CHDP, which would be increased from $20 million to $43 million.[2] AIM provides medical care to pregnant women and their young children by subsidizing private insurance coverage. Because AIM pays a higher reimbursement rate to providers than does MediCal (California's version of Medicaid), it is more popular with medical providers and more expensive than MediCal.[21]

The March 26, 1991, issue of *Capital Correspondence,* the ALA's newsletter to activists, urged them to support AB 99 as it had been introduced by Isenberg, with across-the-board reductions, which meant continued support for diverting Health Education Account funds into CHDP. Among the "writing/speaking points" was the comment that "the provisions of AB 75 (now AB 99) set forth a reasonable and fair system to improve health care and health education programs."[22] The strategy of the voluntaries was to move AB 99 through the Assembly and Senate as fast as possible so the Conference Committee could work at resolving differences among the groups and between AB 99 and the governor's budget. AB 99 passed in the Assembly Health Committee by a 12-0 vote on March 5, 1991, in the Assembly Ways and Means Committee by a 19-0 vote on March 20, and on the Assembly floor by a 68-0 vote on March 21.[23]

The health groups continued to ignore the original mandate for how the Proposition 99 money was to be spent, and they abandoned any interest in framing the issue as "obeying the will of the voters." Isenberg again chaired the legislative conference committee that was to draft new legislation. The bill to appropriate the Proposition 99 funds was AB 99. He was joined by the other original AB 75 Conference Committee members. A conference committee is very much an "insider" forum, often featuring bipartisan negotiation. When political parties engage in collusive or "bipartisan" policy making, especially when both are financed by the same special interests, the public is often excluded from the process, with no knowledge of what is being done and no chance to influence it.[24] The voluntaries had thus agreed to a fast-track process that gave them limited power. By sending the bill to a conference committee, tobacco control advocates lost the advantage of public debate and review, their chief source of power to protect Proposition 99.

THE TOBACCO INDUSTRY'S STRATEGY

Within RJ Reynolds, the governor's budget was welcomed as "the first positive news we have received relative to diverting funds from the Proposition 99 Tobacco Education Account."[25] According to a company memo, "In view of Governor Wilson's action, we anticipate a funding frenzy developing on the part of counties, health groups, and others to divert even more of the funds."[25]

An RJ Reynolds strategy memo of January 29 viewed the governor's budget as a window of opportunity and discussed what the company could do to "provide legislators with an additional reason to support the Governor's proposed budget shift." [26] The company's legislative strategy was twofold: provide the Legislature with evidence that a budget shift would be "consistent with the desires of voters" and would not "materially undermine the state's overall smoking and health efforts given industry and RJR initiated programs." [26] The memo reported on a company survey showing that only 33 percent of voters believed the media campaign was effective and that 37 percent felt they learned nothing from the advertisements.

The industry also explored the feasibility of shifting anti-tobacco education money away from the anti-smoking advertising campaign and into the schools, which the industry considered less threatening. The RJ Reynolds memo observed, "School education and increased parental involvement are seen as the most effective ways to discourage underage smoking—35% and 19% respectively. While this does not speak directly to Prop 99 advertising, it does speak to the importance of 'traditional' forms of education." [26] The plan was to mount a credible campaign to demonstrate that the industry could handle the youth issue itself, because "underage smoking is widely perceived as the most critical problem and single largest impediment to industry credibility." However, the memo concluded with the comment that "any credible attempt to address the youth smoking issue must include a school/youth group program given public opinion on the importance of school education." [26]

THE FINAL NEGOTIATIONS

By June 1991, the CMA's board of directors had endorsed a resolution supporting the governor's proposed reallocation from the Health Education Account to AIM, thus ending any pretense to preserve the status quo. They also supported the reallocation of money from the Physician's Services Account to AIM because those funds "would be used for insurance programs that are likely to pay much higher reimbursement levels to physicians than the maximum of 50% of amount billed that is authorized under Prop 99. There are also significant surpluses being accumulated in Prop 99 Physician Service Accounts which are dedicated to paying for emergency, pediatric and obstetrical services." [27]

On June 13, 1991, Senator Diane Watson wrote to the Legislative Counsel, the Legislature's lawyer, asking whether Health Education Account monies could be used to fund the new AIM program for expanded medical care for low-income women. The Legislative Counsel replied that Proposition 99

> specifically limits the use of the funds in the Health Education Account for programs for the prevention and reduction of tobacco use, primarily among children, through school and community health education programs. . . . *These funds cannot be used for purposes other than programs for the prevention and reduction of tobacco use.* A program for expanded prenatal care is not a program for the prevention and reduction of tobacco use, through school and community health education programs, except to the extent that the program might involve education to prevent or reduce the use of tobacco by prospective parents.[28] [emphasis added]

The Legislative Counsel advised that the Legislature could divert Health Education money to medical services only by returning to the voters with a new statute; a four-fifths vote of the Legislature would not suffice because such diversions were not consistent with the intent of Proposition 99.[28]

The legislative process was not disturbed by this legal opinion pronouncing the diversions illegal, nor by subsequent opinions requested by Isenberg and Elizabeth Hill, the Legislative Analyst.[29,30] The CMA, the Western Center for Law and Poverty, the California Nurses Association, and CAHHS wrote to the Conference Committee on June 30, 1991, suggesting language to strengthen the rationale for funding AIM through the Health Education Account. To make these medical programs appear to be anti-smoking education programs, the organizations wanted to add the clause "Health Education Services, smoking prevention, and where appropriate, smoking cessation services also shall be required." [31]

The voluntaries ended up supporting the diversion into AIM. The ALA argued, as it had done with CHDP, that it would be "a one-time grant of $27 million to provide tobacco related services to this population. Authorization of AIM incorporates and specifies the services to be provided. We believe this will be a one time allocation." [32] Both the ALA newsletter and an earlier Action Alert sent from all three voluntaries emphasized that this was a legal and appropriate compromise:

> With the support of some important allies, the tri-agencies developed a counterproposal to the governor's AIM proposal. Our proposal honors the governor's desire to provide perinatal care to low-income women, yet most importantly, presents an alternative funding mechanism which *does not inappropriately or illegally use Health Education Account monies.* Our proposal

provides a coordinated and integrated approach to a perinatal community-based program with an anti-tobacco health education component.[33] [emphasis in original]

In addition, the voluntary health agencies continued to support funding for CHDP. The ALA newsletter summarized their position:

Our agreement also committed us to support the full caseload of services to young children in the Child Health and Disability Program (CHDP). We have in the past, sponsored most of this service ($20 million annually) in order to provide anti-tobacco services and referrals to these children and their families. Our expanded CHDP responsibilities are expected to total $35 million a year. This is an ongoing commitment, though AB 99 required much closer auditing of the CHDP program in order to assure that needed services are being provided.[32]

The statement is noteworthy in its reference to CHDP as "an ongoing commitment" and in its reference to CHDP funding as "our expanded CHDP responsibilities," implying an agreement that CHDP would be a Health Education Account expense.

The voluntaries agreed to the diversion on June 30.[34] John Miller later recalled that, during the negotiations, "the legislative leadership came down on me and demanded that I give up $20 million, and I looked at the program and figured, 'What can I give up that's least harmful?' And I came up with Local Leads because they weren't always the wonder boys we all think of them now."[35] The Sacramento insiders had been leery about giving money to the local level in 1989 under AB 75 and were willing to reduce their funding now to get a compromise. The tobacco industry would not have objected. The local programs were costing the industry considerable time and money, and stopping the local programs had already become an industry priority.

AB 99 EMERGES

The legislature eventually adopted AB 99, which authorized expenditures from the Health Education, Physician Services, Medical Services, and Unallocated Accounts until 1994. The final version of the bill diverted increasing amounts of Health Education Account money into medical services. The Legislature took $27 million out of the Health Education Account for the AIM program, and CHDP's budget went from $20 million to $35 million a year. In an action that was to have a major impact at the local level, the LLAs were required to spend one-third of their allocation on perinatal outreach programs in their counties. Known as Comprehensive Perinatal Outreach (CPO), this county-based program identifies pregnant women who should be receiving medical care and brings them into the medical care system. The program itself does not offer any services; it merely performs outreach activities. All three of these programs—AIM, CHDP, and CPO—were supposed to have a tobacco education component. The closest any of them came to meeting this requirement was a CHDP form with three questions about tobacco use.

The voluntaries supported using some of the LLA money for outreach to pregnant women "in exchange for the provision of anti-tobacco education."[32] But CPO did not provide anti-tobacco education; it took LLA money that had been used to deliver tobacco programs and shifted it to an outreach effort (like AIM) that would bring women into medical services. The immediate result was fewer tobacco programs because of the redirection of LLA funds; there would be fewer still if AIM needed more money, because AIM had "protected status."

The protected status stemmed from another move that would have a major impact on the anti-tobacco education programs. A clause known as Section 43 was added to AB 99 to guarantee funding for five medical services programs—MediCal Perinatal Programs, AIM, the Major Risk Medical Insurance Program (MRMIP), CHDP, and the County Medical Services Program. Thus, these programs were guaranteed money "off the top" to fund them in the face of declining revenues; the other Proposition 99 programs were cut to support the "protected" ones. This provision, combined with the overall decline in Proposition 99 revenues because of its success in reducing tobacco consumption, promised to wipe out the anti-tobacco education programs over a period of a few years.

Neither the voluntaries nor Miller noticed the Section 43 language when it was added. When they were later interviewed about AB 99, Miller and Najera both expressed bitterness about Section 43. According to Miller, "The Section 43 crap . . . we all come to agreement, we divide the money up, we settle it all. The bill goes out to print, and it's before the Legislature, it goes most of the way through the system and Department of Finance said, 'Oh, oh, one little thing more. We need to stick in this provision to protect it or the Governor doesn't go along with this deal.' We look at it and it says, 'We need to tinker with the numbers to make it come out right. We need to protect some programs.' Okay, do it."[35] Najera added, "We didn't understand what Section 43 was until after it happened and the Department of Finance started coming after that. . . . It just happened, it was just one thing that was thrown in there." [35]

The voluntaries were at a significant disadvantage in staying abreast of important technical details like Section 43, especially compared with the medical care groups, because of the size and depth of their lobbying staffs. Proposition 99 was generating around $500 million a year, making the voluntary health agencies major stakeholders, but they had not expanded their policy analysis capabilities or lobbying presence in Sacramento since the passage of Proposition 99. The devastating long-term effects of Section 43 emerged from policy research and analysis at UC San Francisco.[4]

After the governor signed AB 99, ALA's newsletter announced, "We are pleased to communicate that all the Health Education Programs are in place, functioning and authorized for three more years." [32] The main virtues of AB 99 were that the sunset date was three years away, and, according to the *Los Angeles Times,* the Wilson administration had promised Najera that it would not try to divert any more funds for at least the next three years in exchange for the deal.[36] The ALA's optimistic statement, however, masked a different reality. Rather than the status quo that the voluntaries expected when they allowed AB 99 to be handled through the Conference Committee process, AB 99 represented significant damage to Proposition 99 anti-tobacco education programs. In 1991–1992, of the $151 million available in the Health Education Account, only about half ($78 million) was actually going to tobacco prevention programs. The voluntary health agencies had completely capitulated to the medical interests. In doing so, they abandoned their strongest argument: that the Legislature had an obligation to appropriate Proposition 99 Health Education funds for anti-tobacco education efforts as directed by the voters. Instead, they accepted the reality of insider horse-trading over the budget.

THE GOVERNOR TRIES TO KILL THE MEDIA CAMPAIGN

Governor Wilson finally gave the tobacco industry what it wanted in January 1992: he shut down the media campaign.

Although Wilson had included the media campaign in his 1991–1992 budget, he imposed increasingly tight political control over it as his first year in office unfolded. According to Ken Kizer, director of DHS, the Governor's Office immediately wanted the advertisements toned down and even started to review them.[37] DHS was no longer able to operate free of political interference in mounting its effective campaign to reduce tobacco use.

In his budget for the 1992–1993 fiscal year, released on January 10, 1992, Wilson went one step further and eliminated the media campaign entirely.[38] Moreover, rather than waiting for the Legislature to act, the governor had already ordered DHS not to sign the just-negotiated contract with the keye/donna/perlstein advertising agency, which had been going to continue the campaign on January 1, 1992.[39,40]

The media campaign went dark.

Dr. Molly Joel Coye, whom Wilson had appointed to replace Ken Kizer as DHS director, defended the decision to kill the media campaign.[41] Coye was a dramatic change from Kizer. Whereas Kizer had been a strong program advocate and defender, Coye was not; she followed the governor's orders and remained aloof from the tobacco control community. According to Jennie Cook, "Molly was different. You could never get an audience with Molly. She was never available."[42] Coye vigorously pushed the administration line that the local programs funded by Proposition 99 were a more effective use of resources and that the smoking decrease following the beginning of the media campaign was actually part of a trend that began in 1987 rather than the result of the anti-smoking advertising campaign.[43–45] In an opinion editorial in the *Sacramento Bee,* Coye claimed that "the revenues from Proposition 99 are being diverted for only one reason: to cope with the worst budget crisis in California's history. . . . If the tobacco industry is pleased with this temporary shift, it couldn't be more wrong."[46] In fact, when the media campaign was suspended, the decline in tobacco consumption slowed.

While Governor Wilson justified the decision to eliminate the media campaign by pointing to the state's fiscal crisis, no one in the public health community believed him. Assembly Member Lloyd Connelly (D-Sacramento), the primary legislative force behind the original Proposition 99, expressed a view that was widely held within the public health community: "During the Proposition 99 campaign and the intense negotiations surrounding the implementation legislation, the provisions most virulently opposed by the tobacco industry were those that created the Health Education Account, including the enormously successful TV and radio antismoking ad campaign. Can it be just a coincidence that—after being wined and dined by the tobacco industry last summer—that it is precisely that account which has been gutted? I do not think so."[20]

The governor was, in fact, more interested in killing the media campaign than in weighing how the money was being spent. At a March 16 hearing on the budget, held by the Senate Budget and Fiscal Review Subcommittee on Health, the Legislative Analyst indicated that the proposed diversions were inappropriate uses of the Health Education monies and that only the voters could make that reallocation.[47] The governor then proposed to shift the money to an AIDS testing program, perhaps hoping to enlist the AIDS lobby in the effort to kill the media campaign. In response, the ALA claimed that "the Governor's real agenda was not to fund needed programs but to gut the media campaign in whatever way possible."[48] Kathy Dresslar, an aide to Assembly Member Connelly, agreed: "The fact that the governor has changed the reason why he wants to divert funds from the media account suggests he is less interested in health priorities than he is in gutting the media campaign."[20]

In any event, both the governor's action and the justification for eliminating the media campaign effectively implemented the tobacco industry's plan, dating from 1990, to work with a variety of minority groups, hospital groups, the CMA, and business groups to divert money from the media program into other health programs.[49] The tobacco industry publicly endorsed the governor's action: the Associated Press reported that "Tom Lauria of the Tobacco Institute, the industry's lobby, applauded the proposed elimination of a campaign that 'focused primarily on ridiculing industry . . . and basically put smokers in a bad light.'"[50]

In addition to citing the state's fiscal problems as the reason for suspending the media campaign, the administration claimed, without presenting any evidence, that the campaign was a waste of money because it did not work and that it was of "secondary" importance.

These claims about the media campaign's lack of importance and effectiveness were contradicted a few days later when John Pierce, a professor from the University of California at San Diego, released preliminary data from the California Tobacco Survey (a large statewide survey conducted under contract to DHS), of which he was director. Speaking at the AHA Science Writers Conference, Pierce said that the survey results demonstrated a 17 percent drop in adult smokers between 1987 (the year before Proposition 99 passed) and 1990. In 1987, 26.8 percent of adults smoked, compared with 22.2 percent in 1990. Pierce attributed this drop to the combined effects of the tax, educational efforts, and the media campaign.[51,52] Since the media campaign was the only part of the California Tobacco Control Program that was active during most of this period, Pierce identified it as the primary factor in this rapid fall.

Pierce's report made headlines. The *San Francisco Chronicle* proclaimed, "Anti-Smoking Program Big Hit—But Governor Seeks to Cut It." [45] Other major newspapers gave the study's results prominent coverage: "California Push to Cut Smoking Seen as Success" (*Wall Street Journal*); "Anti-Smoking Initiative Called Effective" (*Washington Post*); "Anti-Smoking Effort Working, Study Finds" (*Los Angeles Times*); "California Smokers Quitting" (*USA Today*).[52–55] Rather than claiming credit for this stunning public health success, the Wilson Administration attacked Pierce's result, claiming that the conclusions were overstated.[43,56,57] DHS's new spokeswoman was Betsy Hite, who had been one of the original advocates for Proposition 99 when she was the ACS lobbyist; now she vigorously defended eliminating the media campaign.

Hite pressured TCS staff members to falsify data about the effectiveness of the programs in support of the administration's claim that the media campaign was not responsible for the state's decline in tobacco consumption. Hite told Jacquolyn Duerr, then head of the TCS media campaign, to back up Hite's assertion that the smoking decline had nothing to do with Proposition 99. Duerr and Michael Johnson, the head of DHS's evaluation efforts, and Pierce's contract monitor, refused to comply.[58,59] Duerr wrote Dileep Bal, the head of the DHS Cancer Control Branch (which includes TCS), saying, "I want you to know that this is some of the most unprofessional behavior I have experienced in my state service tenure"; Johnson wrote, "I hope that something can be done very soon to stop this falsification of results." [59]

THE FIRST LITIGATION: ALA'S LAWSUIT

Shutting down the media campaign was too much for the ALA to swallow. In 1991 the ALA had been promised that, in exchange for accepting AB 99's diversion of funds, there would be no further diversions for the life of the legislation, which would not expire until June 1994. When asked why the agreements of previous years were not being honored, Kassy Perry, the governor's deputy communications director, responded, "That was last year. This is this year." [36]

Rather than allowing the media campaign to be shut down, the ALA filed a suit against Wilson and Coye on February 21, 1992, arguing that by refusing to sign the contract with the advertising agency, they had violated AB 99, which said that the DHS "shall" run an anti-tobacco media campaign. Significantly, ALA did not challenge the diversion of funds on the grounds that this move violated Proposition 99 itself. Bringing such a case might have been difficult since ALA had agreed to the diversions.

Neither AHA nor ACS joined ALA in its lawsuit, although ANR attempted to file a friend of the court brief. ACS was willing, if asked, to state privately its position that the cuts were illegal and a flagrant violation of the will of the people, but it refused to join in the suit. ACS thought it could achieve more working behind the scenes.[20] This view was surprising, since the evidence to date had indicated that health groups won in public venues and lost behind the scenes.

Jennie Cook, ACS lobbyist Theresa Velo, and AHA lobbyist Dian Kiser met with Bill Hauck, the governor's assistant deputy for policy, and Tom Hayes, the director of finance, while the lawsuit was in progress. Whereas ACS and AHA wanted to talk about the anti-smoking program generally, the administration officials seemed to care only about the lawsuit. According to Cook, "The first item on their agenda was the lawsuit. After we explained that our two organizations were not involved, the mood instantly changed and became much more positive."[60] Cook, Velo, and Kiser attempted to discuss the merits of the program, but Hauck and Hayes wanted to discuss budget problems. Cook continued, "They expressed concern regarding the media's interpretation that the Governor is proposing this [sic] cuts for the tobacco industry. They asked our organizations to help clarify these erroneous statements."[60] The ACS and AHA did not do so.

Hauck and Hayes apparently recommended that the ACS and AHA representatives talk to Russ Gould, the secretary of health and welfare. They did so, meeting with Gould and Kim Belshé, the deputy secretary for program and fiscal. (In 1993 Belshé would be named director of DHS, where she would be responsible for implementing Proposition 99. In 1988 she had been a spokesperson for the tobacco industry's No on Proposition 99 campaign.) According to Cook, "We informed them that we are not involved in the pending lawsuit, at which time their apprehensions dissipated."[61] As Cook reported to the ACS leadership,

> Gould explained California's fiscal dilemma and assured us that all accounts were looked into along with the Proposition 99 accounts. The decision was made to preserve only direct service funds (i.e., community-based programs). They felt that while the media campaign is a worthwhile program it does not provide direct services; same for the education and research accounts.
>
> They went into some depth explaining the devastating cuts they have to make and that they are uncomfortable with having to make these choices. They asked for an opportunity to reach out to our organizations to explain

the tight spot that the State is in at this time. Gould offered to attend an ACS Board of Directors to do just that.

Finally, we requested that we keep an open channel of communication with the Agency through one knowledgeable individual. They both indicated that Belshe would fulfill that role; Belshe invited us to call her to discuss the issue on an on-going basis.

In conclusion, this meeting was very productive in establishing a direct line of communication with the Health & Welfare Agency.[61]

Administration officials were happy to communicate with ACS and AHA. But the communication did not lead to any policy changes.

When asked in 1998 about ACS's decision not to join the 1992 ALA lawsuit, Cook, who was by then the national chair of the ACS board and the chair of TEOC, said, "Cancer and Heart were still a little timid to get into lawsuits. Lung led the way and I think the fact that Lung won it with no real big problem made the other two feel that, 'maybe it's time we spoke up.' It wasn't that we didn't want to, it's just that—the old saying about, 'we were using public funds and we felt that that's not what the public gave us money for was to sue the governor.' Today, it's a little different [laughter]."[42] In 1992 ACS was unwilling to confront the Wilson Administration in a public forum where the ACS's high public credibility gave it strength. Cook commented that ACS's preference was to avoid confrontation, to "maneuver it, consider it, talk it out, be diplomatic. What we discovered is where tobacco is concerned, you can't be that way."[42]

On April 24, 1992, the ALA won in court when Judge James Ford of Sacramento Superior Court ruled that Wilson did not have the authority to take funds appropriated for one purpose and use them for another; Ford ordered that the money be used for the authorized media campaign. The big question following the ALA victory was whether the governor would appeal the Superior Court's decision. An appeal would freeze the status quo and keep the media campaign off the air while the case made its way through the courts—possibly for a year or more.

Wilson had appointed Molly Coye director of health services, effective May 29, 1991. Under California law, she could serve for up to one year before she was confirmed by the Senate. If, however, the Senate did not confirm her by the so-called drop-dead date, she would have to leave office. Because of unrelated controversies, the Senate was taking up the matter of Coye's appointment as the litigation over the media campaign was coming to a head. The AHA, which had declined to join the lawsuit, then entered the world of hardball politics.

The AHA convinced the Senate Rules Committee to hold up Coye's confirmation until the deadline for filing an appeal in the media case had passed. At a tense hearing regarding Coye's confirmation, the administration lined up around fifty witnesses to support her, including the CMA, CAHHS, and many other medical organizations. (ALA and ACS took no position on Coye's confirmation.) In the face of this support, Kiser, the AHA's lobbyist, attended the hearing and read a prepared statement that she and Glantz had written, urging the Senate to delay action on Coye's confirmation.[62] The statement read:

> Dr. Coye is responsible for overseeing the Health Education Account, including several key components such as the media campaign, the California tobacco survey, and various grants programs to community-based organizations.
>
> The American Heart Association has serious reservations regarding the way these components are being implemented.
>
> These concerns have led the American Heart Association to seriously consider questioning Dr. Coye's confirmation. However, we would like to suggest a positive alternative and that would be to defer her confirmation until she has had an opportunity to remedy the problems that have been created in the implementation of Proposition 99.[63]

That statement went on to stipulate that Coye "execute the media contract that had been awarded, and see that the contractor can continue the campaign free of political interference."[63]

At her May 6 hearing Coye pledged, "I make the commitment and the Governor makes the commitment. We do not plan to appeal the decision."[64] The governor did not appeal the court decision, Coye was confirmed, the media campaign resumed, and tobacco consumption started to drop again in California. By the end of the 1993–1994 budget period, Californians had consumed 1.6 billion fewer packs of cigarettes (equaling $2 billion in pretax sales) than they would have if historical pre–Proposition 99 consumption patterns had been maintained (figure 13).

The episode demonstrated once more that the anti-tobacco groups exercised the most power in public forums outside of legislative back rooms. In contrast to the tobacco industry and medical interests, which provide substantial campaign contributions to politicians, the health groups get their power from public opinion and public pressure. ALA, which had led the movement to work around the legislative process when it developed Proposition 99, once again succeeded by going outside the Legislature, this time to the courts. AHA solidified ALA's victory by publicly confronting the administration over Coye's confirmation. Pro-

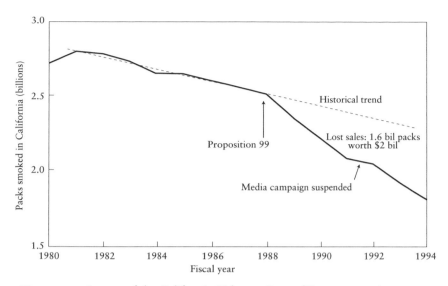

Figure 13.   Impact of the California Tobacco Control Program on cigarette consumption through 1994. Passage and implementation of Proposition 99 was associated with a rapid decline in cigarette consumption in California. During 1991, the year that Governor Pete Wilson took the media campaign off the air and blocked many local programs, the decline stopped. It resumed when the program started up a year later.

gram advocates would eventually use the courts again to leverage the legislative process.

THE 1992–1993 BUDGET FIGHT

In his budget for fiscal year 1992–1993, released in January 1992, Wilson again ignored the deal that he had made with the health groups by diverting the $16 million allocated to the anti-tobacco media campaign into medical care.[38,65] He also proposed to eliminate the school-based anti-tobacco programs.[20] In the first attack on the Research Account, he ignored Proposition 99 and the implementing legislation (SB 1613) by cutting the Research Account from 5 percent to less than 3 percent of tobacco tax revenues. Like the other "temporary" shifts, the ones proposed by the governor in 1992 were part of a continuing downward spiral in the amount of money allocated to Proposition 99's Health Education and Research programs.

The Budget Conference Committee agreed to $80 million of the $123 million allocation for education and research that the governor proposed to divert into medical services during fiscal years 1991–1992 and 1992–1993. The cuts for 1992–1993 completely eliminated the $26 million for school-based programs, cut the media campaign in half to $7 million, and reduced the research program by $12 million.[66] The public health groups opposed these cuts.[67]

The ALA asked its attorney, George Waters, for a formal legal opinion regarding the diversions of Health Education and Research money into medical services. In an extensive opinion that mirrored those offered earlier by the Legislative Counsel, Waters advised the ALA that such diversions were illegal:

> We conclude that funds in the Health Education and Research accounts cannot be used to fund health care programs. . . .
>
> The drafters of Proposition 99 obviously paid a great deal of attention to how the Tobacco Fund would be divided up. The language is very specific. The intent of the drafters, and by extension the intention of the electorate, was to make a fixed percentage of the Tobacco Fund available for specific purposes and specific purposes only.
>
> This conclusion is buttressed by the Voters Pamphlet description of Proposition 99. The Voters Pamphlet is an approved source for the determination of the legislative intent behind a ballot measure. . . . [and] contains the following analysis of the Legislative Analyst:
>
>> The measure *requires* the revenues from the additional taxes to be spent for the following purposes:
>>
>>> Health Education. *Twenty percent must be used for the prevention and reduction of tobacco use,* primarily among children, through school and community health education programs.
>
> Given the above, we are reasonably confident that we can set aside in court any attempt to use monies in the Health Education and Research accounts for any purposes other than health education and research.[68] [emphasis in original]

The ALA chose not to sue. Instead, it made another deal.

On July 15, 1992, ten senators and twenty-seven assembly members signed a letter to Senator Alfred Alquist (D-San Jose), the Budget Conference Committee chair, protesting the committee's action in redirecting Health Education and Research monies to medical service programs. According to the letter, the redirection of these funds violated the public trust, violated the constitutionally protected statutory provisions of Proposition 99, and would disrupt the programs wrongfully receiving the money when it had to be returned to appropriate uses. On July 17, however, the Budget Committee reaffirmed its decision to divert the money.[69]

In opposing the diversions, the health groups created a procedural problem for the forces seeking to dismantle the Health Education and Research programs. This issue had not come up in earlier budget bills because the health groups supported the diversions; the associated legislation, passed by lopsided majorities, had gone unchallenged in the courts. The ALA had gone to court once—over the media campaign in 1992—and won. This time, the health groups were opposing the diversions.

On August 7, 1992, Peter Schilla of the Western Center for Law and Poverty wrote to Assembly Speaker Willie Brown to urge him to separate the Proposition 99 diversions from the remainder of the budget on the grounds that it would be difficult to get a four-fifths vote on the entire state budget.[70] The budget needed only a two-thirds vote to pass, and Schilla and others were arguing that the money could be diverted because of the language in the initiative that permitted the Legislature to enact amendments to Proposition 99 by a four-fifths vote, so long as the amendments were "consistent with its purposes." (Critics were arguing that any reductions in the Health Education and Research programs below 20 percent and 5 percent would not be "consistent with the intent" of the initiative.) Brown followed Schilla's advice, removing the Proposition 99 accounts from the budget bill and placing them in separate bills that would be easier to pass under the four-fifths requirement.[71]

In the end, the bills did not come to a vote. The health groups agreed to a last-minute compromise in which most funding for the media campaign, competitive grants, and schools was restored. The LLA programs, however, took a major cut—from $24 million to $12 million. According to Najera, "In assessing where to amputate, the politicians had to make flash comparisons of the relative return between the different parts of the anti-tobacco program. One strong argument on cutting local leads was that much of the county funds were already spent on direct medical services, and thus the loss of local funding was diminished by whatever amount went to non-tobacco services."[69] From the standpoint of a county's total revenues, this statement might have been true. But the cuts to the LLA would not be offset by money for local medical services. Moreover, the requirement that one-third of LLA money be diverted into the CPO medical services program remained, which amplified the effects of the LLA cuts. The local programs would be forced to absorb large cuts just as they were hitting their stride.

The LLAs were eventually rescued because of the fallout from an unrelated political battle between the Legislature and the governor over funding for community colleges. It turned out that the Legislature did not need the Health Education money to pay for medical services; they instead diverted $21 million from the Health Education Account to community colleges. The governor vetoed this appropriation, and on October 1, 1992, the Department of Finance issued a letter returning this money to CDE, competitive grants, and the LLAs, as specified in AB 99.[72]

The attacks on the LLA budgets in both 1991 and 1992, along with the 1992 attack on the media campaign, were consistent with the tobacco industry's strategy to reduce Proposition 99's effectiveness. The LLAs were costing the tobacco industry time and money with their local ordinance work. Further, by educating minority communities about tobacco issues and bringing them into the tobacco control network, the LLAs and the competitive grants were weakening an industry power base.

The erosion of Proposition 99 continued.

POSITIONING FOR 1994

The continuing failure of CHDP and CPO to provide tobacco use prevention services was becoming an increasing irritant for tobacco control advocates. CPO was, in fact, mainly being used to get federal matching funds. At the county level, CPO programs were supported from two sources: Proposition 99 Health Education Account money and federal matching funds. This money had to be used exclusively for outreach; none could be used to deliver services. Counseling services, which included smoking cessation, did not qualify for federal matching funds.[73] Dr. Rugmini Shah, the director of the state-level DHS Maternal and Child Health (MCH) program, which administered CPO, defined outreach as "finding individuals who are not accessing services and bringing them into the service area system." Cessation classes could not be funded because "the women are already in here for the classes, so it's not outreach."[74] Thus, any Proposition 99 dollars that generated federal matching dollars could not be used for tobacco-related services.

At the November 1992 TEOC meeting, the CPO program was on the agenda. TEOC was concerned that the money was being used illegally to meet a federal match for perinatal outreach services and that the federal rules prohibited the use of state matching funds for any anti-tobacco activities.[75] At the January 1993 TEOC meeting, MCH was able to tell TEOC that $7 million of the Health Education dollars given to MCH went to the federal matching program and that only nine of the fifty-eight counties provided cessation training components.[76] By the March 1993 meeting, the dollar figure for matching had gone up to $8 million, with only $216,000 not qualifying for matching funds. TEOC chair Carolyn Martin called this "a gigantic rip-off of the Health Education Account dollars."[76]

In contrast to their earlier positions, the health groups and their representatives on TEOC were now openly challenging the appropriateness of using Health Education funds for medical services. In submitting the 1993–1995 Master Plan for California's Tobacco Control Program to the members of the Legislature, Cook and Martin wrote to the legislators on behalf of the TEOC:

> We are particularly alarmed by the fact that funding for the CHDP Program continues to expand, yet we have little idea of what CHDP is doing with these funds and no evaluation of its impact. Physicians in CHDP respond to three vague and inexact questions related to tobacco use, second-hand smoke and counseling. The data generated through this protocol is essentially useless. Improving the protocol, which the California Department of Health Service has indicated its willingness to do, might help. However, to date as far as we can ascertain, despite the large funding provided to it, *the CHDP Program has contributed nothing to tobacco control.*
>
> In addition, the one-third of the money set aside in the Local Lead Agency grants for tobacco-related Maternal and Child Health activities *is being used for outreach, without any tobacco education component, despite the legal requirement in Proposition 99 that funds be used only . . . for programs for the prevention and reduction of tobacco use.*[77] [emphasis added]

Tobacco control advocates were beginning to be openly critical of the diversions from the Health Education and Research Accounts to medical services.

Coye resigned as DHS director in September 1993. On November 9 the governor named S. Kimberly Belshé as her successor. Although Belshé had been working in the administration since 1989, she was not a physician, as both Coye and Kizer had been. At thirty-three, she had worked primarily in public relations. More alarming to tobacco control advocates was the role that Belshé had played in 1988 as the tobacco industry's Southern California spokeswoman against Proposition 99.[78] Belshé defended her past association with the tobacco industry, saying that she had opposed Proposition 99 for fiscal reasons.[79] Her proposed appointment did little to reassure advocates of the Health Education and Research programs that they would receive the protection for which Kizer had fought. Her lack of medical credentials notwithstanding, the CMA supported her appointment.[80]

AB 99 continued in force for the 1993–1994 budget year, and the governor's budget for 1993–1994 contained no major raids on the Health Education Account except for those required by Section 43. Section 43, however, led to three cuts to the anti-tobacco program during 1993–1994. Tax revenues ultimately fell by 8 percent between 1992–1993 and 1993–1994, but expenditures for anti-tobacco education fell by 31 percent.[81] The discrepancy between the funding allocation in Proposition 99 and the actual expenditure of funds continued to widen.

While turning a blind eye to the needs of the Tobacco Control Program, the Legislature acceded to pressure from breast cancer research advocates to increase the tax on cigarettes by two cents a pack. The new tax funded a breast cancer research program administered by the University of California similar to the Tobacco Related Disease Research Program. The tobacco industry did not seriously oppose this tax. Aside from the modest increase in price, it did nothing to reduce tobacco consumption. It did, however, offer some political cover for Speaker Brown, Governor Wilson, and the CMA when they were criticized for failing to implement Proposition 99 as the voters intended.

Even though Proposition 99 created a large constituency in the field through the LLAs and local coalitions, these people and organizations were not involved in the dealings in Sacramento throughout AB 99. The Sacramento lobbyists made only a minimal effort to engage these new players in the legislative process, and the local activists were preoccupied with getting the anti-tobacco program up and running. According to ANR co-director Robin Hobart,

> There was still some sort of incursions into the Health Education Account, but they still, at that point, seemed small and not worth spending the kind of political capital that you would have to spend to deal with it. We were busy passing hundreds of local ordinances by that time in California and emphasized our role as helping the local lead agencies get their coalitions in order and start working on grassroots organizing around local ordinance campaigns. We were probably doing trainings about every other month, especially during the first two years, sometimes multiple times in a month. That's where a lot of our energy and emphasis was going.[82]

But the people in the field who were implementing the Health Education program were growing tired of the way the money was being taken away and tired of the rules under which they were forced to operate. Meanwhile, no anti-smoking components had been added to CHDP, CPO, or any other health service programs. Moreover, no evaluations were conducted to test whether CHDP, CPO, and AIM had anything to do with tobacco control, despite pressure from TEOC chair Carolyn Martin.

THE GOVERNOR KILLS THE RESEARCH ACCOUNT

In 1989 the Research Account had been authorized by separate legislation, SB 1613, which did not expire until December 31, 1993. The governor had made several proposals to reduce funding for tobacco-related research in his budgets, but the Research Account did not surface in the battle over AB 99, which dealt only with the Health Education Account and the medical services accounts. In 1992 and 1993, Wilson tried to cut the Research Account but withdrew the proposals when it became clear that they lacked support in the Legislature.

As SB 1613 stipulated, the University of California managed the Research Account using a peer review process modeled on the National Institutes of Health. Applicants from qualifying public and nonprofit institutions (not just the University of California) submitted proposals for research projects that were judged and graded by committees of out-of-state experts. The university funded the projects in order according to their grades.

The university chose to define "tobacco-related research" broadly. As a result, most of the money went to traditional biomedical research with little or no direct connection to tobacco.[83] The university's failure to concentrate more directly on tobacco angered tobacco control advocates, who wanted a more tobacco-specific program. Some of the research was very closely tied to tobacco, however, and became the target of attacks by the tobacco industry, its front groups, and their allies.

In particular, Glantz had won a grant in the first year of the program to study the tobacco industry's response to the tobacco control movement. This research had evolved into a detailed analysis of how the tobacco industry was working to influence the Legislature as well as how Proposition 99 was being implemented. With funding from this grant, Glantz and his coworkers published a series of monographs detailing campaign contributions to members of the Legislature and other politicians as well as documenting the erosion of Proposition 99 funding for anti-tobacco education.[3,4,81,84,85] The monographs highlighted the diversions of Health Education Account funds to medical services and the long-term implications of Section 43.

These reports infuriated the tobacco industry, the Legislature, and the CMA. The industry and its allies vigorously attacked Glantz and his work as well as the University of California for funding the studies. They claimed that this work was "politics" rather than "research," despite the politics that controlled passage of Proposition 99's implementing legislation. The reports that regularly documented the accelerating campaign contributions to Assembly Speaker Willie Brown particularly enraged Brown (who by 1993 had received $474,217 in campaign contributions from the industry, more than any other state or federal legislator). At one point Brown found himself in an elevator with the director of UCSF's Institute for Health Policy Studies (which was located in the same San Francisco office building as Brown's district office), and Brown demanded that something be done to silence Glantz. In a meeting with the university's vice president for health affairs, Cornelius Hopper, Brown again attacked Glantz. A journalist who was writing a profile of Brown observed, "One morning in a sudden burst of temper, Brown pitilessly dressed down top executives of the University of California because a researcher at UCSF had written a report that Brown didn't like about the political influence of tobacco companies. The university officials had come to see him on an unrelated matter, but the Speaker used the opportunity to launch his attack anyway. 'You're going to have trouble with me on *every* single appropriation!' Brown said, jabbing an index finger. 'If that guy gets one more cent of state money, you'll have trouble with me!'" (emphasis in original).[86] Hopper responded that the university believed in academic freedom and would not interfere with Glantz's work or the peer review process.

The process of reauthorizing the Research Account proceeded without much public controversy during 1993. There was some sparring between health advocates and university officials in an attempt to force the university to focus more specifically on scientific and policy issues that were directly related to tobacco, but the university successfully opposed this effort. Before SB 1613 expired on December 31, 1993, the Legislature had unanimously passed SB 1088 to continue the program until 1997. The governor surprised everyone when he vetoed the bill, stating, "This program should not be extended for four years when expenditure authority for all other Proposition 99 funded programs pertaining to health and research will be reviewed during the 1994 legislative session. This program should be reviewed and re-evaluated in the context of all Proposition 99 funded programs and activities to insure the most effective use of those funds."[87]

Wilson's veto effectively shut down the research program. Many were suspicious that Wilson's action was making good on Brown's earlier threat to punish the university if it did not quiet Glantz. Ironically, by the time Wilson killed the Research program, Glantz was being funded by the National Cancer Institute, not Proposition 99.

The governor's veto also meant that the funds allocated for research in the first six months of 1994—$21 million—suddenly became available for other programs. The Research Account money was soon put into play in a manner that would make it easier during the next legislative fight over Proposition 99 authorization to divert the funds into medical services.

CONCLUSION

As memories of the Proposition 99 election faded, legislators could more readily ignore public opinion and the public will unless the voluntary health agencies and other guardians of Proposition 99 found ways to activate and use public opinion. Instead, the groups attempted to play the insider game and were not successful. For five years tobacco control advocates, using an insider strategy, had tried to protect their programs against the tobacco industry, the CMA, other medical service providers, the Western Center for Law and Poverty, and the governor. This approach of working within the Legislature meant abandoning the health groups' most potent weapon: public opinion. In general, the years of AB 75 and AB 99 were characterized by a series of struggles testing the resolve of the guardian groups and by their general unwillingness to fight back.

During the period 1990–1994 the issue of money for health education and research had increasingly been framed as a budget battle, which was damaging for the voluntary agencies trying to maintain these programs. California's economic recession provided a cover for those who wanted to take the money out of the Health Education Account. When Assembly Member Richard Katz (D-Panorama City), a tobacco control advocate in the Legislature, was asked in 1997 if this had really been a budget fight, he said "not really":

> I think all along they [the administration] wanted to help big tobacco. I think it's obvious from the last couple of years in terms of their desire to muzzle or censor some of the advertising that Health Services had done. I think in their

desire to screw with the research that the University of California does that they have been fronting for big tobacco. The budget issue made it convenient. In terms of the overall budget, it's not a lot of money. . . . I don't know who came up with it, it was a very, very clever strategy that helps big tobacco under the guise of providing indigent health care.[88]

In agreeing to the use of Health Education funds for medical services, the voluntary health agencies made this problem worse for themselves. Rather than standing for implementation of Proposition 99 as enacted by the voters, the question became whether the diversions were too large —hardly one that would rally public support.

The one major move outside the Capitol—when ALA filed a lawsuit in 1992 over the media campaign funding—did generate publicity and protection for this program. Significantly, the lawsuit was based on the governor's refusal to implement AB 99 rather than on the broader issue of AB 99's inconsistency with Proposition 99. As parties to the AB 99 compromise, insiders at the ALA were not yet ready to make the more fundamental policy argument: that the governor and the Legislature had violated the voters' mandate and acted illegally in diverting Health Education Account funds into medical services.

The environmental movement, through the Planning and Conservation League and Gerald Meral, had been instrumental in creating Proposition 99. As part of the deal made in 1987 when Proposition 99 was being written, the Public Resources Account was to receive 5 percent of the Proposition 99 revenues for public lands and resources. In 1990 the environmentalists decided to increase their share of revenues by securing part of the Unallocated Account for environmental purposes. They passed Proposition 117, which set up protections for California mountain lions and directed that funding from this program come from the Unallocated Account, so environmental programs began to receive more than 5 percent of tobacco tax revenues. Throughout the fights to save the Health Education and Research programs, neither the Legislature nor the governor touched the Public Resources money—for medical services or anything else. The tobacco industry, after all, had no interest in diverting money from the Public Resources Account. In March 1992 John Miller observed, "[While] health education is more central to the initiative than the 5 percent that went to the environmental stuff," the Legislature "realized they could kick the hell out of the voluntary health organizations. . . . they don't have the political clout of the Sierra Club."[89] Ironically, voluntary health organizations such as AHA, ACS, and ALA consistently rank among the most trusted organizations in the public eye and could presumably muster political clout of their own.

The difference between these health organizations and the environmental groups, however, was in their willingness to confront politicians in the public arena; once Proposition 99 passed, the voters—the grassroots—were not involved. Proposition 99 had become a legislative game. As an LLA staff member and then as co-director of ANR, Robin Hobart conceded that, especially from Tony Najera's perspective, "the ends justified the means" in the early phase. She explained,

> If you have to give up a little bit to get relatively decent funding, then that was an okay deal to make. I don't know if he [Najera] was wrong about that or not the first year . . . but there was never really an attempt at any point in time to really seriously mount grassroots support for the reauthorization issue —the authorization issue and then the reauthorization issue. It always really was done inside Sacramento. We'd send out action alerts and the local units of the Lung and Heart and Cancer would send out Action Alerts, but it wasn't really a serious grassroots campaign. That doesn't really equal a serious grassroots effort.[82]

In 1989 the Legislature and the governor did not harm the Health Education and Research programs because the election was still close enough for the will of the voters to be felt. In subsequent years, the election would fade in the legislative and public memory. Without other efforts to bring public attention to the Proposition 99 expenditures, the preferences of the skilled, the experienced, and the powerful in the legislative insider game asserted themselves.

Between passage of Proposition 99 and the end of the 1993–1994 budget period, a total of $190 million that voters had allocated to anti-tobacco education was diverted into medical services. Despite these cuts, the anti-tobacco education program continued to depress tobacco consumption in California. While impressive, this reduction in tobacco consumption would likely have been even greater had there been no program disruptions (such as suspending the media campaign) or funding diversions.

CHAPTER 11

Battles over Preemption

The combined effects of existing local tobacco control ordinances and Proposition 99's resources for educating the public about the dangers of secondhand smoke dramatically accelerated the rate at which clean indoor air and other tobacco control ordinances were passing at the local level. By 1994, one or two local ordinances were passing every week in California, and the pace of activity was accelerating. The efforts to pass ordinances had raised public awareness about the health dangers of passive smoking, and the issue of clean indoor air was mobilizing the general public to support a broader tobacco control agenda.[1] As a result of this activity, by 1993, nearly two-thirds of California's workers were protected by local laws mandating entirely smoke-free workplaces, and more than four-fifths (87 percent) were subject to some restrictions on workplace smoking.[2-5] Not only did this trend lead to ordinances and other tobacco control policies that protected nonsmokers from secondhand smoke, but the very battle for these protections engaged the community in a way that undercut the social support network for tobacco use that the tobacco industry had spent decades and billions of dollars building.

The tobacco industry viewed this development with great alarm. As early as January 11, 1991, in its plan entitled *California: A Multifaceted Plan to Address the Negative Environment,* the Tobacco Institute's State Activities Division set as one of its long-term strategies "Adopt a reasonable statewide smoking law, with preemption."[6] Preemption is the process whereby a state legislature (or Congress) takes away the right of lesser political subdivisions to enact laws in a certain policy area. Preemption has been the tobacco industry's central strategy for stopping public health activities since 1965, when it convinced Congress to preempt state and local regulation of cigarette labeling and advertising. By December 1990, the industry had succeeded in getting six states to pass legislation preempting communities from passing ordinances pertaining to clean indoor air, youth access to tobacco, and other tobacco control measures.[7]

In the early 1990s there were three major battles over preemption in California: in 1991 with Senate Bill 376 and in 1993 with Assembly Bills 13 and 996. SB 376 was the tobacco industry's first attempt to get the Legislature to pass a preemptive state bill. Tobacco control advocates stopped it. In 1993 Assembly Member Terry Friedman (D-Santa Monica), a friend of public health, introduced a smoke-free workplace law as AB 13; while generally acceptable to health groups, it included preemption of local clean indoor air ordinances.[8] The tobacco industry responded with a competing weak bill, AB 996. Despite divisions in the public health community on the wisdom of AB 13, it eventually passed. At the same time, the public health community stopped the tobacco industry's AB 996. Motivated by the accelerating pace of local ordinance activity and the possibility that AB 13 would pass, Philip Morris, followed reluctantly by the rest of the tobacco industry, tried to overturn all of California's local (and state) tobacco control ordinances with a statewide voter initiative, Proposition 188, masquerading as an anti-smoking measure. The public health community put its differences over AB 13 aside, unified, and defeated Philip Morris and the other tobacco companies at the polls.

SB 376: THE FIRST THREAT OF PREEMPTION

The tobacco industry recognized that it had a serious problem in California because the advocates of local tobacco control were well aware of the industry's strategy of preemption, and they were watching the Legislature carefully. To get advice on how to deal with this problem, Philip Morris flew Assembly Speaker Willie Brown and several other legislators (and their escorts) to New York for a secret meeting in November 1990.[9-11] Brown suggested a three-part strategy. First, the proposed legislation should preempt local tobacco control efforts. Second, since tobacco control was popular in California, the "perception" of a comprehensive regulatory scheme would be essential for preemption of smoking restrictions to pass. Third, the tobacco industry should give the impression of opposing the bill.[9]

The speaker's approach was spelled out in a June 28, 1991, memo from Michael Kerrigan, the head of the Smokeless Tobacco Council (the Tobacco Institute's counterpart for spit tobacco), to his management committee summarizing his conference call with representatives of Philip Morris, RJ Reynolds, the Tobacco Institute, and their lawyers and lobbyists to discuss a proposed Comprehensive Tobacco Control Act in California:

> Kurt opened the call stating the purpose was to have a dialogue on policy questions that have arisen from the Philip Morris/Reynolds approach to seek preemption of public smoking restrictions within the state of California. Kurt positioned this issue by stating the 45 local battles that the T.I. [Tobacco Institute] is fighting concerning smoking restrictions in California, and that they have dealt with them by compromise, not by killing them. Therefore, he was trying to establish *the need for preemption of smoking restrictions* in the state of California and position, at least his concurrence, with the need for a preemptive strike in the state legislature. . . .
>
> Joe Lange reported on "where they are" and stated that while there were some technicalities still open for discussion, he had done a great deal of work on this matter. He stated Speaker [Willie] Brown and Assemblyman [Dick] Floyd visited a cigarette company in New York City last fall and met with the key executives of that company. At that time the Speaker made clear *a significantly more proactive tobacco control effort would be needed to secure preemption.* Out of those discussions the notion of a comprehensive Tobacco Control Act (that would provide preemption) evolved. In order to gain preemption, the Speaker wanted "a Comprehensive Tobacco Control Act along the lines of the alcohol model." The Speaker believes the trick to doing this would be that *such an act would have to have the "appearance" of a comprehensive scheme.* Joe stated that leadership in both chambers are aware of and support this effort. Joe stated that the chances for success, in his judgment are very good because the key players have all been involved. However, *the chances of success depended upon the "perception" that the act was comprehensive.* . . .
>
> The conversation shifted to Joe stating Speaker Brown and Chairman Floyd would attempt to *make the Tobacco Control Act as close as possible in "appearance" to the concepts that the anti-tobacco groups were fostering.* Amazingly, that shuddering thought had no discussion.[9] [emphasis added]

Whatever the Smokeless Tobacco Council ultimately decided about Brown's proposal, it is clear that the cigarette companies worked to implement it. On July 11 SB 376 was amended to propose weak preemptive smoking restrictions following a Tobacco Institute draft. Brown was delivering for the tobacco industry. SB 376 cleared the Assembly Government Organization Committee, a committee that had been historically friendly to the tobacco industry.

The industry's effort was derailed when the Smokeless Tobacco Council memo appeared mysteriously at the offices of the voluntary health agencies and several media outlets. The resulting storm of media criticism killed SB 376.[12-14]

THE VOLUNTARY HEALTH AGENCIES
ACCEPT PREEMPTION

In February 1992 Assembly Member Terry Friedman (D-Santa Monica), one of only 8 legislators (out of 120) who refused to take tobacco industry campaign contributions and a supporter of tobacco control efforts in the Legislature,[15] introduced AB 2667, a nonpreemptive statewide clean indoor air law that would have ended smoking in all enclosed workplaces. Friedman promoted the bill as an alternative to local tobacco control ordinances.[16] Because AB 2667 dealt with labor law, Friedman designated as the enforcement agency the California Occupational Safety and Health Administration (CalOSHA) in the state Department of Industrial Relations instead of the Department of Health Services (DHS). The voluntary health agencies—American Lung Association (ALA), American Heart Association (AHA), and American Cancer Society (ACS)—supported AB 2667, as did the California Medical Association (CMA) and the California Labor Federation (AFL-CIO).[17,18] Despite its lack of enthusiasm for state legislation on clean indoor air issues, Americans for Nonsmokers' Rights (ANR) also supported Friedman's efforts as long as his bill did not contain language that preempted local ordinances.[19,20]

Despite support for AB 2667, it had only a very slim chance of passing because the hospitality and tourism industries, not simply the tobacco industry, were unlikely to allow the bill to go forward.[21] Because the odds against the bill were so great, neither the state voluntary health agencies nor ANR saw any practical reason to engage in broad discussions over the desirability of a state law versus local ordinances or the conditions under which preemption of local ordinances would be an acceptable compromise to obtain a state smoke-free workplace law.

The prospect of enacting statewide workplace smoking legislation improved dramatically when Friedman negotiated support for his bill from the California Restaurant Association (CRA). The CRA was concerned about the growing body of scientific evidence that linked secondhand smoke with illness and the potential liability for tobacco-induced diseases through worker compensation and Americans with Disabilities Act claims.[22] In previous years, the CRA board had taken the position that there should be a single statewide standard regulating smoking in all public places, including restaurants, and that the CRA would continue to oppose local ordinances due to concerns about unfair competition.[23,24]

Because of the CRA's concerns about secondhand smoke, the organization was open to endorsing the Friedman bill. But it was unwilling to do so unless the CRA goal of a uniform statewide law was also met, and it made its support contingent on inclusion of preemption of local ordinances.[25] Friedman amended AB 2667 to include a preemption provision that would "supersede and render unnecessary the local enactment or enforcement of local ordinances regulating the smoking of tobacco products in enclosed places of employment."[26] The CRA immediately endorsed the amended bill.[25] This was the first time an important business lobby in Sacramento had supported tobacco control legislation; the coalition of health groups supporting AB 2667 were ecstatic.[27,28]

By continuing to support AB 2667 after it was amended to include preemption, however, the state voluntary health agencies adopted a position that conflicted with their national organizations' policies against preemption. In 1989, in response to preemptive legislation that had been proposed by the tobacco industry and enacted in a growing number of states, the national voluntary health agencies, acting through the Coalition on Smoking OR Health, took a strong anti-preemption position.[29] It advised affiliates that "it is better to have no law than one that eliminates a local government body's authority to act to protect the public health" and suggested informing the appropriate legislator that "unless the preemption is removed from the bill . . . your organization can no longer support the bill."[29] Despite this national policy, the state voluntary health agencies and Friedman defended the preemption language by arguing that because the bill would make all workplaces 100 percent smoke free, any local standard would be weaker, making the preemption issue moot.[30–32]

ANR representatives, on behalf of many local tobacco control advocates, did not accept this compromise. They believed that local legislation was a better device to educate the public, generate media coverage, and build community support for enforcement and implementation of tobacco control ordinances.[33] ANR also believed that any preemption language would set a bad example for other states. Friedman's supporters countered that it would take years to advance the policy agenda on smoke-free workplaces in some parts of the state. More important, ANR worried that by accepting preemption in principle, it would create a situation in which the tobacco industry would hijack the bill and weaken the tobacco control provisions while maintaining the preemption.[34] In deference to Friedman, however, ANR took a neutral position, stating its opposition to the preemption clause and raising concerns about Cal-OSHA's ability to enforce the law effectively.[35]

Trying to allay these concerns, Friedman modified the severability clause in the bill to limit preemption if the bill was weakened: "In the event this section is repealed or modified by subsequent legislative or judicial action so that the (100 percent) smoking prohibition is no longer applicable to all enclosed places of employment in California, local governments shall have the full right and authority to enact and enforce restrictions on the smoking of tobacco products in enclosed places of employment within their jurisdictions, including a complete prohibition of smoking."[26] Friedman and the bill's supporters argued that this language would protect local ordinances because the preemption clause would "self-destruct" if future legislation weakened the smoke-free mandate.[30,36]

Friedman's attempt at compromise fell short, however, when in April he solicited an analysis from the Legislative Counsel regarding the severability clause. The Legislative Counsel concluded that the severability clause offered no legal protection because the current session of the Legislature had no authority to bind future sessions of the Legislature.[37] Nevertheless, the state voluntary health agencies continued to support the bill because of its 100 percent smoke-free workplace mandate.

Even with the support of the restaurants, labor groups, and voluntary health agencies, AB 2667 failed to pass the Labor and Employment Committee in June 1992.

THE BIRTH OF AB 13

Friedman reintroduced AB 2667 as AB 13 in the next legislative session in December 1992, and it was assigned to Friedman's Labor and Employment Committee in February 1993. The bill was cosponsored by the CRA, AHA, AFL-CIO, and CMA.[38] The AHA, ALA, and ACS supported the bill because they wanted smoke-free workplaces. Groups representing the tourism and hospitality industries and the Tobacco Institute opposed AB 13.[39] ANR opposed the bill because of objections to preemption. ANR was also concerned that CalOSHA would be a less responsive enforcing agency than local health departments or similar agencies that enforced local ordinances.[40] The anti-tobacco activist group Doctors Ought to Care, the City of Lodi, and the California State Association of Counties also opposed the bill because of preemption.[41–43] Trying to address ANR's concerns over enforcement, Friedman amended the bill to remove "appropriate local law enforcement agencies" (police) as the enforcement agency so that local health departments could enforce the law, including levying fines for violations.[44]

These differences of opinion still appeared moot. Despite the broadened support for the bill, it was still viewed as unlikely to pass. AHA lobbyist Dian Kiser wrote her local affiliates, "Frankly, the chance of passage of AB 13, like AB 2667, is minuscule."[21] Rather than treating preemption as a policy issue, supporters of the bill fell back on the argument that since AB 13 was "100 percent smoke free," the issue of preemption was not important.

AB 13, unlike AB 2667, passed out of the Labor and Education Committee. Newspapers credited AB 13's passage out of committee to a 1992 EPA report on secondhand smoke as well as Governor Pete Wilson's decision in early 1993 to end smoking in all state government buildings.[39,45]

At the first hearing of the Ways and Means Committee, Friedman added two amendments in a continuing effort to respond to concerns about preemption and enforcement. The first clarified the severability clause to insure that, if AB 13's smoke-free mandate were weakened, communities could pass and enforce future ordinances as well as enforce existing ordinances. The other was his amendment to allow local governments to designate a local agency to enforce the law rather than specifying local police.[46] While AB 13 was being considered by the Ways and Means Committee, the League of California Cities, which had remained neutral on AB 2667, changed its position and announced support for AB 13 on the grounds that the bill would allow local governments to pass restrictions on tobacco in areas not covered by the bill.[47]

THE TOBACCO INDUSTRY'S RESPONSE: AB 996

The tobacco industry pursued three major strategies to counter AB 13. First, working through its front groups (including the Southern California Business Association) and the California Manufacturers Association (of which Philip Morris was a member), it lobbied against the bill on the grounds that AB 13 would be detrimental to California business.[39] Second, the tobacco industry tried to have the bill amended to weaken the smoking restrictions while maintaining the preemption, as ANR feared and as it had done successfully in other states.[39,48] Third, the tobacco industry proposed a weak law to compete with AB 13 that would preempt local regulation of smoking.

On April 19, 1993, Assembly Member Curtis Tucker (D-Inglewood) amended an unrelated bill, AB 996, to preempt all future tobacco control laws. AB 996 permitted smoking in workplaces when employers met the ventilation standard defined by Standard 62-1989 of the American Society of Heating, Refrigerating, and Air Conditioning Engineers (ASHRAE), although the ASHRAE standard stated that it was not strict enough to protect workers from secondhand smoke.[49] The use of the ASHRAE standard, while sounding official, was already incorporated into most building codes in the state and would have had little effect on restricting smoking in the workplace. The tobacco industry has heavily influenced ASHRAE over the years.[50]

The tobacco industry also used AB 996 to preempt emerging local ordinances restricting youth access to cigarette vending machines. Rather than eliminating vending machines as health advocates wanted, AB 996 proposed electronic locking devices that had proven ineffective in controlling youth access.[51,52] AB 996 was assigned to the Assembly Committee on Governmental Organization, chaired by Tucker, where it passed by a 9-0 vote. The bill was then referred to the Assembly Committee on Ways and Means, where AB 13 was also being considered.

AB 996 was supported by the tobacco industry and its allies in the business community; it was opposed by the same coalition of health, local government, and business groups that supported AB 13 in addition to those who opposed AB 13 because of its preemption clause.[53] The CRA opposed AB 996 because, in protecting current local clean indoor air laws with a grandfather clause, it would not lead to a uniform smoking policy around the state. The CRA also feared that it would not protect restaurant owners from lawsuits and that the ASHRAE ventilation standards would be prohibitively expensive for small restaurants.[22]

The introduction of AB 996 changed the debate over state smoking restrictions. Prior to AB 996's emergence as a competing bill to AB 13, media coverage of AB 13 included the debate among tobacco control advocates over the merits of AB 13, particularly ANR's concern with preemption. When AB 996 started moving in tandem with AB 13, media coverage framed the debate as a good bill (AB 13) versus a bad bill (AB 996). Supporters of AB 13 were successful in garnering support for AB 13 and opposition to AB 996 from editorial boards throughout the state. The fact that AB 996 preempted future local ordinances was an important point in rallying public opposition to the bill.[54,55] Newspapers described AB 996 as a bill whose real purpose was to prevent local communities from approving their own tough anti-smoking ordinances.

THE VIEW FROM OUTSIDE SACRAMENTO

The potential effect of AB 13's preemption provisions on local ordinances created controversy and confusion among local tobacco control advocates over whether to support the measure. Local coalitions, composed of people from local affiliates of the voluntary health agencies, local medical associations, departments of health, and individual activists, received inconsistent information on the state debate over AB 13 and AB 996. While opposition to AB 996 was unanimous, the state voluntary health agencies urged support of AB 13 while ANR continued to urge opposition. Many individuals who participated in these local coalitions were members of both a voluntary health agency and ANR, and so were receiving conflicting action alerts from different organizations.

Some activists at the local level questioned the effect of AB 13 on local legislation and remained skeptical that a workable bill would emerge from the Legislature.[33,56] Of special concern was how the preemption language would affect nonworkplace provisions of local ordinances (such as those mandating public education) or nonretaliation clauses (which would protect employees who complained about noncompliance with the smoke-free workplace requirement). Questions from those communities about AB 13 were interpreted by lobbyists at ALA and ACS as efforts by ANR to undermine their authority, and they complained of having to devote time and resources to respond to what they perceived as ANR's misinterpretation of the bill.[27,31] ANR saw its activities as a legitimate way to present its opposition to preemption to the people most affected.[19]

As controversy over the bill intensified and communication broke down between state players, a hostile exchange occurred, with local activists caught in the cross fire. One LLA director later described the atmosphere: "Oh my God. We were on the record of telling our coalition that it was preemptive and that it was not a good thing. And because we had had these conversations, some individuals wrote letters. I got nasty calls back from Friedman's office just saying, 'It is not preemptive! Who told you this? That's wrong!' And they would call us. I mean these are individuals who English is not necessarily their first language who did not know how to, like, argue back. The whole process of that was real divisive." [57] In a public demonstration of the growing conflict among former tobacco control allies, the presidents of the state voluntary health agencies and the CMA circulated a letter warning, "ANR's opposition is unsound and could have dangerous effects." [36] This letter was a modified version of one that Friedman had written to ACS earlier, claiming that ANR authored "a shocking opposition letter which seriously distorts AB 13." [30]

AB 13 AND AB 996 ON THE ASSEMBLY FLOOR

AB 13 and AB 996 were considered in tandem by the Assembly Ways and Means Committee. Although contradictory in intent and effect, both bills passed the committee, with several members voting for both bills. The bills next moved to the Assembly floor, where AB 13 was amended on May 24, 1993, to exclude hotel guest rooms from AB 13's definition of "place of employment." Since AB 13 preempted only local regulation of "places of employment," local governments would be permitted to regulate hotel guest rooms.

Both AB 996 and AB 13 came to a floor vote in the Assembly on June 1, 1993, and both failed. Just days later, AB 996 was taken up again, while reconsideration for AB 13 was delayed until the following week by a technicality. The tobacco industry's bill, AB 996, passed by a 42-34 vote. The Assembly members who voted for AB 996 had received a total of $964,740 (average $22,970 per "yes" vote) in tobacco industry campaign contributions during the years 1975–1993, compared with only $193,567 for opponents (average $5,693 per "no" vote).[15] Newspapers reported that campaign contributions from tobacco interests to legislators were buying votes against AB 13 and for AB 996.[55,58,59] Friedman denounced passage of AB 996 as "an example of the absolutely disgusting power the tobacco industry wields in the Legislature." [60]

In the debates over local tobacco control ordinances, it had become routine for the tobacco industry, acting through surrogates, to claim that smoking restrictions would cause economic problems. On June 6, the day after AB 996 passed the Assembly but before AB 13 was reconsidered, several Southern California "business" groups, led by the Southern California Business Association, a group with tobacco industry connections, released an economic study by the accounting firm of Price Waterhouse.[61,62] (Price Waterhouse conducts negative "economic impact" studies for the tobacco industry throughout the nation.) The study, sponsored by the San Diego Tavern and Restaurant Association, claimed that AB 13 would jeopardize 82,000 jobs in California and cost the state more than $3.5 billion.[63]

The CRA immediately hired another accounting firm, Coopers and Lybrand, to review the Price Waterhouse report. Coopers and Lybrand said the Price Waterhouse results were biased because the respondents had no previous experience with a statewide smoke-free law, so their impressions would not accurately reflect potential business loss.[64] The survey also produced bias in its results by giving respondents misleading information regarding the scope of areas affected by AB 13. Coopers and Lybrand noted that Price Waterhouse omitted "a key conclusion, if not the key conclusion, that over 61% of respondents thought that there would be no impact or positive impact on sales from the proposed ban."[64] This prompt response by the CRA neutralized the effects of the Price Waterhouse study.

AB 13 was granted reconsideration on June 7 and passed the Assembly with a 47-25 vote. Members who voted for AB 13 had received $363,823 in campaign contributions from the tobacco industry between 1976 and 1993 (average $7,741 per "yes" vote), and those who voted against it, $711,405 (average $28,456 per "no" vote).[15] Friedman hailed his success as a "spectacular turnaround," attributing the change in votes to "the outpouring of spontaneous public support for AB 13 all over the state, and the outrage expressed by the voters at the passage of the industry-sponsored measure."[65] Several members of the Assembly expressed discontent with both AB 13 and AB 996, saying one bill was too strict and the other was not strict enough, and voiced the hope that a compromise bill could be created in the state Senate or in a conference committee.[66]

ON TO THE SENATE

In the Senate, AB 13 and AB 996 were assigned to both the Senate Health and Human Services Committee and the Judiciary Committee. AB 996 died in the Senate Health and Human Services Committee, chaired by Senator Diane Watson (D-Los Angeles), as a result of effective lobbying by tobacco control advocates and senators friendly to tobacco control.

Tucker never brought it up for a vote, presumably because it did not have enough votes to pass.[67] In a November 1993 memo, David Laufer of Philip Morris noted that it was unlikely that the tobacco industry could move AB 996 out of the Senate committee.[68]

AB 13 passed the Senate Health and Human Services Committee on its second hearing after being further amended to exempt hotel and motel lobbies, bars and gaming clubs, and some convention centers and warehouses. Once again, these exemptions were created by excluding these venues from AB 13's definition of "places of employment." Since AB 13 applied only to places defined as "places of employment," these exemptions from the smoke-free mandate were also exempted from the bill's preemption clause, leaving them open to local regulation. Friedman admittedly accepted the amendments to exempt these areas so as to move the bill through committee; he declared the bill's passage to be a victory against the tobacco industry.[69]

The AB 13 coalition continued to support the bill, even though it was no longer "100 percent," the rationale initially used by several members of the support coalition to justify their acceptance of the preemption language. Between the first and second committee hearings, in response to a question from a reporter, Friedman argued that "AB 13 creates one uniform protective statewide law and *preempts* the patchwork of local ordinances around the state with which businesses must currently comply. It protects all workers from environmental tobacco smoke and all employers from claims related to environmental tobacco smoke" (emphasis added).[70]

After passing the Health and Human Services Committee, AB 13 was referred to the Judiciary Committee, chaired by Senator Bill Lockyer (D-Hayward), the author of the "Napkin Deal" (see chapter 3). At AB 13's first hearing in the Judiciary Committee, on August 19, it was clear AB 13 did not have the votes to clear the committee.[67] Over the next several weeks, Lockyer proposed several amendments that would further weaken the bill's smoke-free mandate, including a request that Friedman relinquish his 100 percent smoke-free requirement in favor of ventilation standards. Rather than accepting Lockyer's proposal, Friedman petitioned to turn AB 13 into a two-year bill, allowing him to bring the bill back to committee for discussion in 1994. His request was granted and Friedman vowed to return in 1994 with a stronger support coalition for the bill.[71]

THE PHILIP MORRIS PLAN

Friedman was not the only one making plans for 1994. In November 1993, conceding that it would likely be unsuccessful at "blowing AB 996 out of Senate Health," [68] Philip Morris started planning an initiative modeled on AB 996:

> Simply filing [a proposed initiative] has some advantages because it may force the legislature to act in a way we can help channel (e.g.: if they believe a less onerous bill would pass on the ballot, we can give them the opportunity to pass something a little more restrictive, but less than a total ban, then not turn in any signatures). Conversely, if we believe we can win with something more moderate than the legislature might pass, we should turn in signatures and go to the ballot.[68]

Thus, the filing of an initiative might give the industry some leverage in the Legislature against AB 13. This strategy was similar to the one that the industry had traditionally used at the local level—the threat of a referendum to force counties and municipalities into more moderate ordinances (see chapter 9).

On November 1 David Laufer of Philip Morris laid out the California "situation." [68] The San Francisco Board of Supervisors had just passed an ordinance similar to AB 13. According to Laufer, "It is no coincidence that the bill resembles AB 13, since Terry Friedman has spent the last several weeks in SF lobbying the Board." He went on to say, "Barring a miracle or a decision to take this to the ballot, it is a done deal." He noted that the smoke-free ordinance in Los Angeles had gone into effect and, "while perhaps not enforced," was "being complied with on the whole." He added that the Tobacco Institute "has no more funds this year to continue to pursue the case, so we will need to decide if we want to continue and pick up the tab." In San Jose, the City Council had directed the city attorney to draft a law making all public places and worksites smoke free (which passed on December 30, 1993), and San Diego was discussing strengthening its ordinance. Sacramento had been smoke free for several years. Laufer offered this summary: "In 4 of the 5 largest population centers in the state, a ban is, or will likely be the reality, making AB 13 (a statewide ban) all the more appealing and easy to enact when session reconvenes in early January 1994. . . . In conjunction with whatever remaining allies we have, I believe we must launch a simultaneous counterattack on several different fronts: legislative, initiative, regulatory and legal." [68] Ellen Merlo, Philip Morris's vice president of state activities, agreed: "If the four largest cities in California go, it is a very dangerous precedent and I think we have to throw as many resources at at least some sort of a compromise that we can live with. Let's do ASAP." [72]

On January 12, 1994, Merlo wrote to Geoff Bible, president of Philip Morris, to bring him up to date on "the steps that we will take in California over the next several weeks in order to achieve state-wide preemption with accommodation for smokers." [73] California clearly warranted attention at the tobacco giant's highest levels. Four steps were outlined:

> 1.   We will file a lawsuit on February 1st against the City of San Francisco over the jurisdictional issue of whether or not San Francisco has the authority to ban workplace smoking. We will be a co-plaintiff along with local business people in this lawsuit and based on precedent and legal advice, we think we have an excellent chance of prevailing.
>
> 2.   At the state level, we will create "a flurry of legislative activity to confound the antis by introducing various bills and measures to put them on the defensive, including asking for an audit of the Proposition 99 trust fund, an investigation of political abuses of the Proposition 99 fund and a resolution to ask U.S. OSHA to establish Indoor Air Quality Standards within the state.
>
> 3.   We will create the same level of local activity in cities like Anaheim, South San Francisco, Stockton, Palm Desert, Rancho Mirage, etc. by introducing smoking accommodation bills.
>
> 4.   Finally, on or about January 17th, we will file a ballot initiative seeking a state preemption bill that provides for smoker accommodation. The Initiative will be filed by three independent business and/or association members. Simultaneous with our filing of the ballot initiative, we will conduct additional polling to ensure that we thoroughly probe voter reaction to this bill, which preliminary polling indicates we have a very good chance of winning. [73]

Merlo added that if the company had the "opportunity to reach a negotiated settlement through the Legislature for preemption and accommodation, we will do so." [73]

RJ Reynolds did not share Merlo's optimism about an initiative. On January 17 Tim Hyde wrote to Tom Griscom and Roger Mozingo about the proposed initiative, saying, "Overall, I think this is a bad approach," referring to a survey conducted for Philip Morris. [74] He offered the following arguments to support his view:

A.   I am doubtful we could prevail on such a ballot question. We haven't seen the whole survey, yet, but Q57 [the head-to-head comparison of AB 996 and AB 13], in the deck, shows that almost as many people would vote for a total ban as for designated areas (44–46%). And that's before the other side has had a chance to propagandize about out-of-state tobacco companies spending big money to protect their interests.

B.   *There are tremendous down sides if we lose. It would establish the official position of the California electorate on this issue, making it much more difficult for legislators and local public officials to resist the anti's call for public bans.* It would also have obvious national fallout.

C.   Even if we should win, it doesn't solve the problem. The real problem is the hundreds of millions that other side has in Prop. 99 money to fight us. I suspect that if they weren't spending their efforts trying to enact local ordinances, as they are now, they would be up to worse activities: such things as harassing private employers, even more egregious studies and pilot intervention programs, and who knows what else.

If we were going to mount a proactive initiative, why not one that would divert these funds to prison construction and emergency rooms? That has immediate public appeal, is a "get" for the voters, and would have precedential value for other states.

I also think we need to be careful with what the other side has identified as "front" organizations. A California chapter of the National Smokers' Alliance, for example, will be quickly seen as PM's grassroots arm. The group we have fostered—California Smokers' Rights—has 8,000 paid members and money of their own in the bank, but the [*sic*] are still frequently accused of being a front for the industry.

Finally, five million dollars is a lot of money.[75] [emphasis added]

RJ Reynolds was clearly not interested in an initiative battle over smoke-free workplace laws, preferring instead to try to kill off the Proposition 99 Health Education and Research Accounts once and for all. Local ordinances were causing problems for the industry, but the root cause of the problem was Proposition 99. Philip Morris ignored RJ Reynolds and continued with its initiative.

THE PHILIP MORRIS INITIATIVE

As Merlo had alerted Bible, on January 17 Philip Morris and a group of restaurant owners submitted an initiative statute, the California Uniform Tobacco Control Act (essentially identical to AB 996) to the California Attorney General with the intention of qualifying it for the November election. The initiative stated that "current regulation of smoking in public in California is inadequate" and that "there is a clear need for uniform statewide regulation of smoking in public to assure those interested in avoiding secondhand smoke have the same protection wherever they go in the state and that those who do smoke have fair notice of where smoking is prohibited."[76] The smoking regulations in the initiative were simply worded as broad prohibitions; the even broader exceptions appeared near the end of the initiative, couched in technical terms. The language that preempted all local ordinances regulating any aspect of tobacco consumption, distribution, or promotion was buried on the last line of page 9.

The initiative would have overturned eighty-five local ordinances that mandated smoke-free workplaces and ninety-six ordinances that mandated smoke-free restaurants (as of January 1994). In addition, because strict workplace smoking restrictions encourage some smokers to quit and others to reduce the number of cigarettes smoked,[77,78] a trend that is reversed when restrictions are relaxed,[2,79] passage of the initiative would have actually increased smoking and exposure to secondhand smoke.[80] While Philip Morris's public statements did not emphasize the potential of the initiative to protect tobacco profits, the company explicitly presented the initiative as a way for tobacco retailers to protect their business: "The adverse impact on retail cigarette sales would be immediate [without the initiative]. Your cigarette sales, along with your profits, could drop."[81]

Organized opposition to the initiative, which was eventually placed on the ballot as Proposition 188, developed slowly. When Philip Morris first proposed the initiative in January 1994, only Carolyn Martin, an ALA volunteer and former chair of the Coalition for a Healthy California and TEOC, and ALA lobbyist Tony Najera, expressed strong concern about it. Most people viewed the Philip Morris initiative as a sure failure because the California public had been educated about the health dangers of tobacco and did not trust the tobacco industry.[82,83]

Martin and Najera hired Jack Nicholl, who had been campaign manager for the Yes on Proposition 99 campaign. The three contacted former Coalition members to alert them to Philip Morris's actions and to mobilize local groups to publicly denounce the initiative as an attack on their local tobacco control ordinances, local autonomy, and public health and to contact editorial boards and secure their opposition. Martin also

TABLE 2. NO ON PROPOSITION 188 CONTRIBUTIONS

Donor/Month	ACS	ALA[1]	AHA[2]	AMA/CMA[3]	Kaiser Permanente	California Dental Assn.	ANR	Other[4]	Cumulative
March	$ 8,171	$ 7,500						$ 100	$ 15,771
April	$ 2,000	$ 0	$ 5,000			$ 5,000		$ 3,500	$ 31,271
May	$ 3,000	$ 1,500						$ 0	$ 35,771
June	$ 6,770	$ 3,822		$ 1,000		$ 1,000		$ 2,500	$ 50,863
July		$ 25,000	$ 2,500					$ 200	$ 78,563
August	$ 26,349	$ 0		$ 20,000		$ 10,000	$ 11,676	$ 11,393	$ 146,305
September	$ 40,706	$ 7,459	$ 25,000			$ 15,000	$ 6,977	$ 15,882	$ 262,028
October	$417,678	$101,220	$125,500	$ 30,000	$ 70,000		$ 4,215	$ 70,323	$1,083,727
November	$ 93,000	$ 26,506			$ 3,750			$ 13,323	$1,224,520
Total	$577,734	$173,007	$153,000	$ 51,000	$ 73,750	$25,000	$22,868	$117,221	$1,193,580

NOTES:

1. ALA includes $100,690 from California Division plus $63,317 from various local affiliates and state affiliates outside California. In-kind contributions of staff time are not included.

2. AHA includes $100,000 from national AHA.

3. AMA/CMA includes $25,000.

4. Table names all donors who contributed at least $20,000.

SOURCE: From H. Macdonald, S. Aguinaga, and S. A. Glantz. The defeat of Philip Morris's "California Uniform Tobacco Control Act," *Am J Pub Health* 1997;87(12): 1989–1996. Reproduced with permission of the *American Journal of Public Health* (copyright 1997 by American Public Health Association).

asked for contributions for a three-month campaign to defeat the petition drive (table 2) and convened former members of the Coalition on February 17, 1994.[84,85]

Meanwhile, ACS funded a poll of California voters asking how would they vote if they knew Philip Morris was behind an initiative that would decrease smoking restrictions in California, overturn local laws, and prohibit cities and counties from making their own smoking laws.[86] This poll also tested various messages that could be used to oppose the initiative, so it provided important marketing research for the public health campaign. The results revealed that 70 percent of those polled would vote against such a law, 24 percent would vote for it, and 6 percent were undecided.

While the proponents of an initiative write the text of the proposed law, the California Attorney General provides the official title and summary, which appear on the ballot. This wording is important because it may be the only material that a voter reads about the measure before voting. The title and summary also appear at the top of all copies of the petitions used to gather signatures to qualify the initiative for the ballot. Given their experience in the Proposition 99 campaign, Martin and Najera realized the importance of not only the initiative's title and summary but also the Legislative Analyst's analysis and ballot arguments, which appear in the Voter Pamphlet. Philip Morris had submitted proposed language emphasizing that the initiative "bans smoking," "restricts . . . vending machines and billboards," and "increases penalties for tobacco sale to and purchase by minors" while downplaying the exceptions.[87] The Coalition hired an attorney who presented a title and summary to the Attorney General that emphasized preemption of local ordinances, relaxation of current restrictions on smoking, and the increase in smoking that the initiative would cause.[88,89] The final title and summary that the Attorney General released on March 9, 1994, reflected the Coalition's concerns; it highlighted the preemption of existing laws and significant exceptions to smoking restrictions.[90] The Coalition's timely and assertive intervention would prove very important as the battle over the initiative unfolded.

THE CONTINUING FIGHT OVER AB 13

As he had promised in November 1993, Friedman was ready to push AB 13 when the Legislature returned in January of the following year.

In February 1994 AB 13 was taken up again in the Senate Judiciary Committee. Friedman amended the bill to expand exemptions for hotels and motels to gain the support of the California Hotel and Motel Association, a previous opponent of AB 13. Friedman also adopted Lockyer's amendment to permit smoking in bars until January 1, 1997, after which time bars would have comply with an as yet unwritten EPA or CalOSHA ventilation standard to protect workers from secondhand smoke. However, Friedman made sure to stipulate that if no standard was written by January 1, 1997, smoking would be prohibited in bars and gaming clubs.[91]

AB 13 was continuing to move through the Legislature. When the Senate Judiciary Committee heard AB 13 again on March 22, two tobacco-friendly amendments were added to the bill.[92] The first, sponsored by Senator Art Torres (D-Los Angeles), extended the phase-in period and ventilation options for bars, gaming clubs, and convention centers to restaurants. The second amendment, sponsored by Senator Charles Calderon (D-Whittier), preempted all future ordinances. Calderon had a history of supporting such preemption language as well as the tobacco industry generally.[93] In proposing his preemption amendment to AB 13, Calderon argued that if Friedman truly wanted to establish a state standard for smoking, he should extend the preemption in the bill to all local ordinances. Friedman objected that his fragile support coalition would disintegrate because many supporters were philosophically opposed to preemption.[94] The Judiciary Committee ignored Friedman and passed the bill by a vote of 6-1, including the amendments.

Once AB 13 was amended to broadly preempt local laws, the health groups, which had been divided about the preemption in AB 13, united in opposing it. The League of California Cities, ACS, ALA, and AHA expressed opposition to the two pro-tobacco amendments and said they would oppose the bill until both amendments were removed.[95-98] ANR continued to oppose the bill.

The weakening of AB 13 was front-page news.[99] The *Los Angeles Times* editorial page called the hearing "a rape in Sacramento."[100] Friedman lobbied to remove the Torres and Calderon amendments from AB 13 in the Senate Appropriations Committee, the last committee before the Senate floor.[101] Torres, realizing he had been misled at the hearing by restaurant owners in his district, worked with Friedman's office to remove the amendment he had suggested as well as Calderon's preemption language.[102] Friedman and his supporters successfully removed the hostile amendments in the Senate Appropriations Committee. The AB 13 support coalition once again backed the bill, while ANR continued to oppose it.

THE PHILIP MORRIS SIGNATURE DRIVE

The flurry of press activity surrounding AB 13 did not extend to the Proposition 188 signature drive. Philip Morris began a quiet effort to qualify its initiative, using the Dolphin Group (which had created front groups for fighting local ordinances) to run the campaign as Californians for Statewide Smoking Restrictions (CSSR). Voters began receiving phone calls inquiring whether they would support a uniform state law restricting smoking. Respondents who answered "yes" received a packet that contained advertising materials and a copy of the petition to be signed and returned. This attractive packet, which cloaked the initiative as a pro-health measure, detailed "strict regulations" that would be implemented by the proposed law and outlined its "benefits":

> Completely prohibits smoking in restaurants and workplaces unless strict ventilation standards are met.
>
> Replaces the crazy patchwork quilt of 270 local ordinances with a single, tough, uniform statewide law.
>
> [Is] stricter than 90% of the local ordinances currently on the books.[103]

Preemption of local ordinances was mentioned only in the Attorney General's summary. Nowhere on the materials, and only in small type on the back of the envelope, did Philip Morris reveal its sponsorship of the initiative.

Using staff resources donated by ALA, the Coalition campaigned to keep Philip Morris from collecting enough signatures to qualify the initiative and sought resolutions from local governments that had already passed strong local tobacco control ordinances in an attempt to create debate and interest the press in covering the story. Even though the Coalition considered this strategy a long shot, any controversy created during the signature gathering might attract early press attention before the general election campaign.

The Coalition also advised voters who had signed the petition in the belief that it would promote health to complain to Acting Secretary of State Tony Miller.[104] On April 8 Miller sent a letter to the restaurant owners who had filed the petition, warning them that deceptive petitioning practices would not be tolerated. He later launched an investigation into CSSR's possibly fraudulent petitioning practices, stating that he would "not certify any measure for any ballot that met the signature requirement only by breaking the law." The Coalition capitalized on Miller's actions, publicizing his warnings and simultaneously instructing voters how to request removal of their signatures from the petition (which turned out to be impossible, for all practical purposes).[105]

On May 9 CSSR submitted 607,000 signatures (385,000 valid signatures were required) to the secretary of state's office. As part of his continuing investigation, Miller asked for court permission to randomly sample the signatures to survey for fraud. The court denied permission on the grounds that it would constitute invasion of privacy.[106] On June 30 the secretary of state certified that Philip Morris had collected enough valid signatures to place the initiative on the ballot for the November 1994 election as Proposition 188.

THE LEGISLATURE PASSES AB 13

Back in the Legislature, AB 13 was continuing to move. After passing the Senate Appropriations Committee, it was sent to the Senate floor. Senator Marian Bergeson (R-Newport Beach), AB 13's floor manager in the Senate, successfully fought off several hostile amendments. However, one amendment was accepted on June 16: smoking areas would be allowed in long-term patient care facilities and in businesses with fewer than five employees so long as all air from the smoking area was exhausted directly outside, the area was not accessible to minors, no work stations were situated within the smoking area, and EPA or CalOSHA ventilation standards were met, once established. The bill passed the Senate on June 30, 1994. The Assembly voted concurrence with the Senate amendments. Governor Wilson signed the bill into law on July 21, 1994.

The final version of AB 13 retained its 100 percent smoke-free mandate as well as its preemption clause. Amendments were worded so any exemption from the smoke-free mandate allowing smoking was also an exemption from the preemption clause. Thus, local entities would be allowed to enforce existing regulations and pass and enforce new regulations restricting smoking in areas exempted from AB 13, despite its preemption clause. Nevertheless, Governor Pete Wilson cited the bill's preemption of local ordinances as a reason to sign the bill into law. He stated that AB 13 protected California's businesses as well as the health of workers because "by providing a uniform, statewide standard which preempts the patchwork of local ordinances around the state with which businesses must currently comply, the law does not give one business an economic advantage over another business." [107]

Wilson continued to press his view that AB 13 preempted local communities from regulating smoking. In 1995 a nursing home resident in San Jose complained that he was being forced to breathe secondhand smoke in the television room at the nursing home; he asked the city, under its clean indoor air law, to require that the room be smoke free. The city complied, and DHS sued, claiming that AB 13 preempted the ordinance. DHS lost in the trial court and appealed. On August 18, 1998, the Sixth District of the Court of Appeal unanimously ruled that the neither federal law nor state law preempted localities from enacting local tobacco control ordinances:

> By disavowing any intent to preempt the regulation of tobacco smoking, and by in fact expressly authorizing local agencies to "ban completely the smoking of tobacco" in any manner not inconsistent with the law, the Legislature clearly indicated its intent to leave to the local authorities the matter of regulating the smoking of tobacco in their respective jurisdictions, provided the regulations so adopted do not conflict with statutory law. In delegating such regulatory power to local agencies and expressing its preference that regulation of tobacco smoking at the local level be made by local governments, the Legislature impliedly [sic] decreed that where the local agencies have stepped in to regulate the smoking of tobacco within their own territorial boundaries, the state's administrative agencies, such as the Department [of Health Services] should step back. . . .
>
> Evidently, the rationale for the Legislature's deference to local governments, equipped as they are with superior knowledge of local conditions, [is that they] are better able to handle local problems relating to regulation of tobacco smoking.[108]

The fact that DHS under the Wilson administration was willing to advocate the position that a nursing home resident had no right to a smoke-free environment while watching television was just one more example of the administration's pro-tobacco position. The result, however, was a resolution of the bitter debate within California's tobacco control community over whether or not state law was preemptive. It was not.

AB 13 AND PROPOSITION 188

For the tobacco industry, Proposition 188—which had started out as a way to finesse legislative behavior and get what the industry regarded as a good preemptive bill—had become essential after passage of AB 13.

John M. Hager, a vice president at American Tobacco, wrote Donald S. Johnston, president and CEO, "AB 13, a virtual smoking ban, is in place for January 1 and Prop 188 is our 'last chance' for reason in California."[109]

In June 1994, before AB 13 became law, the tobacco industry commissioned a public opinion poll on Proposition 188. The poll, conducted by Voter/Consumer Research of Houston, showed that the initiative was running even among voters (43 percent for, 43 percent against). Its supporters were primarily people who wanted to strengthen smoking restrictions, and opponents were primarily smokers, people who opposed government regulation, and people who disapproved of Philip Morris's sponsorship of the measure.[110] The poll also revealed that Proposition 188 faced two other problems. The first problem was that the initiative was confusing to people (especially with tobacco control advocates and the media attacking it), and confusion leads to "no" votes. The other problem was that the industry was asking for "yes" votes, which are historically harder to get.[110] As RJ Reynolds recognized, "Since the signing of AB 13, the effect of P[roposition] 188 would be to relax restrictions. In other words, the whole electorate will probably reconfigure on this issue."[111] Those who wanted smoking restrictions would likely shift to support the new status quo, AB 13, which meant they became "no" votes, while those who opposed Philip Morris sponsorship would stay on "no." Only smokers and opponents to regulation would stay where they were. The only hopeful news for the tobacco industry from the poll was that while Californians preferred smoking bans to nothing, they preferred restrictions to bans, and that while tobacco sponsorship was not a plus, it was not a killer.[111]

THE STEALTH CAMPAIGN

After the initiative qualified, CSSR avoided the media and public debates on the initiative and instead began an expensive direct mail advertising campaign to reach voters. Proposition 188 was promoted as a tobacco control law, a tough but reasonable alternative to AB 13. Although virtually all the money for Proposition 188 was coming from the tobacco industry (table 3), CSSR downplayed the industry's role in the campaign and, in typical fashion, presented itself as a coalition of small business owners, restaurants, and concerned California citizens.

Lee Stitzenberger of the Dolphin Group ran the campaign for Philip

TABLE 3. YES ON PROPOSITION 188 CONTRIBUTIONS

Company/Month	Philip Morris[1]	RJ Reynolds	Brown & Williamson	Lorillard	American Tobacco	Tobacco Institute	Other[2]	Cumulative
March	$ 491,213						$ 480	$ 491,693
April	$ 1,246,955						$1,852	$ 1,740,500
May	$ 100,000							$ 1,840,500
June	$ 150,000							$ 1,990,500
July	$ 2,513,000							$ 4,503,500
August		$1,617,150	$ 628,500	$130,000	$364,260			$ 7,243,410
September	$ 432,188			$130,000			$5,657	$ 7,811,255
October	$ 7,499,152	$1,773,506	$ 676,695	$574,110	$392,220		$1,822	$18,728,760
November	$ 144,708			$ 10,594		$30,000	$ 5	$18,914,068
Total	$12,577,217	$3,390,656	$1,305,195	$844,704	$756,480	$30,000	$9,816	$18,914,068

NOTES:

1. Philip Morris includes $786 from Miller Beer and $1,740 from Kraft General Foods.

2. Table names all donors who contributed at least $20,000

SOURCE: From H. Macdonald, S. Aguinaga, and S. A. Glantz. The defeat of Philip Morris's "California Uniform Tobacco Control Act," *Am J Pub Health* 1997; 87(12):1989–1996. Reproduced with permission of the *American Journal of Public Health* (copyright 1997 American Public Health Association).

Morris. RJ Reynolds's Roger Mozingo and Tim Hyde described Stitzenberger's plan to Tom Griscom and B. Oglesby on August 4:

> It calls for no television, 15 m pieces of mail, the ol' slate-card extortion,
> earned media, some newspaper ads, and a couple of weeks of radio at the
> end. *Basically, it is a kind of stealth campaign: much of it will fly under radar
> cover.* The first phase of the campaign, between now and Labor Day, will hit
> the sponsorship head on. "If you think this is a ploy by the tobacco compa-
> nies, read the proposal. Here it is. Read it." The next phase will attempt to
> use allies, broaden the base with coalitions, and the use of spokespeople for
> earned media. The final phase will be targeted radio and the slates.
>
> *The primary message, other than "we don't have anything to hide," will
> be that AB 13 goes too far, we need severe restrictions, not bans. The other
> side won't have any money, but they will have almost universal editorial sup-
> port. The campaign will monitor their use of Prop 99 monies and is prepared
> to challenge any use thereof in court.*
>
> They [CSSR] have a $9 m budget for the remainder of the campaign. We
> guess PM has put about $1.5 [m] in so far. Ellen [Merlo] said that PM has
> budgeted $6 m, so they are looking for $3 [m] from the rest of the industry.
> *In addition, National Smoker Alliance will do two statewide smoker mailing
> [s] (which, of course, PM will pay for). . . .*
>
> What they want from the rest of the industry, in addition to $3,000,000,
> is the use of some of our outdoor boards, help with point-of-sale distribution,
> smoker lists, and spokespeople (such as Danny Glover).
>
> We speculate that PM is interested in full industry participation for rea-
> sons beyond money. We suspect they want to share the negative pr this effort
> is taking in the media and among elected officials.
>
> Lee said that there is not a 50-50 chance that we will win this, but it isn't
> far off. Their main point (and that of the entire California team, including
> O'Mally) was that *this is the only chance we have of making progress in that
> state.*[111] [emphasis added]

The CSSR attempted to present Proposition 188 as an anti-smoking measure. In doing so, the organization departed from previous tobacco industry election campaigns by emphasizing anti-tobacco themes: limiting
youth access to tobacco, protection of nonsmokers, and accommodation
(figure 14).

Yet Proposition 188 represented a rollback of existing California tobacco control laws. Philip Morris used the industry's usual rhetoric only
in emphasizing that restrictions on tobacco represented unwarranted
government intrusion into people's private lives; targeted mailings to its
National Smokers' Alliance and other smokers' rights lists portrayed
Proposition 188 as a chance to "preserve your right to smoke."[112]

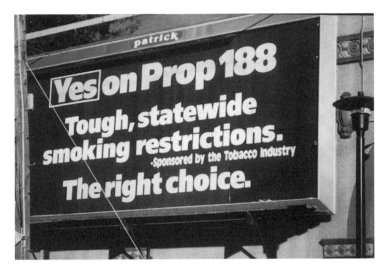

Figure 14.   Tobacco industry billboard promoting Proposition 188 as a "tough" anti-smoking measure. The statement "Sponsored by the Tobacco Industry" was added by a graffiti artist. As originally displayed, the billboard did not disclose who was financing the campaign. (Photo courtesy of Julia Carol, Americans for Nonsmokers' Rights)

THE "NO" CAMPAIGN

The Coalition for a Healthy California chose "Stop Philip Morris" as its campaign theme. Polls dating back to 1978 had consistently shown that the tobacco industry had very low credibility among voters.[86,113,114] For example, a 1982 poll prepared for the Tobacco Institute as part of its effort to defeat a tobacco control initiative in Bakersfield revealed that "knowledge of tobacco company [opposition to a measure] *does* move a significant number of respondents into the 'yes' column."[113] The Coalition concluded that simply educating the voters about the tobacco industry's involvement with Proposition 188 would convince them to vote "no."

By mid-September, the formal No on 188 campaign was launched. The ALA and ACS were actively working together, with Martin sharing the CHC chair with ACS volunteer Gaylord Walker. The Coalition held press conferences around the state, and press events aimed at informing the public that Philip Morris was behind the initiative. Following the press conferences, the tobacco industry received telephone calls from media in only San Francisco and Sacramento and considered the extremely quiet press "good news." [115]

Despite strong grassroots support for its position, the Coalition was having difficulty raising money to counter the tobacco industry's direct mail campaign. Knowledgeable observers—who knew Philip Morris was behind the campaign—could not believe that the voters would support Proposition 188 after several years of anti-tobacco public education funded by Proposition 99. According to Nicholl, Proposition 188 "was viewed as such an extreme and aggressive tactic by the tobacco industry that it couldn't possibly win." [116]

Philip Morris's strategy, however, was working. The independent Field Institute California Poll in mid-July had shown the initiative ahead: 52 percent for, 38 against. [117] By mid-September, polls conducted by the Field Institute and the *Los Angeles Times* showed that voters were evenly divided. [118,119] Proposition 188 had a good chance of passing.

Media attention is generally attracted by controversy, and reporters usually seek to represent both sides of an issue. The tobacco industry was so committed to staying out of the public eye that CSSR had an unlisted telephone number and actively avoided journalists and public debates. [120,121] For example, when the League of Women Voters scheduled a debate to be broadcast in the Bay Area (the second-largest media market in California), CSSR refused to send a representative. Unable to take a formal position opposing the initiative due to its bylaws (which required equal consideration of both sides before taking a position on an initiative), the league canceled the debate. [122] When the Senate Health Committee and the Assembly Governmental Organizations Committee held the public hearing required by law to present issues raised by Proposition 188, CSSR refused to participate. [123] By shunning the spotlight, CSSR successfully minimized controversy over Proposition 188, clearly part of Stitzenberger's stealth strategy. The strategy allowed Philip Morris to control the message through direct mail advertising while denying the opposing camp the free forum that would have accompanied media coverage.

On October 21, 1994, John H. Hager of American Tobacco again wrote to Donald S. Johnston to brief him on the Proposition 188 campaign. He enclosed an analysis of Proposition 188. [109] A notable strength of Proposition 188 was low awareness of the measure, especially compared with two high-profile initiatives that were on the ballot ("three strikes," which required long prison sentences for repeat offenders, and anti-immigrant measures). Other strengths included support now among smokers, high-turnout groups (such as the elderly), and those who favored the initiative's youth focus. The weaknesses were, however, significant: support for the measure declined when voters were somewhat informed; AB 13 had strong support (48 percent preferred it to Proposition 188); the health groups had substantial credibility; and Philip Morris's sponsorship of the initiative was a distinct liability. The strategy for the last month of the campaign was to identify and mail to likely smoker households, exploit populist themes, and keep buying media.

American Tobacco knew something that the Coalition did not know. The California Wellness Foundation, a large California foundation, was thinking about launching a large nonpartisan voter education project to make sure that the public understood exactly what Proposition 188 meant—and who was supporting it and who was opposing it. While strictly neutral from a content perspective, this educational campaign would effectively smoke out the tobacco industry's involvement and expose its stealth strategy.

American Tobacco's analysis presented four major concerns:

Wellness Foundation. While the official "NO" campaign has only $90,000 cash on hand as of 9/30, the nonprofit Wellness Foundation may spend anywhere from $1 million to $3 million in "non-partisan" radio spots. . . . They are being quoted non-profit rates, so this would also extend the reach of their buy. While we may be able to counter a $1 million buy, an effective $3 million buy to raise awareness of 188 sponsorship virtually dooms our campaign.

Prop 99 ads. Even though they do not mention 188, the extent of these new ads pose[s] a real threat, especially if the NO campaign or the Wellness Foundation helps voters relate the theme of the 99 ads (lies and deceit) to the initiative.

Media. The media could accomplish the above connection with little difficulty.

C. Everett Koop. If the NO campaign has any money to put him on TV ads, we're in trouble.[109]

The tobacco industry did not have to worry about the Proposition 99 ads. Sandra Smoley, Governor Pete Wilson's secretary of health and welfare, had been one of two votes against the Sacramento County smoke-free ordinance in 1990 when she was a member of the Board of Supervisors. As secretary of health and welfare, she forbade DHS from doing any public education about AB 13, despite the fact that educating the public before such laws are implemented greatly smooths the process.

In anticipation of a major media blitz by CSSR, the Coalition laid out a strategy for utilizing paid advertising to get out its message. Nicholl produced television and radio advertisements highlighting the deceptive nature of CSSR's advertising. The Coalition ads featured former surgeon general C. Everett Koop, one of the signers of the ballot argument against Proposition 188.[116,124] But there was no money to broadcast the advertisements. With the discouraging September poll results indicating that Proposition 188 would win, the California voluntary health agencies approached their national organizations for money.

The AHA and ACS national organizations responded with substantial donations in late October, which represented a major shift in policy for these organizations. In the past they had considered measures like Proposition 188 as state matters to be handled by the state affiliates. National AHA and ACS leaders recognized that a victory for the tobacco industry in California, which had been regarded as a pioneer in tobacco control efforts nationwide, would not only have national repercussions but also help the industry pass preemptive statewide smoking regulations elsewhere.[125,126] The national ALA continued its past practice of not providing financial assistance to individual state campaigns,[127] but four ALA state affiliates (in Oregon, Maine, Nebraska, and Wisconsin) saw Proposition 188 as a national issue and sent a total of $32,800. The American Medical Association gave $25,000. The Kaiser Permanente health maintenance organization donated $50,000 and ran full-page newspaper advertisements opposing Proposition 188. These last-minute injections of cash allowed the Coalition to run the Koop advertisements for the last week of the campaign. The tobacco industry has long understood that local and state campaigns make an important contribution to national policy and has always treated these tobacco battles from a national perspective. The Proposition 188 campaign marked a growing, but still limited, recognition by the national organizations supporting tobacco control that state and local issues are strategically important.

THE WELLNESS FOUNDATION

The tobacco industry's fears were confirmed when the California Wellness Foundation initiated a nonpartisan educational campaign to give voters accurate information about Proposition 188. The Wellness Foundation was concerned that Philip Morris and the other tobacco companies were controlling the public's perception of Proposition 188. On October 17 the Public Media Center, a nonprofit advertising agency in San Francisco, launched a unique $4 million campaign, funded by the California Wellness Foundation, to educate the public about Proposition 188. The campaign was designed to "provide California voters with objective and balanced information on a ballot question that many voters are uncertain or confused about."[92] The Public Media Center print, radio, and television advertisements presented the ballot arguments, signatories, and major donors to both sides of Proposition 188. The campaign also presented a toll-free number (1-800-KNOW188) that voters could call for more information. A voter calling the number was sent the Voter Pamphlet (containing the proposition's title and summary, the Legislative Analyst's report, and arguments for and against the proposition). To ensure neutrality in designing its campaign, the Public Media Center did not confer with advocates or opponents of Proposition 188; it relied entirely on publicly available, official information. The Coalition's victory months earlier in securing accurate Voter Pamphlet language proved to be crucial to innovative advertising strategies used by the Public Media Center.

After meeting with representatives of the Coalition and CSSR, the Legislative Analyst stated that Proposition 188 was weaker than the protection most Californians enjoyed. CSSR then sued the Legislative Analyst, Attorney General, signers of the ballot arguments against Proposition 188, and the Coalition, claiming the initiative's ballot label, title, summary, ballot arguments, and Legislative Analyst's statement did not present the public with nonprejudicial statements of the initiative's content and potential effects. On August 12, 1994, the Superior Court ruled in favor of the defendants and allowed the Voter Pamphlet to stand.

Despite the fact that the Public Media Center campaign did not support or oppose Proposition 188, the center's attorney received an inquiry from a deputy attorney general, investigating a complaint lodged against the California Wellness Foundation for supporting the educational campaign.[128] (California Attorney General Dan Lungren had close ties to the tobacco industry and the Dolphin Group, which managed his unsuccessful bid for governor in 1998.[129]) The deputy refused to specify who had lodged the complaint, but the Public Media Center interpreted it as a "clumsy attempt to intimidate us" by tobacco industry lawyers.[130]

By presenting the facts in a clear way, this educational advertising campaign focused media and public attention on the role of the tobacco industry in the Proposition 188 campaign, which forced CSSR to abandon its low-profile campaign strategy. CSSR supplemented its direct mail with broadcast advertising using formats almost identical to those of the Public Media Center, with the same visual presentation and voice-over techniques, but presenting only arguments in favor of Proposition 188 and urging a "yes" vote. The Public Media Center sued in federal court, requesting that the copycat ads be taken off the air. The judge granted the Public Media Center's request, but later that same evening an appellate court stayed the restraining order, citing infringement of free political speech.[131] Despite the loss in appellate court, the legal challenge to the copycat ad was well documented in the media, bringing attention to CSSR and the tobacco industry's role in Proposition 188.

Another CSSR advertisement, which featured middle school vice principal Nancy Frick claiming that Proposition 188 would benefit children, backfired in the last week of October. (Frick's husband had appeared in one of CSSR mailings.[132]) The Coalition sharply criticized the advertisement, emphasizing the industry's deceptive practices.[133] Two days later, the Coalition persuaded Frick to retract her comments and widely distributed the retraction, in which she stated that she was unaware Proposition 188 would overturn 300 local laws.[122,134–136] She also demanded that the advertisements be taken off the air.

THE FEDERAL COMMUNICATIONS COMMISSION

ANR decided to use the truth-in-advertising provisions of the Federal Communications Act to force the tobacco industry to clearly disclose its sponsorship of Proposition 188 in radio and television advertisements. ANR reasoned that requiring disclosure of tobacco industry funding would reduce the effectiveness of the Yes on 188 advertisements, and perhaps even make them counterproductive. ANR had used a similar tactic successfully during the Proposition P campaign in San Francisco in 1983 (see chapter 2). On October 20 ANR sought help from the Media Access Project, a nonprofit telecommunications law firm in Washington, DC.[137] Since CSSR had filed with the California secretary of state as "Californians for Statewide Smoking Restrictions—Yes on 188, a committee of Hotels, Restaurants, Philip Morris, Inc. and other tobacco companies," as required by California law, the Media Access Project believed the Federal Communications Commission (FCC) would likely agree that all CSSR's advertisements should reveal the entire committee name.[137]

On October 21 ANR informed all radio broadcasters running CSSR's advertising that their failure to reveal CSSR's complete legal name at the end of all commercials was in violation of FCC regulations and that unless the advertisements were corrected by October 24, ANR would file a complaint against the station with the FCC.[138] Many stations immediately changed the commercials.[139] On October 25 ANR filed a complaint with the FCC against several stations who had refused to comply.[140] In addition to forcing many stations to change the Yes on 188 advertisements, the controversy surrounding the FCC complaints focused the media on Proposition 188.

ANR's actions took place the same day that the Coalition held a press conference unveiling its Koop advertisement, with the hope of generating free media attention. (At that point the Coalition still did not have money to purchase air time to run the advertisements.) Although the other Coalition members failed at first to see the value of the ANR strategy, once the complaint proved useful, they cooperated with ANR. Ten days later the Coalition joined ANR in a new complaint to the FCC against television broadcasters who refused to modify CSSR's advertisements to disclose the tobacco companies' involvement.[141] On November 1 the FCC made an informal determination that proper disclosure after CSSR's commercials should include the information about tobacco industry sponsorship.[142]

By November 2, 1994, the tobacco industry's tracking polls showed that Proposition 188 was losing, along with these findings:

> As voters become more aware of the initiative's sponsorship, they tend to become opposed to Proposition 188.
> We have learned the opposition has doubled their air time purchase for the remainder of the campaign using Wellness Foundation money.
> We have targeted mailings, television and radio spots dropping during the next three to five days. Unpaid media continues to be manageable, but the infusion of Proposition 99 ads and Wellness Foundation funded ads are responsible for the shift in poll numbers.[143]

On November 8, Proposition 188 was defeated by a vote of 71 percent against to 29 percent for—the widest spread of any measure on the ballot. Thirty-eight percent of the people who voted against Proposition 188 stated that they did so to protect smoke-free public places, and another 22 percent voted against it because it was sponsored by the tobacco industry.[144] Seventeen percent of the people who voted for the initiative did so because they still felt it was an anti-smoking measure. Proposition 188 lost in every county in California, liberal and conservative, urban and rural. As Philip Morris's overwhelming defeat at the polls demonstrated, tobacco control had become a popular issue that cut across all demographic, geographic, and party lines. According to Peter Hanauer, one of the original tobacco control activists from the Proposition 5 campaign of 1978, "That was the icing on the cake in terms of showing the extent to which the tobacco industry had fallen out of favor." [145]

AB 13 was implemented on January 1, 1995. Restrictions on smoking in bars were to take effect January 1, 1997. The following year the tobacco industry convinced the Legislature to delay the smoke-free bar provision until January 1, 1998; the public health groups, who thought that the state was not ready for smoke-free bars at the time, put up only token opposition. In the fall of 1997 the tobacco industry tried to delay the effective date again. This time the health groups mobilized and beat the industry. Senate president pro tem Bill Lockyer shifted sides and helped the health groups defeat the tobacco industry. On January 1, 1998, all bars in California became smoke free.

CONCLUSION

In California 1994 was a busy year for tobacco control. By bringing together business, labor, local government, and health organizations, Friedman and the AB 13 support coalition successfully transformed public sentiment against smoking into statewide legislation that the tobacco industry did not like. The voluntary health agencies disseminated information about the adverse health effects of secondhand smoke, the CRA helped dispel fears that state smoking restrictions would hurt the restaurant business, and the League of Cities lent support to arguments that the bill would not limit the power of local governments to pass stricter restrictions than those contained in the bill. The coalition prevented the tobacco industry from taking control of the bill and passing a blatantly pro-industry version in the guise of tobacco control.

However, there was no consensus among California's tobacco control advocates on whether it was acceptable to compromise on preemption. Tobacco control advocates in Sacramento viewed the preemption clause in AB 13 as an acceptable compromise because of its 100 percent smoke-free mandate. They did not consider players outside Sacramento relevant, an attitude that damaged efforts to build support in the field for state-level legislative efforts. When asked about the disagreement within the California tobacco control movement over AB 13, a representative of the ACS's Sacramento Public Issues Office responded, "Organizations that are interested in tobacco control and have Sacramento-based lobbying offices were in agreement, and worked together regarding AB 13." [146]

In 1994 the tobacco industry was nearly successful in tricking California voters into repealing their own tobacco control laws. If the tobacco industry had been able to maintain its original strategy of a stealth campaign, its effort might well have succeeded. By limiting itself to direct mail, the industry would have stayed within a medium where it could control the message and deprive the health community of a platform. However, once the industry was forced out into the more public realm of mainstream advertising, it lost control over the public discourse about Proposition 188.

The Proposition 188 battle reunified tobacco control advocates as they put the fights over AB 13 behind them. According to one LLA director, "The whole process of that [AB 13] was real divisive. You know, we had members on our coalition who were saying, 'No, this is great and although it's not perfect, it's better to have something than nothing.' And it's like, 'But is it good to have something that's a piece of trash? That's going to eliminate ever doing anything better?' . . . Huge arguments. Once it finally passed and then Prop 188 came along, it was interesting, everybody sort of banded back together in the fight against Philip Morris." [57] California's tobacco control community was able to unify against and defeat Philip Morris.

But the passage of AB 13 and defeat of Proposition 188 significantly distracted the health groups from the fight to reauthorize the Proposition 99 programs. The legislation authorizing expenditure of Proposition 99 funds expired on June 30, 1994, at the height of the AB 13 debate and shortly after Proposition 188 had qualified for the ballot. AB 13, in particular, dominated the tobacco control agenda in California, draining the resources of health groups and commanding attention by the press and public.[147] So in what was a critical year for Proposition 99, its chief defenders were largely occupied elsewhere, which did not bode well for reauthorization. In addition, AB 13 and Proposition 188 would give the CMA and other medical groups cover for diverting Health Education Account monies. Proposition 99 was destined for another hard year in the Legislature.

CHAPTER 12

The End of Acquiescence

By the beginning of 1994, California's tobacco control movement had become a national and international model of how to use community-based programs and media to reduce tobacco consumption and exposure to secondhand smoke: 334 communities had passed local tobacco control ordinances, and the Legislature was close to passing AB 13, which would require virtually all workplaces in California to become smoke free. California had the third-lowest per capita consumption of tobacco of any state, and the reduction in smoking in California was costing the tobacco industry hundreds of millions of dollars in lost sales every year. Despite the diversion of money from the Health Education Account and the Wilson administration's lack of enthusiasm for implementing the anti-tobacco program, there was no longer any question about the effectiveness of Proposition 99's programs.

But the Health Education and Research Accounts were hardly secure. The 1988 election approving Proposition 99 was over five years old, and the strong public support for those programs, as reflected in the vote, was no longer as obvious as it had been when AB 75 had passed in 1989. The June 30, 1994, sunset of the legislation that authorized Proposition 99 expenditures—AB 99—meant that new authorizing legislation for Proposition 99 would have to be passed in 1994. Thanks to the governor's veto of SB 1088 late in 1993, both the Research Account and the Health Education Account were at risk in 1994. Indeed, Assembly Member Phil Isenberg (D-Sacramento), who had chaired the conference committees that crafted AB 75 and AB 99, referred to the unspent $21 million that had accrued in the Research Account as a "pool of opportunity."[1] Without a concerted effort by tobacco control advocates to activate public support, the Legislature was again likely to spend the Proposition 99 dollars as the politically powerful tobacco and medical interest groups would prefer—on medical services.

   Program advocates had three important things working in their favor: the success of the program (and thus a growing confidence in those who were running this major anti-tobacco campaign), the continuing popularity of anti-tobacco policies and programs, and the existence of a program constituency that had been created in the field. Success at the legislative level required the ability to rely on all three. But 1994 was a bad year for tobacco control advocates to be dedicating either staff or funds to a campaign to preserve Proposition 99. They were stretched thin by the spring battle over AB 13 and the looming fall battle over Proposition 188. Despite the inability of the health groups to protect the integrity of Proposition 99 in the conference committee setting in previous years, they once more agreed to a conference committee, again headed by Isenberg. Reauthorization was to be another insider deal.

THE GOVERNOR'S 1994–1995 BUDGET

Repeating the pattern he had established in prior years, Governor Pete Wilson drew up a budget that again called for diverting Health Education and Research funds to medical services, only at a higher rate. Perhaps in response to the bad press that the administration received when the American Lung Association (ALA) won its case over the media campaign, Wilson proposed giving the media campaign Section 43 protection, which meant that the media campaign would not be cut to get money for the protected medical programs. This decision would mean, however, that the local lead agencies (LLAs) and other local programs would be hit even harder by any Section 43 reductions. Following caseload adjustments and diminishing revenues, the governor's budget cut LLA funding from $20 million in 1993–1994 to $15 million in 1994–1995, competitive grants were dropped from $15 million to $10 million, and funds for schools from $22 million to $16 million. In total, the governor proposed that Health Education programs get only 12.7 percent of the total tobacco tax revenues instead of the 20 percent required by the initiative. In one of the few instances in which the Public Resources Account was threatened, the governor proposed a redirection of some Public Resources funding to the Child Health and Disability Prevention Program (CHDP). The governor proposed full funding for the Research Account, although there was no mention of the six months' worth of funds that had not been spent in the prior year.

In the governor's budget summary under "Preventive Services" the tobacco education program was not mentioned, despite its success. Instead the governor mentioned Healthy Start, Access for Infants and Mothers (AIM), and Education Now and Babies Later, among others. In describing the need for perinatal substance abuse services, alcohol and other drugs were specifically mentioned, but not tobacco.[2] The Wilson administration had no desire to draw public attention to tobacco.

Wilson also tried to quiet opposition from the ALA and Senator Watson's office. A top Wilson administration official held a secret meeting in which she threatened to "cripple" the implementation of the Proposition 99 programs if Najera and Miller did not accept the diversions demanded by Wilson. Wilson's representative threatened to seek out "the most stupid, incompetent, belligerent bureaucrats" she could find and put them in charge of tobacco education. Further, all the committed and effective members of the TCS staff would be reassigned to a regulatory "Siberia."[3] In fact, although the TCS staff was not replaced, the Wilson administration had already slowed the media campaign and would continue to hobble the program administratively until Wilson left office in 1999.

The hypocrisy of the argument that the state's budget problems made it necessary to divert money from the Health Education Account to medical services was exposed when the Legislative Analyst reviewed the governor's proposal for AIM. The analyst noted that AIM, the program which provided subsidized private health insurance for poor pregnant women, cost more money than providing the same services through MediCal, the state's Medicaid program. Moreover, AIM yielded worse clinical outcomes than MediCal.[4] Thus, the state was paying more money to get worse outcomes in terms of serving this population. The analyst proposed that AIM be discontinued and the services be provided by expanding MediCal eligibility.

Implementing the Legislative Analyst's proposal to switch from AIM to MediCal would have saved $74 million dollars, more than was being diverted out of the Health Education Account. Thus, changing programs could give better pregnancy outcomes and save enough money to avoid diversions from the Health Education Account for medical services. AIM, however, was to be preserved. It paid higher reimbursements to providers and involved the private insurance sector, which meant that it had powerful friends, especially the California Medical Association (CMA).

THE CREATION OF AB 816

Isenberg had generally been able to win consensus over the expenditure of Proposition 99 funds in prior years. In January 1994 he telephoned ALA lobbyist Tony Najera to discuss the reauthorization. Isenberg wanted Najera's viewpoint on whether he should again chair the conference committee that would handle Proposition 99 reauthorization through a bill named AB 816. According to Najera,

> Phil Isenberg called me personally. I can just remember the day so clearly in the first week in January. He said, "Tony, I've been encouraged to carry the ball and to chair a conference committee and to carry the bill on reauthorization. What do you think I ought to do?" I encouraged him to do it because I remembered my days with AB 75, that he was in fact one of our champions. He also had been the chief engineer in previous reauthorizations which I thought were a fair process. The process really really broke down during the AB 99 process and it was never recaptured for AB 816. So for me I encouraged Isenberg . . . and I said, "I think what you need to do is have a conference call with me, CMA, Western Center [for Law and Poverty]," and I did. That was to me the turning point in terms of what role I saw he was going to want to play for this.[5]

According to Najera, Isenberg was willing to chair the committee if there was "agreement amongst all of us," which meant that the principals agreed to the status quo.

When interviewed later, several of the principals had differing views of what this "agreement" had been. To Isenberg, "status quo" meant that everyone agreed to use the process that had been used with AB 75 and AB 99—a conference committee and behind-the-scenes deal-making.[6] Thus, while "status quo" also likely meant continued dwindling of funds for Health Education and Research programs and another "insider" deal, this deal had not been explicitly struck. When asked if she perceived that a deal had been made early with Isenberg, Elizabeth McNeil, the CMA's chief lobbyist on Proposition 99 in 1994, said she thought the status quo which had been agreed to included the maintenance of the AB 99 funding pattern. According to McNeil,

We had lots of meetings with Tony [Najera] and John [Miller], the hospitals, us, and the Western Center about Prop 99 reauthorization. *At the time, we all felt going in that pretty much trying to do status quo and make sure it was reauthorized was kind of the program.* And later on, the Lung Association and others decided no, they didn't want to fund CHDP. They wanted it out and they wanted increases for their programs. So we do feel like that was not the plan that we all went in with when we asked Isenberg to sponsor the bill. That's strongly how I felt about where we went in. . . . I don't know if there was miscommunication. It wasn't articulated strongly where his groups were really coming from. I think he [Najera]'s sensitive too because he was part of the group that authorized the original CHDP expenditure and was criticized for doing that, and I think was really feeling that criticism. So the tune changed and it was a problem amongst all of us.[7] [emphasis added]

The ALA's name appears with the CMA, California Association of Hospitals and Health Systems (CAHHS), and the Western Center for Law and Poverty as supporting the version of AB 816 that the Senate and Assembly voted into the Conference Committee. The bill extended the sunsets for both the program authorizations and the program appropriations to July 1, 1996, and also authorized the expenditures from the Research Account.[8] Senator Diane Watson (D-Los Angeles), the longtime champion of the Health Education Account and John Miller's boss, voted for AB 816 at this stage.

According to Najera, he and Miller had agreed to a quiet strategy of letting the Legislature make its decision and then taking the issue to court. He said, "We were not demanding [full] 20% [funding for Health Education] initially. We were prepared to do what we had to do in order to get it out of here and take it to the courts, and let the battle be there and not in here."[9] The voluntaries hoped that Wilson would not win reelection and that a new Democratic governor would be more sympathetic, ignoring the fact that opposition to the anti-tobacco education and research programs in the Legislature was spearheaded by Speaker Willie Brown, a Democrat. In any event, Wilson won reelection later that year.

OBJECTIONS TO CHDP

The early commitment by Najera and Miller to maintain the status quo and accept continued diversions of funds from the Health Education Account to CHDP and other medical services ran into trouble with the constituency that Proposition 99 had spawned. The Sacramento-based lobbyists were not used to considering the grassroots in their thinking.

The Sacramento lobbyists were used to compromising in the Legislature whereas local grassroots activists were used to winning pitched battles with the tobacco industry.

These two cultures clashed in October 1993 at the California Strategic Summit on the Future of Tobacco Control, a two-day meeting funded by the California Wellness Foundation to develop recommendations for the Legislature regarding reauthorization. Four major recommendations emerged from this conference: (1) the new legislation should authorize the program until the year 2000, (2) the diversion of Health Education monies into medical services should stop, (3) the Health Education Account should receive 20 percent of the tax money, as the voters mandated, and (4) Section 43 should be dropped.[10] The program constituency was tired of compromise. There was a strong feeling that Najera and the chair of the Tobacco Education Oversight Committee (TEOC), Carolyn Martin, who argued against the meeting's recommendations as being unrealistic, had already agreed to maintain the status quo in 1994. The conference forced the issue of demanding the full 20 percent of revenues for anti-tobacco education. There was pressure to fight a hard and public fight.

The public health groups also came under pressure from a study commissioned by the Department of Health Services (DHS) to examine the structure of the Proposition 99 program.[11] The committee preparing the study was chaired by Dr. Thomas Novotny of the federal Centers for Disease Control and Prevention (CDC) and the School of Public Health at the University of California at Berkeley. The central conclusion of the report was that the greatest threat to the tobacco education program was the "lack of will on the part of the government to implement the Health Education Account as originally mandated by the voters."[12] (The draft of the report went to DHS in December 1993, but it was not released until February 1994. Health groups suspected that the release of the report, which was critical of the governor, was delayed until after Kimberly Belshé was confirmed as head of the DHS.[13]) The second threat was the "failure of key constituent groups to hold the government fully accountable to the will of the voters."[12]

The ALA's position on Proposition 99 hardened. In an Action Alert sent by ALA on February 16, 1994, ALA urged recipients to write the members of the Conference Committee and request the following:

1. the removal of Section 43.
2. the removal of CHDP funding.

3.   removal of the requirement that ⅓ of LLA money go to perinatal funding.

4.   full 20% funding of health education.[14]

The boards of the ALA and the California Thoracic Society (a related medical association) adopted motions that they would not accept less than 20 percent funding for the Health Education Account.[15]

But taking a firm stand did not necessarily translate into an effective strategy. Paul Knepprath, who was working for ALA-Sacramento/Emigrant Trails during the 1994 fight, was advising the state-level ALA on media strategies and was urging them to be more public and confrontational. On March 18 he wrote to Miller and Najera to alert them that "time is running short on our opportunity to generate media on the Health Education Account." Knepprath continued, "Taking the offensive is critical. To do so, we need to create some waves, and plant the seed in the minds of conferees and other members that 'hey something's going on with that tobacco tax conference committee.' . . . *It may not be comfortable, but we have got to raise a stink if we want anyone to pay attention. Without the controversy, we don't have much hook and all the letter-writing will fall on deaf ears*" (emphasis added).[16] In spite of Knepprath's advice, ALA did not pursue a more aggressive public stance. Mary Griffin, a contract lobbyist who had been at the state Health and Welfare Agency during the debates over AB 75 and was paid by Americans for Nonsmokers' Rights (ANR) to monitor the 1994 process, criticized this approach. When asked about the failure to stop the diversions in AB 816, she replied, "Dragging their briefcases through the Capitol building does not constitute lobbying. Sitting in a legislator's office saying, 'Well, we really want this and blah, blah, blah,' it doesn't do it. Let me tell you, it doesn't do it. You need to lobby. That means using every resource at your command. It means getting your folks to give. Don't put out a letter and think your alert is going to go drum up the word. It doesn't work that way."[17]

As the process proceeded, the health groups began to vigorously object to CHDP and the other diversions from the Health Education Account. They were, however, hampered by their previous agreements to divert funds out of Health Education and into medical services. When asked about the CHDP compromise, Cathrine Castoreno, a lobbyist with the University of California, made the distinction between the CHDP compromise and other compromises that are typically done in the legislative arena:

Precedent is a powerful thing. . . . There are some cases where you compromise on stuff that you care about and it presents no tremendous risks. But they weren't just compromising the program, they were compromising the integrity of that statute. And once you agree to disregard the law, you're sucked in because there's no one who has greater disregard for the law than the legislators. And it's impossible for you with any credibility to go back and say, "Well, I agreed to break the law last year, but I don't want to do it this year." [18]

Isenberg was perceived by many parties to have been more hostile to the Health Education and Research Accounts in 1994 than in prior years. In a 1997 interview, Isenberg said that what really irritated him in 1994 was that representatives of the voluntary health agencies tried to argue that they had never supported the diversions into CHDP:

The part that I found most objectionable from the non-profits is they . . . said, "We never agreed to the first allocation, we didn't agree to the second allocation. You did it over our dead bodies." That is not true . . . and one of the problems with that posture, which has served them politically in many ways, . . . is that . . . this was not a case of a fifteen-year-old memory where nobody was left. This is where all the active participants were still there, and goddamn it, they were so angry, so bitter, so disappointed that they were misrepresenting the fact they signed off on the first deal. Well, in retrospect, *they shouldn't have signed off on the first deal, although they would have been ignored had they not participated.* There would have been other undesirable consequences that flowed from that. . . . If everybody knew then what they know now, that fight would have been exactly that issue.[6] [emphasis added]

The voter mandate of specific allocations to the Health Education and Research Accounts was no longer an issue. It was all about who was willing to deal.

Other key players also had some opinions about why Isenberg seemed so much more hostile in 1994. ANR's Robin Hobart observed,

He historically . . . had been very supportive of the health education efforts and then just totally turned about and was furious. And I really believe it's because he thought he had made a deal with Tony [Najera], that they were going to make that appropriation that way. Tony probably thought it was okay because it was going to be short term until the budget got better. And then when it turned out Tony couldn't really speak for the rest of the now many many players out in the field who were saying, "This is not acceptable," I think Isenberg was just furious. He felt a deal had been made and now it wasn't being delivered on.[19]

Peter Schilla, the lobbyist for the Western Center for Law and Poverty whose priority was finding money to pay for health services for poor people, continued to be an extremely influential lobbyist working against the tobacco control programs. Although his organization did not give campaign contributions, Isenberg listened to Schilla. According to John Miller,

> Somebody asked [Isenberg] in all the conflicting claims of the different sides on this dispute who did he believe. He said, "Peter Schilla is who I believe." And Peter was a very credible figure, very highly regarded around here in the health care field. And CMA moves huge muscle on these things and I think I, in [AB] 816, underestimated who was driving this thing. I believed it was the tobacco industry with the medical providers along for the ride. And I think it was just the opposite now. But while the CMA has huge weight with certain members, Peter's influence was greater. CMA couldn't have moved Phil, but Peter could. . . . Most politicians understand that when the industry comes to them and asks them to do something, that it's in the interest of that industry. But when the Western Center, good guy/consumers'/poor peoples' defenders, comes and says this is the right thing to do, they tend to do it.[20]

In the face of a hostile Isenberg and concerted and talented opponents, tobacco control advocates had a difficult authorization fight ahead. One of Schilla's sources of power was his ability to both raise and solve problems, based in part on his in-depth knowledge of health programs and budgets. The voluntaries' lobbying staffs never developed the same level of expertise on these important technical details.

Isenberg was correct in pointing out that the voluntary health agencies had acquiesced in the previous diversions of Health Education Account money into medical services, including CHDP. They were now trying to change course five years into the program, which meant that they needed to account for the shift. A May 9 memo from the ALA Government Relations Office explained the change in ALA's stance: "CHDP's costs have grown so large that they now jeopardize the very existence of the Health Education Program. We can now support CHDP only by sacrificing the anti-tobacco education effort. Straight line projections indicate that the Health Education Program would be ineffectual in two years and disappear entirely in four years if it is forced to sustain CHDP. We simply have no choice but to insist that the Medical Services appropriation support CHDP—not Health Education."[21] ACS's Don Beerline echoed this philosophy when he was asked in 1996 why the voluntary health agencies decided to refuse to accept diversions in AB 816: "We said that this is destroying the program at this point. In the previous diversions, the money did go to indigent care, that's consistently where it went. But it was such a smaller percentage, we felt that the programs could be carried out. But in '94–'95 that was obviously the point where we felt that the programs were becoming ineffective. So that's the reason that we decided to go along with drawing the line in the sand."[22]

But the tough stance in 1994 was about more than just the size of the diversions from anti-tobacco programs to medical services. One of the reasons why the Coalition came down so hard against the diversions in 1994 was that for the first time they acknowledged how little was being done for tobacco use prevention within CHDP. When asked about the decision to try to halt the diversions, TEOC chair Carolyn Martin explained, "The TEOC had worked very diligently to try and get information on what was going on in CHDP and, believe me, it was not easy. Dr. [Lester] Breslow especially and I were down there pounding on their door and eventually we figured out there was nothing to give us because they weren't doing anything. So I think that made a huge difference, plus the extent of the diversion. Suddenly we're talking about huge percentages and big drops in programs."[23]

Martin was supported in several quarters on CHDP's lack of effectiveness as an anti-smoking program. Bruce Pomer, executive director of the Health Officers Association of California, wrote to Isenberg on June 21, 1994, protesting the planned diversions. He specifically criticized the latest effort to put Health Education Account money into CHDP:

> Our concern is the deceptive nature of the proposal. The current health provider protocols ($150 million in CHDP) have never had their effectiveness assessed. The last assessment of medical anti-tobacco protocols found no demonstrable effect what-so-ever from physician provided anti-tobacco advice. We find it ironic that the medical industry now proposes expanding physician assisted anti-tobacco education, which has been found to be largely ineffective. Likewise, it should give one pause that these amendments are supported exclusively by the medical industry and that not a single health education organization considers the suggestion to have any merit.[24]

The California Tobacco Survey, the large survey of tobacco use in California conducted by John Pierce of the University of California at San Diego for DHS, failed to demonstrate any impact on smoking by CHDP.[25] In contrast, the survey found large effects from much smaller programs, such as the media campaign and the creation of smoke-free workplaces.

THE HIT LIST

The passage of Proposition 99 and the infusion of millions of dollars into anti-tobacco education gave public health advocates in California the means to embark on a comprehensive public health program that was far more aggressive than previous anti-tobacco campaigns. Instead of running cessation classes that emphasized the health effects of tobacco use, DHS and the county LLAs funded innovative programs that battled the tobacco industry in the arenas where it pushed tobacco use. For example, since the industry targeted auto racing, DHS funded a race car to carry the anti-tobacco message to the racetrack. This program disrupted tobacco industry use of auto racing as a promotional medium and led patrons to demand smoke-free areas at racetracks. A grant to the Kirkwood Ski Foundation was used to counter tobacco sponsorship of and advertising at ski events over a period of two and a half years. The project hosted athletic magnet events that included both competitions and tobacco-free presentations and ultimately displaced tobacco sponsorship. Another program sought to reach poor women by sponsoring smoke-free baby showers. According to Carol Russell, who oversaw these programs for TCS, "We're going where the companies are and they hate us for it."[26] And the program was showing results. Tobacco use in California declined faster than it did in the rest of nation and at a rate three times faster than it had in California prior to Proposition 99.[27]

The tobacco industry peppered the program with public records act requests to collect detailed information on every aspect of Proposition 99, then used this information to prepare a "hit list" of unconventional Proposition 99 programs that distorted and ridiculed these programs.[28] Californians for Smokers' Rights (CSR), an organization fostered by RJ Reynolds and headed by Bob Merrell, objected to the programs as frivolous. He also accused the state of building and operating a "statewide political organization" that illegally spent tax dollars to lobby.[26] The CMA distributed a similar list to the Legislature and journalists.[29] And the promoters of the hit list were successful in getting their message out. Conservative *San Francisco Chronicle* columnist Deborah Sanders echoed the list's message with this jibe: "Pretend for a minute that you are a legislator—just for a minute, I'll try not to make this too painful. You are given a choice. You can spend $175,000 on prenatal care, or you can spend $175,000 on a 'Ski Tobacco-Free' weekend at Kirkwood Meadows in Tahoe."[30] A highly innovative, two-and-a-half-year program was, with the stroke of a pen, reduced to a boondoggle weekend. Another list made fun of some projects funded by the Research Account, such as a study of smoking and facial wrinkling in women. These lists became major tools for the tobacco industry and its allies in the 1994 reauthorization fight.

A similar hit list turned up in Massachusetts in 1992 and Arizona in 1994, where the tobacco industry was fighting initiatives modeled on Proposition 99.[31-35]

THE ANR-SAYNO LAWSUIT

Two players entered the debate over the future of Proposition 99 with the explicit goal of forcing the debate out of the Legislature and back into the public arena and the courts: ANR and the new organization Just Say No to Tobacco Dough (SAYNO).

ANR was increasingly critical of the approach that the voluntary health agencies were taking in Sacramento, which ANR viewed as gutless. ANR director Julia Carol described the voluntaries' AB 816 reauthorization effort this way:

> Nobody was willing to fight. They're all still asking nicely. . . . the CMA was still eagerly grabbing the money and none of the voluntaries were willing to publicly slap their hands about it or to use any sort of clout. You know, in advocacy you have two tools. You have a carrot and you have a stick. The really good advocates figure out when to use which and how much, and whether you use both. What the voluntaries were using mostly was the carrot. They said they were doing an aggressive fight, but they didn't really know what that meant. . . . I think it means [to them] that every now and then they write a sort of tough letter that they don't publicize in any way. And that they speak up kind of boldly behind the scenes in closed-door sessions.[36]

If ANR was to get involved, it would be outside the Legislature's back rooms.

Attorney A. Lee Sanders, who had been executive director of California Common Cause in the 1970s, wanted to do something to discourage politicians from taking money from the tobacco industry. He had just formed SAYNO to encourage candidates for office in California to refuse such contributions. When he contacted Stanton Glantz for information on campaign contributions by the tobacco industry, Glantz expressed frustration that none of the health groups had sued to restore the integrity of Proposition 99. When Sanders expressed interest, Glantz put him in touch with ANR, which joined with Sanders because of the organization's belief in the power of outside strategies.[37] On February 2, 1994, SAYNO and ANR sent formal demand letters to the California State Treasurer and Controller, asking for the return of funds already diverted from the Proposition 99 Health Education Account and threatening to

sue if the money was not returned. ANR invited ALA and the other voluntary health agencies to join their effort, but they "would have nothing of it at the time." [36]

On the morning of March 23, just hours before the Conference Committee was scheduled to meet to consider AB 816, ANR and SAYNO
held a press conference in Sacramento to announce that they had filed a
lawsuit against the governor, the Legislature, and others seeking restoration of the $165 million that had been diverted from the Health Educa-
tion Account into medical services under AB 75 and AB 99 and attempt-
ing to stop future misappropriations. The lawsuit (*ANR et al. v. State of
California*, Sac. Super. Ct. No. 539577) derailed the plan for a quick
passage of AB 816.

Najera and the other lobbyists were furious. They believed that the
ANR lawsuit made the AB 816 fight more difficult because the legislators
did not separate ALA from ANR. Najera tried to distance himself from
the suit, and an April 8 ALA press release announced that the American
Lung Association of California "is not currently a party to, or involved
in any way with, a lawsuit filed by Americans for Nonsmokers' Rights
(ANR) and Just Say No to Tobacco Dough (SAYNO)." [38] Najera was still
hoping for success at the inside game that ANR was disrupting.

THE CONFERENCE COMMITTEE HEARING

The Conference Committee held its hearing on AB 816 on March 23,
but most of the program advocates observing the process thought that
they had little ability to affect the outcome. Isenberg used the hit list that
CSR and the CMA had prepared and widely circulated (without attri-
bution) to ridicule the program. According to Miller, those who wished
to protect the Health Education Account were not given much of an opportunity to do so:

> It was a fairly perfunctory hearing. . . . I mean, after berating us, they didn't
> take any evidence. Then Phil announced the findings that he intended to move
> the money out of Health Education into these other programs. And I remem-
> ber Ken Maddy [Republican minority leader] was sitting next to him and Ken
> turned to him and said, "But we all agreed that that was not possible." And
> Phil said something to the effect that "things are different now." And I real-
> ized that that was the first Maddy knew they were going to go for four-fifths
> and that they were going to change it. It was a Democratic initiative, 816
> was. . . . Maddy quickly realized what was going on and got on board in a
> hurry.[20]

Supporters of the health education programs were surprised to find that
Isenberg was a leader in attacking the programs. Isenberg sought to paint
the health advocates who were seeking to protect Proposition 99 as being just another special interest now addicted to public funding. Isenberg pointed out to a *Los Angeles Times* reporter that many of the same
groups who were now fighting the use of Health Education Account
funds for health screening and prenatal care programs had agreed to this
use in the past. According to Isenberg, these groups "have taken on the
garb of a religious crusade." [1]

Martin, responding on behalf of the ALA, wrote that they were
"shocked" by Isenberg's comments.[39] She pointed out that Proposition 99 funds distributed to ALA represented less than 4 percent of ALA's
budgets from around the state of California and was only .001 percent
of the 1993–1994 tax revenues. She argued that the appropriation
should be made, not only because it was a voter mandate but also because the program had demonstrated its effectiveness. She pointed out
that "criticizing a few programs cannot erase the tremendous total impact of this complex prevention program." Neither ACS nor AHA took
Proposition 99 money.

The University of California had generally been quiet about the Research Account, reflecting its position as a public body whose board of
regents is chaired by the governor. This stance sometimes frustrated the
university's allies. For example, in 1992 AHA officials had written to
University of California president Jack Peltason to express their disappointment at the university's failure to oppose diversion of the Research
Account funds and the hope that "the University of California will take a
leading role in opposing such attempts." [40] Put to the test again in 1994,
the university would again play a cautious role.

UC lobbyist Cathrine Castoreno was frustrated trying to protect the
Research Account in the 1994 hearings. University representatives testified on behalf of the Research Account—but without drawing any lines
in the sand—and, in fact, worked to accommodate Isenberg. According
to Castoreno,

> I gave explicit testimony about what was most definitely illegal versus what
> they might possibly be able to do. This is a point in the proceedings towards
> the end of the Conference Committee on 816 where it was clear that there
> was going to be a diversion of Research Account monies. The issue was how
> much and how. We were pretty well beat up by that time . . . so, in an effort to
> try and keep the program from being completely defunded and to keep them
> from making a move that would be wholly illegal, I worked with our coun-
> sel and Dr. [Cornelius] Hopper [UC's vice president for health affairs] to put

together an analysis of 99 and see, given their goal to divert money, how they
might do it legally. . . . We made it very clear that simply using the money
straight out of the Research Account for health services or any other purpose
was obviously and clearly illegal and challengeable in court. And they thanked
us very much for that [laughter].[18]

The university even provided a written proposal on how the Research Account might legitimately be used for other purposes, such as by explicitly amending the initiative to put the diverted money into the Unallocated Account instead of directly funding medical care from the Research
Account. The university's official position on reducing the Research Account from 5 percent to 3 percent was "neutral."[41]

The schools were also subjected to a harsh review by Isenberg, who
was frustrated by the lack of tobacco programming there. By March
1994, after the program had been running for four years in the schools,
the evaluation conducted for the California Department of Education
(CDE) by Southwest Regional Laboratory reported that 41 percent of
youth in grades 7 through 12 reported at least one tobacco lesson and
activity event.[42] This finding also meant, of course, that 59 percent did
not, despite the fact that the schools had received a total of $147 mil-
lion in Proposition 99 funds in the 1993–1994 fiscal year.[43] Through
the spring of 1994 all schools were getting entitlement money based on
average daily attendance. The report also pointed out that "the DATE
[Drug, Alcohol, and Tobacco Education] program needs clear definition of the model and its components in order to standardize and focus
prevention and reduction efforts targeting school youth."[42] The health
groups generally agreed with Isenberg's criticisms of the schools.[20]

THE CMA

In 1992 Steve Thompson, who had served as Assembly Speaker Willie
Brown's chief of staff and the head of the Assembly Office of Research,
had moved to the CMA to become its vice president and head lobbyist.
This job change put him in a powerful position from which to continue
to advocate for the diversions out of the Health Education Account into
CHDP, a program he had helped design years earlier while working for
Brown. Brown and the tobacco industry were both interested in shifting
Health Education and Research monies into other programs.

The CMA continued to portray its position as a painful choice between taking care of poor children and funding prevention programs
that have a longer-term benefit. In the end, of course, providing money

for medical providers always took priority. A CMA Executive Committee report stated, "While CMA policy supports the funding of the medical research program and health education, it generally gives funding priority to health care programs for the uninsured. In 1990 and with agreement from the health education community, CMA supported the proposal to fund CHPD [*sic*] screens for California's poor children from the health education account. Later CMA supported the addition of AIM, MRMIP and OBRA perinatal services."[44] The statement reflects the CMA's long-established position that the program allocations among the different accounts in Proposition 99 are not binding. The framing of the issue as a choice between women and children on one hand and health education on the other had relieved the tobacco industry of the need to take overt measures against the Proposition 99 Health Education and Research programs. Legislators were not voting for the tobacco industry; they were voting for pregnant women and poor children. The CMA supported this view from the right, and the Western Center for Law and Poverty supported it from the left.

The medical interests and counties warned the ALA that they intended to pursue a four-fifths vote in the Legislature to divert the Health Education and Research money into medical programs. In a private meeting hosted by the County Supervisors' Association, the CMA, the CAHHS, and the Western Center for Law and Poverty, among others, informed ALA and Miller that passage by a four-fifths majority vote would occur and threatened that, if the voluntaries did not accept the terms they offered, the health community would take the entire Education and Research Accounts. Najera and Miller refused and promised there would be "blood on the walls."[3]

Whereas the Health Education Account had been under siege in previous authorization battles, the Research Account had been reasonably well protected. But in 1994 the CMA had the Research Account in its sights. Among other things, the program had funded studies on campaign contributions by the tobacco industry to members of the California Legislature as well as an analysis of the implementation of Proposition 99 highlighted the pattern of diversions of funds. This work angered Willie Brown, who demanded that the University of California stop this work.[45,46] Soon after the university refused, the CMA began attacking the Research Account as a waste of money and agitating to use the money for medical services.

Elizabeth McNeil, one of the CMA lobbyists, said that the CMA had neither prepared nor circulated the hit list of Health Education and Re-

search Account projects. She declined to speculate about who had prepared them and went on to say,

> Research by far got the most criticism and they didn't do a good job at de-
> fending themselves . . . and they [the Conference Committee] took those dol-
> lars to balance the budget basically and fund some kids' health programs that
> I have to say are very worthy. And that was a tough call, but we did support
> the overall dynamics because of the political pressures on getting the budget
> and with budget deficits and the importance that we place on some of these
> indigent programs and when there was some frivolous research projects go-
> ing on perhaps. . . . We really didn't support that shift being made, but in the
> end we supported the whole deal, felt like it was the best compromise we were
> going to get.[7]

Steve Scott of the *California Journal* reported, however, that he got the
list from the CMA. More important, he saw CMA's support of the diversions as important to getting them through the Legislature:

> The California Medical Association got successively more brazen in its ap-
> proach and its willingness to kind of undermine the tenets of the education
> fund. I remember in the Conference Committee meetings on [AB] 816, As-
> semblyman Isenberg started rolling out the horror stories about the Research
> Account and how the Research Account was being used for these . . . ridicu-
> lous grants. And I got a list of those ridiculous grants from the California
> Medical Association. It was leaked to me through the CMA. . . . You talk to
> their lobbyist and she'll deny that they were openly advocating the diversions,
> that it was an unfortunate necessity that they had to agree to the diversions to
> make the tradeoff. But in truth they were right in there pitching subtly on the
> whole question of, and not so subtly, increasingly less subtly, on the issue of
> the problems with the Research Account. . . . So a lot of the pushing against
> the Research and Education Account, or in favor of more money going to di-
> rect medical services, was coming from the California Medical Association.[47]

In addition to attacking the Research Account, a May 1994 CMA report justified the use of Health Education Account monies for CHDP
"due to the anti-smoking education component of the program."[29] It
reported that the administration offered "education representatives" a
compromise—capping CHDP at $30 million a year—but were turned
down. The report comments that some "questionable 'education' projects," such as anti-tobacco sponsorship of a ski program ($175,000), a
race car ($200,000), and a high school rap contest ($175,000), led
"many" conferees to believe that there was adequate funding of both
the Health Education Account and CHDP. The projects that the CSR
and the CMA used as examples of frivolous expenditures were some of
the most innovative programs spawned by Proposition 99.[28,29]

Physician Roger Kennedy, a CMA member who worked throughout the nineties to get the CMA to support health education and the chair of Santa Clara County's tobacco control coalition, believed that the doctors had talked themselves into a bad position:

> When the diversions occurred, I had a number of discussions with some very highly responsible people that I respect and have known for a long time . . . people who were in significant roles, people on the board, who were of the view that this money was so crucial to provide care for the kids in California. . . . But I think they fooled themselves into thinking that they couldn't take care of kids without this money. . . . This allowed them to overlook the fact that AIM program was, by everybody's analysis, extremely inefficient and was money that could have been covered in another way; MediCal would have been a much better way.[48]

Kennedy believed that the CMA should have been willing to call Wilson's bluff and saw two key reasons for the CMA's unwillingness to spend political capital on this issue. First, the CMA needed the governor's support on other important matters and did not want to alienate him on this issue. According to Kennedy, "It was the easier path to go that didn't require pushing Wilson and angering Wilson. The CMA leadership wanted to work with Wilson on other issues, and they felt that to push him on this would compromise their ability to work with him. At this point, he really had his heels just dug in. So they felt he wouldn't move on this or, if they forced him to move on this, it would harm them in other ways."[48] Second, the CMA gives priority to the pocketbook issues of its members. As Kennedy explained, "The CMA has already been in trouble for a number of years in terms of membership because doctors' incomes are dropping and they don't see the value. So if the CMA isn't using its political clout to ward off the optometrists and instead is going along with making sure that the money from Prop 99 goes to fund tobacco education instead going into doctors' pockets, the CMA is going to look like they're not really supporting their members."[48] Thus it was in the CMA's interests to support the same agenda that the tobacco industry had: further diversions of Proposition 99 anti-tobacco Health Education and Research money into medical services.

LAST-MINUTE EFFORTS TO STOP AB 816

There were some last-minute efforts to attract publicity to the Proposition 99 reauthorization fight. On June 2 the Coalition had a press conference featuring Senators Art Torres (D-Los Angeles) and Tom Hayden (D-Santa Monica) and Assembly Member Delaine Eastin (D-Fremont) to "expose the budget 'smokescreen' being used by opponents of the successful community-based anti-tobacco education."[49] It attracted little coverage. A June 6 Action Alert, issued in both English and Spanish by the Coalition to Save Proposition 99, tried to generate pressure on the Legislature.[50] On July 6 Joe Holsinger, a deputy superintendent at CDE, wrote a letter cosigned by representatives of a variety of education organizations and school districts to Assembly Speaker Willie Brown and Senate President pro tem Bill Lockyer, asking for their help in stopping the diversion of funds.[51,52] ALA issued a press release containing a statement from Spencer Koerner, the chairman of the board of ALA, that explicitly confronted the medical lobby:

> Today marks the beginning of the end of the world's most successful tobacco use prevention and education campaigns. . . . AB 816 destroys that program by diverting money earmarked by the voters for education (20% of the revenues of the tobacco tax) into medical care programs. This in spite of the fact that over 70% of the Proposition 99 revenue is already being spent on medical care. *Organized medicine represented by the California Medical Association and California Association of Hospitals & Health Systems, and community clinic providers led by the Western Center on Law & Poverty has successfully hijacked California's tobacco education funds as well as the five percent designated for research.*[53] [emphasis added]

ALA wrote members of the Legislature urging them to vote against AB 816, warning that "with the passage of AB 816, California's popular anti-tobacco research and education program will die a slow, painful death."[54]

The governor personally intervened to kill the tobacco research program. According to Castoreno, she was abruptly ordered to halt the lobbying efforts: "I was busily conveying the university's opposition to the measure along with the voluntaries. The director [of the university's Sacramento lobbying office], Steve Arditti, came running into the hallways with a look on his face like somebody vital had died. And it shot a pain through my heart and he conveyed that the governor had just called the [UC] president—Peltason, at the time—to say that AB 816 was part of the budget package. It's absolutely important to him, he wanted it and we needed to stop opposing it."[18] The CMA wrote legislators supporting the bill and presenting its passage as a routine extension of the status quo: "Except for the cuts to the research account, which were part of the

overall state budget agreement, the bill distributes Prop 99 funds much
the way they have been apportioned since the inception of Prop 99."[55]

THE FLOOR FIGHT

The tobacco and medical interests could control when AB 816 would be
heard in the Legislature. ALA anticipated they would schedule the hearing just before the summer recess, when Legislators were eager to return
home and unlikely to think much about proposals before them. The voluntary health agencies, knowing they lacked the clout to stop even a
four-fifths vote in the Assembly, decided to concentrate their efforts
on stopping the bill in the Senate. Miller believed that the core of liberal Democratic senators who truly cared about the issue would be tobacco control's best—indeed only—chance against the allied tobacco
and medical interests.[3]

Isenberg took up AB 816 in the Assembly on the day before the summer break, describing the bill as a routine fiscal bill necessary to balance
the budget and fund important health programs. Few members bothered
to read the bill, only a handful abstained, and the measure passed out of
the Assembly with the necessary four-fifths vote.

About two o'clock that same afternoon, Senator Mike Thompson (D-
Santa Rosa) took up the bill in the Senate without ceremony—and it
was immediately defeated. Thompson could not even achieve a majority,
to say nothing of a four-fifths vote. The bill failed by a vote of 18-12.
Thompson was dumbfounded, and he immediately left the floor to notify AB 816's sponsors and author.[3] The tobacco and medical interests
and county governments were galvanized into action, and the next four
hours saw a dramatic legislative conflict.

The three voluntary health agencies, public health officers, public
schools, and the independent universities had stunned the multi-billion-
dollar tobacco and medical industries in a remarkable upset. Watching
the defeat on television in Senator Diane Watson's office, the dozen or so
Proposition 99 proponents could not believe their own success. Minutes
after the defeat of the bill, the Democrats withdrew from the floor for a
closed caucus. Watson returned to her office and warned the celebrating
tobacco control advocates that they could not relax; they were about to
witness the full fury of the medical providers, the tobacco industry, and
local governments.[3]

Back in session, the Senate violated its own procedural rules, granting

AB 816 immediate "reconsideration" and another vote. More than fifty lobbyists spread through the Capitol building with promises or threats or demands of support from the senators. On the floor, a passionate debate was underway, pitching the interests of the ill and enfeebled against the obligation of the Legislature to honor the will of the voters.

In a remarkable political event, Governor Wilson left his office (which is also located in the Capitol building) and met with Senator Marion Bergeson (R-Newport Beach), a conscientious Mormon and the only Republican determined to resist the tobacco-medical coalition. This incident was the first and only time during his tenure that Governor Pete Wilson left his office to influence a vote on the floor of the Senate. Senate Republican minority leader Ken Maddy demanded that every member of the Republican caucus support AB 816 and refused to permit any Republican to exit the caucus without a commitment. The speaker of the Assembly, Willie Brown, appeared on the Senate floor with Phil Isenberg and pressured senators to vote for AB 816. Bill Lockyer, a Democrat, moved from desk to desk demanding Democratic votes for AB 816. For three hours, the contest continued as other business was carried out on the floor. Slowly, gradually, inevitably, the governor, legislative leadership, and county and medical lobbyists moved vote after vote. A core group including Senators Art Torres (D-Los Angeles), Diane Watson (D-Los Angeles), Tom Hayden (D-Santa Monica), and Nicholas Petris (D-Oakland) refused to compromise. With only one necessary vote remaining, Lockyer and Maddy threatened to fly in Senator Bill Craven (R-San Diego), who was seriously ill with lung disease, to conclude the contest, and a last holdout conceded, giving AB 816 the necessary four-fifths vote.

THE FINAL BILL

The governor signed the bill, which contained cuts in anti-tobacco health education and research that were approximately what he had originally proposed (figure 15). Over the two fiscal years 1994–1995 and 1995–1996, AB 816 appropriated only $94 million for anti-tobacco education (as opposed to the $157 million required by the initiative) and $8 million for research (as opposed to the $44 million required by the initiative, plus the $21 million left unexpended from the previous year).[56] AB 816 brought the total amount of diversions from the Health Education and Research Accounts to medical services to $301 million since Proposi-

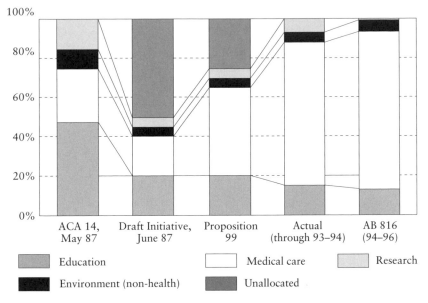

Figure 15. Proposition 99 funding allocations for AB 816. The legislation substantially accelerated the shift of money away from anti-tobacco education into medical services and now shifted funds from research too. It represented the most drastic diversion from the terms of Proposition 99 to date.

tion 99 had passed, or about 34 percent of the total allocated by the voters to anti-tobacco education and research.

The outcome in 1994 thus continued the downward spiral for the Health Education and Research Accounts that began in 1989 with the first CHDP compromise. There was one important difference, however: in 1994 all three voluntary health agencies actively—if unsuccessfully —opposed *any* diversion from the Health Education and Research Accounts to fund medical services.

Assembly Member Terry Friedman (D-Santa Monica) abstained rather than voting against on AB 816.[43] A "no" vote would have deprived AB 816 of a four-fifths vote in the Assembly and stopped the diversions. In spite of all the work that the voluntary health agencies had done to pass his AB 13, which had barely made it through the Legislature in June 1994, Friedman did not support them on the AB 816 vote. Ironically, AB 13 was presented by some as an alternative to full funding of the Proposition 99 anti-tobacco education and research programs. For example, the *Los Angeles Times* editorialized in May 1994 that "the continuing diversion of [Health Education] funds is regrettable, if seemingly unavoidable, but the gains against cigarette smoking . . . need not be lost. The best strategy, in our opinion, is passage of AB 13, which would make smoking illegal in most workplaces throughout the state."[57]

AB 816 contained three significant program changes. First, more controls were put on the schools. Schools would receive money based on Average Daily Attendance only for grades 4–8, while high schools would have to apply for competitive grants. In addition, evaluation of their programs would be conducted by evaluators in the DHS Tobacco Control Section (TCS), and the deadline for becoming tobacco free was moved from 1996 to 1995. Miller was less critical of Isenberg's stance on the schools than of his stance on the health departments and the Research Account. According to Miller, "The kinds of changes which had been proposed, indeed what Phil proposed for the schools, I think were long overdue and appropriate. I would still have an in-school program . . . [and] restrict it to those schools which express an interest."[20] Second, public policy research was added as a priority area for the Research Account funding because it was "an area of compelling interest" to the Legislature. Third, the Tobacco Education Oversight Committee had oversight of the Research programs added to its mission and was renamed the Tobacco Education and Research Oversight Committee (TEROC). These changes were all consistent with positions the health groups had been advocating.

While the Health Education and Research Accounts took heavy hits from the Legislature, the governor's proposal to redirect some of the funds from the Public Resources Account was dropped, so this account again got more than its required minimum of 5 percent of the Proposition 99 dollars. According to Miller, the Legislature "gave about ten minutes to thinking about ripping off the mountain lion money and walked away from that" because "the environmentalists will kick their ass."[9,20] The CMA's lobbyist, Elizabeth McNeil, had a similar response: "I think . . . fighting the environmentalists was a whole other realm, and a whole other fight, and I think that a lot of people made the assumption that that was a fight that was not even winnable. And that here was an arena where you had all health care organizations, who you could hope could help prioritize health care interests."[7] There were important lessons here for the tobacco control advocates. The Public Resources Account was able to resist raids on its funds, and its advocates apparently had to do very little to protect it because everyone knew they were willing to "kick your ass."

CONCLUSION

By 1994, there was no question that Proposition 99 had succeeded in achieving the goal its framers had in mind: to create a large anti-tobacco education and research program that would accelerate the decline in tobacco consumption in California. Through the end of fiscal year 1993–1994, the Proposition 99 programs (combined with the impact of the price increase that accompanied the tax) had roughly tripled the rate of decline in cigarette consumption in California and prevented about 1.6 billion packs of cigarettes from being smoked, worth about $2 billion in pre-tax sales to the tobacco industry.

Over this period of time, however, the Legislature and the governor had diverted a total of $301 million out of the anti-tobacco programs, about 34 percent of the total that the voters had set aside for these activities. Assuming a proportional drop in program effectiveness, these diversions probably resulted in an additional 530 million packs of cigarettes being consumed, worth about $800 million to the tobacco industry. Viewed from this perspective, the $23 million that the industry spent on campaign contributions and lobbying between 1988 and 1994 yielded a good return on investment.[56,58]

Until 1994, full funding of anti-tobacco education had been withheld with the consent of the agencies who were responsible for lobbying for the Health Education and Research programs—ALA, ACS, AHA. The passage of AB 816, however, was different; it passed despite the strenuous objections of the three organizations. While the confrontation over the diversions in AB 816 did not put an end to them, the dispute did achieve two other objectives. It began to engage the media and the public, and it set the stage for a legal test of the diversions.

CHAPTER 13

The Lawsuits

By the conclusion of the AB 816 fight, the principled position that the voluntary health agencies had taken left them free to pursue relief in the courts. The fact that the American Lung Association (ALA), American Cancer Society (ACS), and American Heart Association (AHA) had agreed to the diversions under AB 75 and AB 99 made it both legally and politically difficult for the organizations to reverse their position and challenge the diversions in court when those bills were passed. The AB 816 fight left them with no such encumbrance.

During the conflict over AB 816, everyone knew that the issue would end up in court. On the same day that the Conference Committee was to vote on AB 816, Lee Sanders and Americans for Nonsmokers' Rights (ANR) had filed the SAYNO suit to derail the early deal that ANR believed ALA and others had made to support AB 816, including the diversions. ANR also wanted to put everyone on notice that there would be legal challenges to any bill that did not comply with Proposition 99. By the end of the legislative debate over AB 816, the health groups were openly threatening to sue if the Legislature and the governor persisted in adopting legislation that was not consistent with Proposition 99. The Legislature attempted to head off or at least weaken a potential legal challenge to AB 816 by the way it wrote the "findings" portion of the bill. All references to the medical problems caused by smoking were eliminated, and instead the bill stated that "the efforts to reduce smoking in California have led to a drop in the consumption of tobacco. Although not on target to meet the goal of achieving a 75-percent reduction in tobacco consumption in California by the year 1999 [established in AB 75], the results are encouraging."[1]

ANR filed the first lawsuit over AB 816 on August 31, 1994, asking the court to block the $128 million in expenditures from the Health Education and Research Accounts during fiscal years 1994–1995 and 1995–1996 for purposes other than health education and research. At that time, ANR withdrew from the SAYNO suit to pursue this new case, since the legal issues in the AB 816 case were similar and its resolution would move more quickly for procedural reasons. (As a result, Lee Sanders and the Attorney General agreed to suspend action on the SAYNO suit until the AB 816 case was resolved.) A week later, on September 6, ALA and ACS filed a similar lawsuit. (AHA refused to join the suit because it thought that the fight would be costly and the plaintiffs would lose.[2]) The two lawsuits were consolidated and heard in Superior Court in Sacramento. At issue was the nature of two programs—Child Health and Disability Prevention (CHDP) and Comprehensive Perinatal Outreach (CPO)—and whether they could legitimately be considered "health education."

CHILD HEALTH AND DISABILITY PREVENTION

AB 75 had mandated that the Department of Health Services (DHS) issue protocols for an anti-tobacco component in CHDP, including protocols dissuading children from beginning to smoke, encouraging cessation, and providing information on the health effects of tobacco use on the user and nonsmokers, including children. DHS used a report produced by the National Cancer Institute, *How to Help Your Patients Stop Smoking: A National Cancer Institute Manual for Physicians,* and a supplement, *Clinical Interventions to Prevent Tobacco Use by Children and Adolescents,* as a model for developing and implementing tobacco prevention programs within CHDP.[3-6]

According to DHS, the department informed local agencies of the anti-tobacco requirement, developed a protocol, added three questions on tobacco to the CHDP claim form, and provided training in the use of the protocol.[7] While training targeted CHDP staff, the screens were actually performed by 4,500 provider organizations, not local CHDP staff.[8] The "train the trainer" model used by DHS assumed that the county-level staff, once trained, would indeed train the actual providers and require that the tobacco use prevention be done. This model assumed a commitment to anti-tobacco programs throughout CHDP that simply did not exist.

Gordon Cumming, the DHS official responsible for CHDP, made his view of the CHDP funds clear when he met with the Tobacco Education Oversight Committee (TEOC) on December 3, 1991. When asked about a formal evaluation, Cumming told TEOC that "tobacco funds were meant primarily to provide for screenings of more children, and that the only evaluation is that entailed in the program management."[9] He also admitted that he had little faith in the data collected on the answers to the three tobacco questions "because of the context of its collection and the difficulty with just getting correct birth dates on the invoices."[9]

Another indication of the level of CHDP's commitment to tobacco use prevention is the nature of its program. The National Cancer Institute (NCI) guidelines are much stronger than those of CHDP, even though the CHDP program was supposedly based on the NCI guidelines. Under the CHDP protocol, the only requirement was an answer to three questions on the reimbursement form:

1. Is the patient exposed to secondhand smoke?

2. Does the patient use tobacco?

3. If the patient does use tobacco, was the patient counseled about/ referred for tobacco use prevention or cessation programs?[10]

The NCI guidelines recommend a much more involved role for the physician and the office staff. In 1994, when asked to critique the CHDP protocol, Marc Manley, chief of the NCI Public Health Applications Research Branch and a coauthor of the NCI guidelines, saw wide variances between those guidelines and the CHDP protocol.[11] For example, while the CHDP protocol makes the creation of a smoke-free office a "suggested" intervention, the NCI guidelines state unequivocally, "Create a smoke-free office" and require a list of six steps for accomplishing this.[4,12,13] Furthermore, the NCI provides detailed guidance on how to deal with smoking by people of different ages. The CHDP protocol simply says, "Reinforce the positive behaviors [and] dissuade patients and parents from beginning to use tobacco."[10]

During the debate over AB 816, Lester Breslow, a former head of DHS and a member of the TEOC, was more direct when he described CHDP: "'Issuing a protocol' on tobacco education, but doing nothing to follow-up on its use; bringing administrators and physician aides into brief 'training sessions"; and requiring checking three 'tobacco points' on the payment claims forms—all for the expenditure of tens of millions of dollars annually, a total of more than 100 million dollars since 1989 —is lampooning public health and Proposition 99." [14] In one county, according to the LLA director, the CHDP staff did pick up brochures, train staff, and refer people to the LLA. But a physician in this county commented, "The fact is, given a busy practice, 15 minutes is probably generous because those pediatric visits are more like 7½ to 10 minutes. . . . So I don't think much was actually happening. I think the idea that was education money was just wishful thinking more than honesty." [15]

COMPREHENSIVE PERINATAL OUTREACH

TEOC had earlier raised concerns about the perinatal diversion. In the fall of 1992, Carolyn Martin wrote the DHS director, Molly Joel Coye, on behalf of the TEOC expressing concerns about how the money was being used and how its use would be evaluated.[16] Coye responded on January 22, saying that spending Health Education money on CPO was appropriate because the expenditure was "formulated through a protracted process involving the various anti-tobacco constituencies, health care professionals, and others. The passage of these bills indicates that both the Legislature and the Administration approve of the appropriations in them." [17] She then indicated that plans were still incomplete for the implementation of the CPO component. The CPO dollars were going to be used by counties to generate their matching funds for a federal program providing outreach to pregnant women.

The program structure and the rules governing it created confusion in the field, compounded by a September 15, 1991, memo from Dileep Bal, the head of the DHS Chronic Disease Control Branch (which included the Tobacco Control Section, TCS), and Rugmini Shah, the director of the state-level Maternal and Child Health (MCH), discussing the CPO program. According to the memo, AB 99 broadened AB 75 to include identifying pregnant women, assessing their health needs, and facilitating the delivery of services to them. The fourth step, according to the memo, was to "provide the necessary resources to help the pregnant woman deal with the negative effects of tobacco use and exposure to cigarette smoke on herself, her baby, and her family." [18] This "provision of resources" step, however, violated the rules for federal matching funds for CPO, which explicitly required that the dollars be used only for outreach, not to deliver services, such as anti-tobacco education.

After a year of trying to get CPO working in the counties, the local lead agencies (LLAs) complained to TEOC. In October 1992 Breslow reported to Coye on the widespread discontent among the LLAs about CPO. These feelings were voiced at a statewide event called the Revolt Against Tobacco Conference, a meeting of approximately 300 leaders of the California tobacco control movement. After the TEOC met with the leaders, Breslow reported allegations of illegal use of Proposition 99 funds to match federal funds, orders from MCH staff to do traditional outreach, refusals to train staff in tobacco use prevention, and responses from MCH staff that were given with "arrogance and insistence that no one can 'take money away from babies.'" He told Coye, "How the department can tolerate, and apparently even encourage, the diversion of such funds to MCH and CHDP without any substantial effort to ascertain what is being accomplished by those services toward tobacco use control is difficult to understand." [19]

Martin also wrote Coye on behalf of the TEOC, which had received San Diego State's analysis of the county CPO plans, drawn up under contract with TCS. The majority of counties (52 percent) did not even include any mention of providing enhanced tobacco use prevention in their CPO plans. She also mentioned the "abysmal response" to the ethnic-specific training workshops and anecdotal reports of county health officers telling units to "spend the money as you wish—don't worry about tobacco." [16]

By July 1993, Jennie Cook, who had become TEOC chair, had written to Coye to again express TEOC's concerns. She specifically asked how much of the Health Education money was being used to educate women about the risks of smoking and secondhand smoke. Coye sent her letter to Stephen Kessler, the deputy director for Primary Care and Family Health, who wrote back, "I believe it would not be the best use of these limited funds to conduct the level of data collection and analysis required to answer your specific question." [20] Not surprisingly, this response did little to assuage TEOC's concerns about how the money was being used. The issue of CHDP and CPO was on its way to the courts.

THE HEALTH GROUPS' VICTORY

On December 2, 1994, Superior Court judge Roger Warren heard the lawsuits against AB 816. The Attorney General argued that the medical programs to which funds had been diverted had a health education component and thus could legitimately be funded from the Health Education Account. For example, the state argued that the diversion of funds to CHDP, a medical screening program for the poor, was appropriate because three questions about smoking were included on the forms and physicians were told to provide cessation advice.

Evidence presented by ANR and ALA/ACS, however, showed that CHDP and CPO were not legitimate anti-tobacco programs: 80 percent of CHDP health screens involved children under six years of age and only 0.4 percent of those eligible for the screens smoked.[21] All county CPO services were funded by Proposition 99 Health Education Account monies, and 86 percent of these funds were used to generate matching funds for federal money. Under federal guidelines, state matching funds could not be used for interventions to prevent smoking or interventions to stop exposure to smoke during pregnancy and after birth. It was therefore impossible for these funds to be used for anti-tobacco education.

On December 22, 1994, Judge Warren ruled that AB 816 illegally diverted $128 million from the Health Education and Research Accounts. He wrote, "In my view, one can't make a cat into a dog by calling it Fido or by putting a dog collar on it. . . . It seems to me that the legislature has called this component of the program an education program and has attached a tobacco-related education component to the health services program, but those two facts do not, in my view, convert this health services program into a tobacco-related education program."[22] The court ruled that the Legislature had violated the specification in Proposition 99 that the funding allocations could be amended only by a four-fifths vote of the Legislature and then only for purposes "consistent with its purposes." The court further ruled that the Proposition 99 ballot arguments assured voters that money allocated for tobacco education and research would be spent for these purposes and that the Legislature could not amend the allocation of revenues until Proposition 99's "finding of fact" (i.e., that tobacco is the number one preventable cause of death and disease and causes pain and suffering) changed. All use of the contested funds was to stop.

At the hearing, Judge Warren had requested that both sides advise him on how to tailor the relief to be granted ANR and ALA/ACS should they prevail. The Attorney General argued that, if no other fund source for the programs could be found, "a great many needy people with serious medical problems will find themselves without access to the health care they require."[23] Alternative funding was a possibility, according to the state, but locating an alternate funding source would require at least

ninety days. If alternate funding was not found, it would require the state
an additional sixty to ninety days after this fact was established to implement the cutoff of the programs. Based on this arithmetic, the state argued that the programs should be allowed to finish the fiscal year.[23]

Lawyers for ANR and ALA/ACS argued that the courts should order
the state to cease and desist immediately from the illegal expenditures.
They argued that the lawsuit had been brought promptly and that the
state had been warned by its own Legislative Counsel—twice in 1991 and
once in 1992—that the diversions were likely illegal.[24-26] Fred Woocher,
ANR's lawyer, specifically argued that

> Respondents [the state] were on full notice well before AB 816 was enacted
> that the diversions from the Health Education and Research Accounts were
> illegal, and that Petitioners [ANR] were prepared to challenge the diversions
> in court. Having elected to violate their legal duty nonetheless, Respondents
> simply cannot now be heard—much less in the name of *equity*—to complain
> that they must be permitted to continue their unlawful activities in order to
> avoid "confusion" or "disruption" to the other programs that they have cho-
> sen to fund with the Health Education and Research Account monies. Any
> such confusion and disruption is solely the result of Respondents's [*sic*] own
> wrongdoing, and they cannot be permitted to use that as a justification for
> violating the people's will under Proposition 99.[27] [emphasis in original]

The fact that a lawsuit had not been filed before 1994, when the CHDP
diversion had begun in 1989 and the CPO diversion in 1991, the lawyers
argued, should not affect the cease and desist order because the health
groups "did everything that they could do to prevent the health education diversions short of litigation."[27] The groups filed suit as soon as
"AB 816 increased the diversions from the Health Education Account
and gutted the Research Account [and] petitioners saw that there was no
recourse short of litigation."[27]

The health groups also argued that the state's claims of harm needed
to be balanced against the harm caused by underfunding the health education campaign. This assertion was based on work done at the University of California at San Francisco by Stanton Glantz, who prepared an
estimate of the health impact of underfunding. One of the state's arguments was that immediate harm would be experienced by those who relied on the state for health care, while those served by the Health Education and Research Accounts would not experience immediate harm.
Glantz demonstrated that, especially in the case of heart disease, there
was immediate harm. Among individuals who stop smoking, the cardiovascular system starts working better by the next day; the excess risk

of a heart attack is halfway back to that of a nonsmoker in a year. Similarly, if a woman quits smoking even two-thirds of the way through her pregnancy, the chance that she will have a low-birthweight baby is substantially reduced. Based on the quit rates achieved by the Proposition 99 programs before they were cut under AB 816, Glantz figured that the short-term hospitalization costs of the additional cases of disease caused by funding the program at 12 percent instead of 20 percent was approximately $28 million in fiscal year 1994–1995. Moreover, this estimate did not include physician fees, subsequent hospitalizations, outpatient care, rehabilitation, disability costs, lost tax income, or the costs associated with passive smoking or fires. California government paid about one-third of this amount, or $9 million.[28]

At a hearing on January 19, 1995, Judge Warren granted the plaintiffs' request for an injunction against further illegal diversions in the 1994–1995 budget. The ruling was memorialized in a written order on January 23, 1995. The court ruled specifically that the $64 million in expenditures for medical services from the Health Education and Research Accounts authorized for 1994–1995 by AB 816 were illegal.

The degree to which the state was allowed to spend money that was illegally appropriated had to be established. Similar diversions that AB 816 authorized for 1995–1996 were also found illegal and enjoined. Judge Warren entered different judgments in the ANR and ALA/ACS lawsuits. In the former case, the state was allowed to spend $83,000 in CPO funds; in the latter, $4.25 million. The ANR ruling blocked all CHDP expenditures, and the ALA/ACS ruling allowed $18.5 million to be spent on CHDP. Thus, the ANR judgment blocked spending of $128 million while the ALA/ACS judgment blocked $105 million. The judge gave ALA and ACS the opportunity to sign on to the ANR judgment, but they declined on the grounds that they sought only prospective relief, following through on their assurances to legislators who agreed to be plaintiffs in the suit. Further, the ALA/ACS lawyer advised them that since ANR was asking for the full amount, they "would not really lose anything if there is a good strategic reason for asking for less" and the lesser judgment might have a better chance of not being stayed by the Court of Appeal.[29] The governor appealed Warren's decision, and the California Medical Association (CMA) and Californians for Smokers' Rights filed friend of the court briefs supporting the state.

On May 24, 1995, the Third District Court of Appeal denied the state's request to issue a stay of the lower court's ruling. A stay would have unfrozen the illegally diverted funds and allowed the governor to spend the money as authorized by AB 816 while the appeal was in progress. The plaintiffs successfully argued that if Judge Warren's order was stayed, the contested funds would be lost forever.

The governor tried to avoid complying with the ruling. In response to the injunction, DHS verbally instructed counties to proceed with business as usual in terms of spending money on health services. The administration claimed it wanted to keep the programs alive while a new source of funds was found for CPO programs. In fact, the state waited three months (until April 21, 1995) before it mailed notices to the local health departments formally notifying them that they could not rely on AB 816 appropriations to fund CPO services.[30]

The state returned to court late in 1995 to request that it be allowed to spend an extra $3.1 million on CPO services in 1994–1995. This move was in response to the portion of the ANR judgment that restricted the state to spending $83,000 on CPO but allowed the state to ask for more. On January 30, 1996, ANR protested the state's application. Specifically, ANR pointed out that the state had not advised the counties in a timely manner to stop using funds for illegal purposes and had not used rollover funds from previous years to fund CPO services. The state, in fact, had used "new" AB 816 monies in 1994–1995 before using rollover funds from the previous years. Using the new money was prohibited by the court while using the rollover funds was not. ANR further pointed out that the state had sufficient funds to reimburse the counties for illegally spent monies. The court denied the state's request to use $3.1 million from AB 816 monies to fund CPO services.

The governor's May revision of his proposed 1995–1996 budget included a request to use $36.7 million in General Fund monies to replace the funds lost because of the lawsuits, although he made it clear he was not giving up on new attempts at diversion of Proposition 99 Health Education and Research Account funds during the 1995–1996 fiscal year.[31] While Wilson sought to keep the medical services programs funded from the General Fund, he did not seek permission to spend the contested funds for anti-tobacco education and research. He was happy to let the money sit in the bank pending appeal. Money in the bank, after all, would not hurt the tobacco industry.

THE LAWSUIT'S AFTERMATH: SB 493 IN 1995

Judge Warren could only block money from being spent illegally. He could not order money to be spent as the voters specified; only the Legislature could appropriate the funds. Thus, the victory in Judge Warren's court for ANR and ALA/ACS was only the beginning of the battles to be fought in 1995 over the illegally diverted funds. The health organizations had to go to the Legislature for a new bill to restore full funding. They did not, however, publicize their victory in the lawsuit or otherwise use it to bring public pressure to bear on the governor or the Legislature. The court victory was viewed as a new piece of ammunition in the insider game, not as a way to involve the public and get the media to frame the issue as "following the will of the voters."

Senator Diane Watson (D-Los Angeles), a longtime supporter of Proposition 99, proposed SB 949, which would have appropriated the frozen Proposition 99 funds for legitimate anti-tobacco health education and research in accordance with Proposition 99 and with the court's judgment. While SB 949 was passed by Watson's Health and Human Services Committee, it was stopped in the Senate Appropriations Committee by the same forces that had supported the use of funds from the Health Education and Research Accounts for medical services: the CMA, CAHHS, and the Western Center for Law and Poverty.[32] Meanwhile, the tobacco industry continued to escalate its campaign contributions to members of the Legislature. In 1995–1996 the tobacco industry spent $10,440 per member, twice its U.S. Congress contributions of $5,044 per member.[33]

Rather than accommodating the court rulings, Governor Wilson worked to get around them. He wrote the Legislature urging it to enact new legislation that continued to divert Proposition 99 funds into medical services but which would pass legal muster:

> I hope that you will agree with me that neither the executive nor legislature [sic] branches of state government can abide the court's decision to substitute its will for that of the elected representatives of the people of California with regard to the allocation of critical state resources. Indeed, the State has met the very requirements of the proposition to make allocation decisions consistent with the Proposition's purposes and done so with the required ⅘ vote of both houses of the Legislature. I therefore call upon you to establish an appropriate structure for immediate consideration of legislative alternatives to resolve this egregious action by the court so that we may minimize the disruption and loss of medical care to uninsured and indigent persons in California.[31]

Wilson was offended that the court had imposed its will on the state's elected representatives; he did not object to elected representatives imposing their will on the expressly stated mandate of the people. On June 27 the voluntary health agencies wrote an angry response to the governor:

> We believe that the intent and effect of your proposal, as stated in your letter, is to circumvent the judicial system, subvert the Constitution, and impose your will over that of the voter. We are unified in our opposition to this action and will pursue every avenue to ensure that Proposition 99 is upheld. . . . The Superior Court made two points very clear. First, funds in the Proposition 99 Health Education and Research Accounts cannot be used to fund medical care. Second, any attempt to divert the Health Education and Research Accounts into medical care will be closely scrutinized.[34]

They did not release this letter to the press or make any effort to marshal public support.

As the governor requested, the Legislature passed SB 493, which contained a funding plan that was identical to AB 816. SB 493, originally sponsored by Senator Cathie Wright (R-Simi Valley), had proposed a minor change in the portion of the health and safety code dealing with radiologic technologies. In this form, it had passed through the committee structure and the Senate and was awaiting final action on the Assembly floor. There Wright was replaced by minority leader Ken Maddy (R-Fresno) as the bill's sponsor, and the old bill was amended in its entirety to appropriate Proposition 99 funds. The section on radiologic technologies was dropped. By using an existing bill in this manner, there would be no hearings on the issue and virtually no deliberation. It was the ultimate insider deal.

In SB 493 the Legislature sought to avoid the legal problems of AB 816 through two actions. First, it presented a long series of "findings" that were designed to convince the courts that the tobacco use situation in California had changed substantially enough to justify major cuts in the anti-tobacco education programs. For example, the Legislature included the "finding" that "the decline in overall tobacco use since 1988, the resulting decline in cigarette and tobacco tax revenues and the decline in the number of Californians with health insurance, such that 6.5 million people are uninsured, make it critically important to reallocate revenue for one year to meet urgent health care needs in a manner consistent with the purposes of the act."[35]

Second, rather than simply using Health Education and Research money to fund medical services, SB 493 amended the percentage allocations of tobacco tax revenues in Proposition 99 to put less money into the Health Education and Research Accounts and put more directly into the Physician Services Account, where it was then appropriated to the same medical service programs that the court had ruled illegal in the AB 816 suit. SB 493 put only 10 percent of the tobacco tax revenues in the Health Education Account (instead of the 20 percent required by Proposition 99) and only 1 percent in the Research Account (instead of the 5 percent required). The Physician Services Account was given 22.5 percent of the revenues (instead of the 10 percent specified by the initiative); the Unallocated Account was given 26.5 percent (instead of 25 percent). This action was taken to deliberately amend the initiative rather than rely on the appropriations process.

By this time every county in California had formed a tobacco control coalition, which had created a network of people who were well informed about tobacco control and who could have been a substantial resource for the reauthorization effort. The lobbyists did not tap this resource. Cynthia Hallett, who at the time was working for the Los Angeles LLA, later described how advocates in the field finally began organizing their own effort: "Where I remember the most amount of activity coming up was SB 493, and that was May of '95. That was a long way down the pike. And what happened was it got to the most dire stage and then finally there was much more communication. But what was interesting was that activities to combat SB 493 did not necessarily originate from anybody out of Sacramento. . . . I mean, that was the first major effort that I can remember people really getting behind." [36] The frustration in the field was clearly growing, but it was not organized and focused enough to influence the events of 1995.

On July 10 the Assembly passed SB 493 on a 67-4 vote and returned it to the Senate, where it was approved, as amended, on a 32-6 vote just five days later. The Governor signed SB 493 into law on July 27, a mere seventeen days after it was "introduced." Once again, the established power structure within the Legislature and administration, in alliance with powerful tobacco and medical interests, pushed through an appropriation designed to reduce the tobacco control program.

Proposition 99's advocates had no chance in this game of political hardball. Carolyn Martin observed that SB 493

> zoomed through the legislature faster than any bill that I've ever seen. I think it was a done deal in four days. The only thing we did to even try and slow down this missile was to require a Senate hearing and by then the Senate was in the last days of the budget session when everyone is so frazzled and tired they can't think anyway. Lots of people in the Assembly told us they didn't even know what they were voting on when they voted on 493. One of our mistakes was we did not have a strong Assembly leader who would just scream

and stomp and carry on to try and expose any chicanery on diverting the money again. We needed that and we didn't have it. And, remember, Willie Brown was still there.[37]

THE SB 493 LAWSUITS

ANR and the voluntaries—this time including AHA—sued again, separately, seeking temporary restraining orders against the implementation of SB 493. They asked that the matter be assigned to Judge Warren, who had presided over the earlier case, on the grounds that he already knew the legal issues. The state contested the application to assign the matter to Warren, and the case was assigned to Judge James T. Ford, who had been the judge in ALA's 1992 lawsuit to restore the media campaign.

The health groups argued that SB 493 was not "consistent with the purposes" of Proposition 99 on its face without presenting any evidence that the cuts were hurting the program, as they had done in the AB 816 case. Even so, the health groups won again. Judge Ford issued a temporary restraining order on August 1, 1995, to stop the contested expenditures and issued a preliminary injunction against SB 493 on September 1, 1995.

As with the rulings on AB 816, none of the litigation surrounding SB 493 compelled spending the $64 million in contested funds from the Health Education and Research Accounts, and the governor again simply let the money sit in the bank. Nevertheless, the health groups' victory represented a shot in the arm for the people working in the field. According to Cynthia Hallett,

> The lawsuits were really when . . . the larger sort of California constituencies started moving . . . the Prop 99 constituency. . . . People finally got the word out, "This is what's happening, and this is what they're doing. Are we going to sit behind and let this happen?" And a lot of that message came from ANR. . . . We were able to clearly communicate with our coalition members. And we were able to help. We were able to say, "They're collecting affidavits or letters of support from previous clients. Can you do it?" And sure enough, people were popping them out. And it was great because then the community agencies felt a part of the process. And that's what it takes because they do so much of this work.[36]

The lawsuits also demonstrated how far away from each other the original Proposition 99 coalition members had moved, with the voluntary health agencies on one side and the medical service providers on the other. As noted in the ALA newsletter, "The beneficiaries of the diverted tobacco monies, the California Medical Association, California Associ-ation of Hospitals and Health Services, medical clinics, the Western Cen-ter on Law and Poverty, and the tobacco companies wielded enough po-litical influence to achieve the diversion and are expected to lend legal support to the State's Attorney General in order to keep the Prop 99 money." [38] The health groups finally accepted that the CMA, CAHHS, and Western Center for Law and Poverty were not even potential allies. They were linked with the tobacco companies.

CONCLUSION

The lawsuits did several useful things for the Proposition 99 programs. They increased the visibility of the Proposition 99 issue, framing it not as sick babies versus prevention but as voter-approved initiatives ver-sus illegal legislative deals. For the constituency in the field, those who worked on the programs on a daily basis, the lawsuits showed a greater level of commitment to protecting those programs than they had seen before in Sacramento. The lawsuits showed that the health groups were willing to fight for the Proposition 99 programs and to fight for them outside the world of Capitol insider politics. The litigation also engaged ANR in the fight over Proposition 99. Although ANR was not working with the voluntary health agencies, ANR's experience in grassroots po-litical fights had the potential to be useful in protecting Proposition 99.

In 1996 new legislation would again be needed to authorize the Propo-sition 99 programs. Regardless of the legality or illegality of AB 816 and SB 493, both were facing a sunset deadline on June 30, 1996. The ques-tion before tobacco control advocates was how they could exploit both their legal victories and their organizational strengths in a way that would make full funding of the anti-tobacco education and research programs a reality.

CHAPTER 14

Doing It Differently

By the fall of 1995, because of the failure of the Legislature to appropriate the Proposition 99 revenues in accordance with the lawsuits, substantial amounts of Proposition 99 money had not been spent for anything. The courts stopped the governor and Legislature from spending the money for medical services, and the governor and the Legislature refused to spend the money for anti-tobacco education and research. The Health Education Account was projected to contain $191 million by June 1996, and the Research Account $82 million. A total of $274 million had been diverted away from anti-tobacco education and $71 million from research, and these cuts were having an effect. The prevalence of youth smoking had increased by 20 percent between 1994 and 1995 (from 9.1 percent to 10.9 percent), and adult prevalence was no longer declining.[1] In fact, adult prevalence appeared to be increasing for the first time since the state began collecting statistics in 1974. Thanks to the governor, the Legislature, and the medical lobby, the tobacco industry was reversing the damage that Proposition 99 had done to it.

As they prepared for the 1996 reauthorization fight, tobacco control advocates had two court decisions on their side. But a favorable court decision had been of little help to them in 1995 when the Legislature passed SB 493. The governor and Legislature seemed more angered than chastised by their legal defeats. The challenge to tobacco control advocates was how to change the outcome of the authorization fight.

THE NEED FOR A CHANGE

The lobbyists from the three voluntary health agencies—American Cancer Society (ACS), American Lung Association (ALA), and American Heart Association (AHA)—organized a series of fall meetings led by AHA to plan a strategy for the Proposition 99 reauthorization fight. They needed focus, energy, and resources. As Paul Knepprath, who had joined Tony Najera as a lobbyist for the state ALA in 1995, explained, "What we needed the next go around was not a pure sort of traditional legislative lobbying campaign but rather a campaign that included other elements that brought the public pressure from the outside more. . . . There was a consensus that we needed to do things differently for reauthorization than what we had done in the past. There was consensus on bringing in new players and new partners, which I'm not sure which ever came to fruition."[2] Beyond acknowledging that something had to be done differently, there was little activity.

This lack of action on the part of the voluntaries was confirmed for the local lead agencies (LLAs) in a monthly technical assistance telephone call hosted by the American Nonsmokers' Rights Foundation (ANRF), the educational arm of Americans for Nonsmokers' Rights (ANR). The service was part of the technical assistance provided by ANRF under contract to the Tobacco Control Section (TCS). ANRF director Julia Carol used this forum to let the LLAs know what was happening on reauthorization. Carol attempted to use an early fall teleconference to bring the LLAs together with the ACS:

> ANR's plan was to have nothing whatsoever more to do with any statewide efforts, we were just doing our work. But I still wanted to look out for the constituency we serve, so I invited the Cancer Society to come on the line and give an update on the plans for reauthorization for Prop. 99. . . . I was trying to get these people to look to the Cancer Society for leadership and not to us and that these people were very mistrustful and that they needed to know that something was going on and they needed to be included. *They needed to be a part; they're tired of being left out. They're suspicious of deals being cut in the dark and of people not telling them things.*
>
> So really there needed to be a frank conversation with them about what the plans were and what they could or couldn't do, what the communities could or couldn't do. So . . . I asked Theresa [Renken, the ACS lobbyist] to give an update and she said, "Well you know, we're going to be forming a coalition and we're going to be talking about blah and we're going to have a big meeting in the fall and we're going to do this and that and by November we'll do the other and the Legislature is gone and they'll come back and blah and blah and blah."

> And I said to her, "What's our plan in the meantime, right now?" And I
> meant for influencing the budget language before the budget comes out, but
> I didn't say that. "What's our plan now?" And she said in a very snotty tone,
> this is a teleconference with over one hundred people on it, "Well, Julia, if
> you understood the legislative process you would know that the Legislature is
> about to be out of session. So there is nothing that can be done until they re-
> turn anyway." . . .
>   So I said to her, "Theresa, it sounds to me like the campaign is going to
> be run much the same way as it has been the past, is that correct?" And she
> said, she paused and said, "Well, yes." And I said, "I see. . . . well then, *if you
> are going to do things the same way, what makes you think you are not going
> to get the same results?"* [3] [emphasis added]

The Sacramento lobbyists who had negotiated the implementing legislation for Proposition 99 over the years still did not appreciate the need to
actively engage the grassroots or the power of doing so.

Tony Najera, who, with John Miller, had headed the "inside" game on
behalf of the health organizations since 1989 and the passage of AB 75,
revealed why the inside game was played the way it was: "Paul [Knepp-
rath] would from time to time criticize me and rightfully so because he
wanted me to include other parties. And I would always say, 'That's nice
to be inclusive and to bring people along. However, there are times where
you have personal relationships and . . . they don't want other people.
They want to be able to confide, quietly tell you what they think.' " [2] Najera was sensitive to his role in the inside game: "I've been accused of
giving away the store by people that don't understand this game. I consider that a false accusation which is very unfounded." [2]

Steve Scott of the *California Journal* observed that the behavior of the
voluntary health agencies' lobbyists was typical of the tendency of the
lobbyists in Sacramento to live in their own world:

> As somebody who covers the Capitol, I can't be too critical of the way they
> [the voluntary health agency lobbyists] approach the Legislature. . . . You
> tend to become a product of the system in which you operate and over time
> I'm sure that these lobbyists are no different from any other lobbyists. Over
> time you become inculcated into the culture and you start to think in incre-
> mental terms rather than in bolder terms. But that's why you have grass-
> roots. . . . Ultimately the lobbyists are employees. And if the people who
> employ them don't look beyond what they are telling them, then they are not
> doing their members any good service either. So I don't think that the grass-
> roots arms of the organizations can be exempted from a share of responsi-
> bility for allowing the Prop. 99 situation to atrophy the way it did. Because
> the repository for all wisdom isn't the lobbyist in Sacramento. [4]

Thanks to Proposition 99, the TCS and ANR leadership, and the LLA directors, the local tobacco control coalitions were getting stronger and more organized. They could not understand why the lobbyists in Sacramento were not reaching out to tap this power.

At the same time, things were changing at the AHA in a way that would lead to a much stronger appreciation of the grassroots. Mary Adams had recently replaced Dian Kiser as AHA's lobbyist. While Adams had been involved in the early Proposition 99 fights as the ACS lobbyist (as Mary Dunn), she had lived in Europe for several years and had only returned to Sacramento in November 1994. She was surprised at how far the Proposition 99 allocations had deviated from the terms of the initiative. In crafting a legislative strategy for 1996, Adams felt that the voluntary health agencies needed to open up the process and involve new people, particularly those in the field who had been fostered by Proposition 99's community-based activity.[5] She also recognized the need for the tobacco control advocates to be more nonpartisan and bipartisan:

> I wanted to have both Democratic and Republican representatives. Because in the past, we'd just always focused on the Democrats and I felt like that wasn't going to get us where we needed to go. . . . I started communicating to my organization after meeting with this group and I hawked the same three points all the way through with this group that I had drawn together and then with my own organization: that we needed to have an intensive grassroots effort, . . . that we had to have intensive use of the media to get the public to focus on the issue, and that we needed to have a contract lobbyist with Republican ties who would be able to work the issue for us in a successful way. And then I shored that up with just my strong feeling that this was all going to take place through the budget, that it was not going to go through the normal legislative track.[5]

Having been absent from the battles in Sacramento over the past few years, Adams had an easier time recognizing strategic errors that the voluntary health agencies had made: "The strategies that had been used in the past . . . had been dismal failures. When I left, there was a ton of money coming. When I came back I saw the whole thing in a real mess. I knew that we had to draw together many more facets, many more approaches than had been used in the past."[5] Adams wanted a more aggressive campaign to defend Proposition 99 that reached well beyond the Capitol building and was determined to get ANR and its past president, Stanton Glantz, on board.

But involving Glantz and ANR was not just a matter of adding their names to a coalition letterhead and proceeding with business as usual.

Neither Glantz nor the ANR leadership had much confidence in pursuing the kind of insider game that had failed for the last several years. They were committed to action with a strong grassroots component based on their experience doing battle over Propositions 5, 10, and P and passing hundreds of local ordinances. They also recognized the central role that the CMA and other medical interests had played in legitimizing the diversion of money out of the Health Education and Research Accounts; they viewed neutralizing the CMA as the crucial first step to restoring Proposition 99. But they doubted that the voluntary health agencies would have the nerve to confront the CMA, much less the governor or the Legislature.

ANR had built its reputation as a grassroots organization by being a confrontational outsider. Even if it could be persuaded to change its focus from local ordinance fights, its preferred strategy, to a state-level one, it would certainly not compromise its style in the process. ANR had its own vision of what was needed in the Proposition 99 fight. According to ANR co-director Robin Hobart,

> One thing that we realized was that the only way you were going to see real reauthorization of Prop. 99 at the full level—and this was based on our experience with [Proposition] 188 in some ways—was that you're going to have to run it like an election campaign, not like just any old bill. It had to really be a campaign with all the attendant grassroots strategy and media strategy and inside-the-Capitol strategy. . . . The other thing that we knew based on how the governor had responded and the Legislature responded to our lawsuits—we were successful in court but having absolutely no effect whatsoever with regards to what the Legislature was prepared to do—was that it was going to have to be a real gloves-off campaign. People were going to have to name names. And the California Medical Association was going to have to be forced to get out of the way.[6]

ANR could envision an effective strategy, but it had no intention of actually getting involved. Hobart continued, "We didn't believe that it ever was going to happen and so to a certain extent, we decided, 'It's really awful, it's really a shame, but ANR has absolutely no ability to do anything about any of this by ourselves and we're done.' We gave at the office, the lawsuit was the last thing that we made a commitment to do to try to save Prop. 99 and after that, we were done."[6]

Glantz also saw the need for a more confrontational strategy but was more willing to get involved. In a 1996 interview he said,

> And what happened last year [in 1995] was I saw the whole program just going down the drain. I think the CMA and the Tobacco Institute were coming

in for the kill. . . . The program was in a complete shambles, because local lead programs had basically been dismantled, because the media campaign was a mess. And the tobacco companies and the Medical Association had succeeded in turning this into a fight about money, and a fight about money is not news in Sacramento. And Tony [Najera] and John [Miller] and the others up there were still pursuing the same old insider strategies where they'd been screwed every time. Just all the tea leaves were looking bad. . . . I sat back and I said, "Now, . . . am I going to sit here and chronicle the demise of this program while watching it and have a nice clean paper where I've written about how the thing went down the drain?" . . . I just decided I could not stand to sit and watch this thing go down the drain because I thought it was just too important.[7]

Meanwhile, as AHA was trying to recruit ANR and Glantz, ACS was engaged in its own discussion about reauthorization. According to Don Beerline, a past chair of the ACS California Division, ACS also recognized the need to do something different:

What the ACS decided early last fall [of 1995] was that we had been unsuccessful. The advocacy in those previous reauthorization campaigns had primarily been carried out by our professional lobbyists. The lobbyists in those previous campaigns have complained somewhat that they didn't feel like they really had the support to do what they needed to do. And given the past history of that failure, the ACS said, "We need to do something different this time." The debate went on within the ACS, and it culminated when our board of directors in November of 1995 committed $120,000 for this campaign plus obligated one individual full time for the first six months of 1996, and this is not a clerical person. This was a middle manager. So that's a significant commitment of personnel and funds compared to the last time, the assumption being with that sort of commitment then we would become, for the first time, the lead agency in this fight. And in the past, it has been other organizations have been considered the lead agency. And that is exactly what happened. . . . Lung Association definitely and their representatives were definitely not happy when ACS took the role of the lead agency in this and decided that we needed to have a different strategy.[8]

Although everyone had the same goal—full funding of the Health Education and Research Accounts—there were no indications that their plans to achieve those goals meshed.

THE DECEMBER MEETING

Adams scheduled a December 13, 1995, meeting at AHA in Sacramento in the hope that it would get the key players together to discuss reauthorization, but she had some difficulty persuading ANR and Glantz to come. Believing that it was impossible for a voluntary health agency to take the kind of strong action necessary to rescue Proposition 99, Glantz told Adams that he would only be willing to attend a meeting after the AHA "did something real."

AHA had its chance to do so when Glantz obtained a copy of a thirty-second anti-smoking advertisement, "Insurance," produced by DHS. After making the point that tobacco companies owned insurance companies that gave nonsmoker discounts, the advertisement ended with the question "What do the tobacco guys know that they are not telling us?" The administration was sitting on the advertisement. Glantz suggested that AHA hold a press conference to demand that the governor put the advertisement on the air. AHA did so, together with ALA and, at the last minute, ACS. The event got media coverage, and Glantz and ANR agreed to attend the December meeting.

Adams's meeting brought together lobbyists from the three voluntary agencies—Adams from AHA, Knepprath and Najera from ALA, and Renken from ACS—as well as John Miller from Senator Diane Watson's office, Carolyn Martin, a volunteer with ALA and past chair of the Tobacco Education Oversight Committee (TEOC), Carol and Hobart from ANR, and Glantz. The morning session featured a briefing by the TCS staff on the substance of the program; TCS left before the afternoon strategy session.

During the afternoon session, Adams announced that AHA had committed $50,000 for the reauthorization effort, $25,000 of which would go to ANR for a grassroots campaign and the rest to do other things, such as hiring a Republican lobbyist. ANR committed $25,000 of its own, ALA committed $10,000, and Glantz wrote a personal check for $1,000—creating a war chest of $86,000. Renken did not mention the fact that ACS had already committed $120,000 to the Proposition 99 effort. The meeting ended with the health groups posturing, not with an action plan. Glantz, Carol, and Hobart, who felt that the pledged money would be enough to mount a substantial campaign, left the meeting demoralized.

The meeting was a watershed. Rather than resulting in a larger, more diverse working group, which had been AHA's goal, the meeting eventually resulted in a divided coalition and two different reauthorization campaigns.

Najera later described his reaction to the meeting:

> We had been planning and planning since October and we had one thing in
> mind, that was a statewide coalition—united we stand together. But we go
> to this meeting in December and that was the telling . . . thing for me, that
> Mary was playing both sides, because ANR and Stan had not been working
> with us necessarily at the October meetings. And consequently when we got
> to the meeting in December, it was very clear that the Heart Association was
> not necessarily interested or concerned about working together with the Coa-
> lition. And they frankly were attempting to tell us that this wasn't going to
> work. It was for me the telling time when it became clear that they didn't want
> Cancer and they were afraid that by contributing the money Cancer would
> take the leadership in this thing. And it wasn't going to work because Cancer
> and the governor were friends.[2]

According to Knepprath, ANR and Glantz were assuming that any ACS
strategy would represent "the old school, the old way of doing things,
Sacramento based, lobbying, an inside play of the game." Knepprath
went on to say, "Stan and ANR were advocating 'we're not doing that
this time. We're doing something different this time,' which is their right
and prerogative. . . . They were definitely thinking fast track, and Stan
by this time had been pitching to all of us, 'Let's utilize the [Proposition]
188 format in which it wasn't centralized; you didn't really have a centralized coalition. Everybody did their own thing and we worked together
and, gee, wasn't that great? So let's do that again.' "[2] Knepprath was seeking basically the same type of centralized coalition that had operated in
the past, except with ACS in charge.

Adams remembered a lot of tension in the room at the December meeting: "Theresa went out in the hall and was talking to somebody, she had
her little nose out of joint and certainly didn't say that they had any
money. . . . But I think that they had already gotten some money put
together as well. But it was clear that Tony was already starting to feel
somewhat threatened. The fact that I had been the one that convened
this meeting with TCS and with the others, that Stan and Julia were
there . . ."[5] For Adams, the philosophical differences could have been accommodated if only the strong personalities had not gotten in the way.
This view underestimated the depth of the philosophical disagreements
that existed over the approach the campaign should take. Adams was
unaware of how much money ACS had committed to the campaign, and
the distrust she, ANR, and Glantz felt about ACS in a leadership role
was aggravated by Renken's failure to mention it when all the other organizations were anteing up their contributions.

If the other organizations had negative reactions to the ANR presence, it was echoed by ANR's response. ANR had not wanted to be involved in the Proposition 99 reauthorization campaign and had not wanted to go to the AHA meeting. Adams convinced them to come. Carol said about the meeting,

> We didn't want to be involved in a big campaign to save Prop 99. However, one of ANR's goals is to separate tobacco money from politicians and to highlight the nefarious connection between the tobacco industry and politicians and their interference in public policy. To that end, the thought of beating up Pete Wilson a little every now and then over his connection to Philip Morris in fact appealed to me greatly. When Pete Wilson appointed Craig Fuller, the former senior vice president of Philip Morris, as his campaign manager [for Wilson's abortive presidential campaign in 1995], we had run a radio spot asking if Pete Wilson was running for president or just wanted to be the next Marlboro Man. . . . And I thought we'd follow it up with a Hall of Shame ad, which I had in draft form at that meeting and we wanted to run. . . . People were starting to put money on the table as far as what they were going to do with Prop 99, and Stan thought it would be great for us to spur them along by saying what we were doing. Stan and Mary both begged us to be there. . . . Mary decided, and she probably regrets it now, but Mary decided that in order to win Prop 99 we had to be a major player. . . .
>
> . . . it was awful. The Cancer Society said nothing, Lung said what they were going to put up, we said what we were going to put up, Heart said what they had to put up. Cancer stayed silent. Theresa only said one or two things, one of which was, "Well, if you beat up the governor, how do you expect him to sign your bill? Why would he sign the bill if you beat him up?" . . . She said nothing about any money.
>
> The next thing I know, Cynthia [Hallett of the Los Angeles LLA] calls me from L.A. and tells me that the Cancer Society has announced the week before in a public forum . . . they had I think it was $110,000 and they were going to run a Save 99 campaign. Now why the Cancer Society would feel free to discuss this publicly, . . . but would sit there in a meeting with her so-called partners—an inside-the-room confidential meeting—and not say a word about it is beyond me.[3]

ANR did not believe that the coalition was prepared to adopt a vigorous grassroots strategy, attack the CMA, or take ANR's advice seriously. Hobart "came away from that meeting really firmly convinced . . . this is not going to work."[6]

At the December meeting Glantz knew about the money that AHA, ALA, and ANR had available, but he did not know about the ACS plan. He later recalled,

> We went into that meeting with $86,000, which I thought, intelligently spent, was enough money, and I went up there all excited. And what happened was

exactly the opposite of what I was expecting, and I think the basic problem was that if normal human beings had been at that meeting, as opposed to voluntary health agency lobbyists and small-minded people, we would have walked out of that meeting excited and with a new leader in Mary. Because she's the one who pulled it together. She had established a working relationship with TCS. She had gotten all the key stakeholders in the room and come up with a significant amount of money.

I would have thought we would have walked out of that meeting with a new fresh face, with a smart woman with some serious resources: I was there with the sort of intellectual stuff, Julia was there with the grassroots stuff, Tony was there with all of his insider stuff, which he's good at, Mary was there. We had Paul Knepprath, who is good with the media. And I think we had the real makings of a good solid campaign. . . .

I think they were tremendously threatened by her [Mary Adams] and the Heart Association. . . . This had been their little sandbox for all these years and all of a sudden, here was a new player. And rather than saying, "Oh boy! We've got somebody else to work with, we can be strong and productive and this and that," they were instantly threatened. . . . And I think the fact that Theresa did not disclose that the Cancer Society had this big wad of money at the meeting was just at the very least, unprofessional, and duplicitous and devious and dishonest and all these other things. And so we came out of that meeting . . . very depressed and Julia had had it. And I was very discouraged.[7]

The only person who did not seem discouraged by the meeting was John Miller. Miller felt that the meeting revealed the divisions between the insiders and outsiders but that, in the end, having an aggressive outside campaign might be helpful.[9]

Whereas Najera and Knepprath suspected that ANR and Glantz were threatened by ACS, Glantz was concerned that ALA and ACS were threatened by AHA. Either way, the questions about leadership and direction, far from being settled by the meeting, seemed to be exacerbated. Despite their differences in strategies, however, all the players believed that three things had to happen in 1996 if they were to secure full funding of the Health Education and Research Accounts. First, the CMA had to drop its advocacy of the diversions. Second, the sole reliance on the inside game had to end and the grassroots constituency had to be involved. And, third, the media attention had to be recaptured with a focus on "following the will of the voters" instead of a budget battle.

THE CMA

California's fiscal problems and the CMA's support of diversions had been the governor's best defenses for diverting the Proposition 99 monies.

Scott emphasized the importance of the CMA to the success of previous diversion efforts, saying,

> I don't necessarily believe that you're going to find secret communiques between the tobacco industry and Steve Thompson [the CMA's chief lobbyist] or anybody with the California Medical Association. I don't think that there is direct contact and I don't think there was intentional collaboration. But what you had was a sort of a symbiosis which was acquiesced to by the Medical Association because it furthered their goals. As this relates to Prop 99, you had the Medical Association that wanted more money for direct medical services, specifically CHDP. You had the tobacco industry that was only too happy to let that happen. The Medical Association in the minds of the legislators who want to support the tobacco industry becomes their astroturf, their front. They say, "Well, I'm just following the views of the California Medical Association, which has always been very strong on tobacco issues, co-sponsors of Proposition 99, co-sponsors of AB 13." Whatever else you want to say about them as a special interest, you can't impugn their reputation on tobacco. You could, but for a legislator who is inclined to vote tobacco's way, that gives them convenient cover.[4]

In fact, there was a much more active and direct engagement between the CMA and the tobacco industry than Scott believed (see chapters 3–5).

An important leadership change in the CMA helped to shift the CMA away from its aggressive opposition to the anti-tobacco education and research programs. In 1995 Dr. Jack Lewin was appointed as the new executive vice president, replacing Robert Elsner. Lewin had headed the public health department in Hawaii prior to his CMA appointment and was personally sympathetic to tobacco control. When asked about finding Proposition 99 on his agenda almost immediately, Lewin said,

> As I arrived on the scene, I was confronted with allegations from Dr. Glantz and others, who told me that CMA had been far from a proponent of anti-tobacco efforts and really had thwarted those efforts by virtue of its collusion with the tobacco industry and many other nefarious scenarios. I knew from my discussions with the leadership, the doctors of the association, that nothing could be further from the truth. And while I was greatly concerned, I knew that there had to be some complex relationship in the competition for funds or in government relations or in strategies and tactics, where you have competing agencies in a very awkward state of working against each other instead of with each other.[10]

At the time, of course, Lewin was not aware of the secret tobacco industry memos documenting its relationship with the CMA. (These memos were not made public until 1998 as part of the State of Minnesota's lawsuit against the tobacco industry.) Lewin recognized that the CMA's history on tobacco control was a problem. He went on to say,

> In the back of the history of CMA, there was clearly a part of the time when Prop 99 came out, where the person who was in charge of our government relations at that time was a wheeler-dealer type of very effective political strategist in Sacramento who was willing to work with whomever he needed to work with to get things done. Sometimes he would make a trade-off that would frankly not please me or the current leadership of CMA. But that was just the way things were then.[10]

Like AHA, ANR, and ACS, Lewin believed that people outside the Sacramento lobbyists' circle needed to get involved in the decision making about Proposition 99:

> If you talk to the constituencies in those [voluntary health] agencies, they're victims in my view because the doctors will be happy to get together with the Cancer, Heart and Lung boards and those constituencies and work on this. You're stuck at the political level of the agency staff and the government relations people that themselves have developed long-standing animosities they're not going to let go. . . . So what we decided to do was try to get out of that loop. That meant telling our government relations people to change the way they were relating to these other groups. If they couldn't do it, then we had to get some other people to make the relationships because the relationships were dysfunctional. . . . We're going to have to get through this whole epic of the past—"you did that to me, you did that to me, why did you do that to me?" Get beyond that and say, "Can we get together this year to go get this money?"[10]

But Lewin could not act unilaterally. There was a strong animosity within the CMA toward the anti-tobacco education and research programs that had built up over the years, dating back to at least the Napkin Deal of 1987. Steve Thompson, Willie Brown's longtime aide, was an especially popular figure within the CMA.

THE GOVERNOR'S BUDGET

The health groups hoped to avoid another battle in the Legislature. They had won two court rulings on the illegality of diverting Proposition 99 Health Education and Research money into medical services. More important, the state's economy had improved, which meant that the excuse for the diversions—fiscal necessity—had evaporated. Indeed, when Governor Wilson released his budget on January 10, 1996, he announced that "solid gains in employment and income will continue for the next two years." [11]

Rather than proposing expenditures conforming with the two court orders, however, the governor's 1996–1997 budget was identical to AB 816 and SB 493. (Wilson cited SB 493 as his rationale, purposely ignoring SB 493's stipulation that, effective July 1, 1996, the allocations of tobacco tax revenues to the Health Education and Research Accounts would conform to those established in Proposition 99: 20 percent and 5 percent, respectively.) Wilson proposed spending only $53 million (of the available $191 million) on anti-tobacco education and $4 million (of the available $82 million) on research. He proposed diverting $57 million into medical services. [12] Wilson was still trying to starve the anti-tobacco programs to death.

The three voluntary health agencies issued a press release immediately after the governor released the budget, saying they were "outraged" at the budget proposal and that "it reveals his latest attempt to thwart the law and steal monies earmarked for anti-tobacco education and research programs by the voter-approved Proposition 99." [13] The press release announced that "the health agencies refuse to let that happen and are launching a statewide campaign to invoke public awareness and put pressure on legislators to reject the Governor's tobacco fund raid."

CHANGES IN THE LEGISLATURE

Not only would the health groups' change in approach have its effects, but the fate of the governor's budget in the Legislature would be different this year because the Legislature had changed too. The Republicans had taken control of the Assembly in the 1994 elections by one vote, thanks in part to a massive $125,000 contribution that Philip Morris made to Republican Steve Kuykendall (R-Long Beach) the weekend before the election, which helped him defeat incumbent Democrat Betty Carnette. [12] By that time, the tobacco industry had shifted from giving campaign contributions in a bipartisan manner to favoring the Republicans. During the 1993–1994 election cycle, 45 percent of the contributions went to the Republicans; by 1995–1996 the share had shifted to 56 percent.

On April 24, 1996, Senators Watson, Hayden, and Petris, three of the strongest advocates for tobacco control in the Senate, wrote a long memorandum to Senator Bill Lockyer, the Senate's president pro tem and a senior Democrat in the Legislature. The subject of the memo was the Democratic "Caucus Position on Tobacco Issues," and the senators argued that it was not only good policy, but good politics for the Democrats to embrace tobacco control:

> Tobacco regulation, a long-standing and contentious political issue, has assumed even greater prominence in recent months, and gives every indication of continuing to hold the media and the public's interest. We would like to encourage the Democratic Caucus to assume a much more aggressive attitude against tobacco. There are sound policy reasons for such a reassessment of our position, but there are also equally sound political reasons for such a change.
>
> . . . Control of tobacco is morally the best policy. It is also a popular issue consistent with Democratic principals [sic], and an issue *with every possibility of becoming an electoral wedge. We believe the benefits to Democrats in terms of the public good will substantially outweigh the anticipated loss of tobacco support.*[14] [emphasis added]

In John Miller's view, the shift in tobacco industry campaign contributions to the Republicans was the key factor that got the Democrats lining up to support the Proposition 99 programs. He commented, "What moved them as a body wasn't our rhetoric or the public's interest or the public's wishes clearly expressed and apparent to everyone. It was the stupid move by the industry in terms of donations."[9]

The new Republican leadership in the Assembly was clear about its pro-tobacco sympathies. Curtis Pringle (R-Garden Grove), who became the speaker of the Assembly on January 5, 1996, accepted $17,250 in tobacco industry campaign contributions in the election cycle from 1995 through the March 1996 primaries; this amount ballooned to a total of $105,750 after he became speaker.[15,16] Pringle believed that "some of the legislative changes [to limit tobacco] swung the pendulum too far in one direction."[17] The chair of the Assembly Health Committee passed to Brett Granlund (R-Yucaipa). In the 1995–1996 period, he accepted $31,750 in tobacco industry campaign contributions and described himself as "a free-enterprise, no-tax smoker. It doesn't matter if I'm chairing the Health Committee. Those [anti-smoking] people don't have a right to tell everybody else how to live."[16,17] A *Los Angeles Times* editorial saw the Republicans as a "Whole New Pack of Buddies for the Cigarette Industry."[18]

The Democrats also had an important leadership change. Willie Brown, the longtime speaker of the Assembly when it was controlled by the Democrats, left the Assembly in January 1996 to become mayor of San Francisco. By then, Brown had accepted $635,472 in campaign contributions, more than any other legislator in the country, including mem-

bers of Congress from tobacco-growing states.[16] Brown had been a
powerful presence and used his power as speaker to protect the tobacco
industry's interests.

Assembly Member Richard Katz (D-Panorama City) replaced Brown
as the Democratic minority leader. In stark contrast to Brown, Katz was
a longtime supporter of tobacco control and had only taken $5,500 in
tobacco industry campaign contributions, none of them since 1991.[15,19]
Katz specifically rejected the claims that the Proposition 99 diversions
were made because of fiscal necessity: "In terms of the overall budget,
it's not a lot of money. . . . I don't know who came up with it; it was a
very very clever strategy that helps big tobacco under the guise of providing indigent health care. . . . The budget was a convenient issue for
them."[20] As Adams observed, "The real hero this year was Richard
Katz. Without a doubt. . . . Since he's the Democratic floor leader, he's
got a lot of loyalty from the other Democratic members on both sides of
the house, so that was really good. . . . it was like they'd all had this con-
version, some sort of 'Come to Jesus meeting' must have taken place in
the California State Capitol because they were all saying how wonder-
ful they thought Prop 99 was."[5] Katz's ascendancy to the leadership
greatly reduced the likelihood that the Assembly could muster a four-
fifths vote to divert Proposition 99 money, regardless of what the Republicans wanted to do. This fact fundamentally changed the political
dynamics surrounding Proposition 99 in the Legislature.

Meanwhile, the Democrats still controlled the Senate, and a shift in attitude toward Proposition 99 diversions appeared to be occurring there,
too. Senator Mike Thompson (D-Santa Rosa) chaired the Senate Budget
and Fiscal Review Committee, which meant that his position on Proposition 99 was also important. According to Diane Van Maren from
Thompson's office, "Mike made it very clear he was not going to vote
for a redirection to that level and that we thought that we needed to talk
about transitioning some of these programs and using some General
Fund monies, in a prudent manner. . . . Mike was very well aware of the
increase in adolescent smoking and thought that if we had the opportunity, we should start using the Health Education monies again and more
fully to mitigate that."[21]

Another change was the decision of Assembly Member Phil Isenberg
(D-Sacramento) not to be involved in Proposition 99 reauthorization.
Isenberg said, "I'm bored with it, I don't want to do it anymore. I've
done it three cycles. I've done enough. I've got other things to do."[22]
Isenberg's absence meant that the dynamic of the previous authorization

efforts would be disrupted, which was potentially advantageous for the tobacco control advocates.

A final major change in the Legislature, according to Richard Katz, was the effect of term limits. Katz felt that they helped the Proposition 99 Health Education and Research Accounts:

> One of the things with term limits is you have a whole bunch of members here who did not vote for that compromise, didn't go through that budget fight. So they said, "How could you do that? Don't you understand, you can't do that now the courts have ruled?" So you lose the historical context that that all took place in and without saying that's good or bad, they bring a different set of criteria to the evaluation. I also think that the folks who are elected now are much more anti-smoking than the group that was here ten years ago.[20]

In January lobbyists from the three voluntary health organizations—Najera, Knepprath, Adams, and Renken—met with Katz to sound out his views on the Health Education and Research Accounts. They proposed several authors for the Proposition 99 reauthorization bill, but Katz decided to carry the bill to restore Proposition 99 himself. He also agreed to let individual members vote their conscience on the bills rather than make this a leadership issue, as it had been in AB 816 and SB 493. When asked why he decided to carry the bill, he said, "I like fights. I like fighting with people that are arrogant."[20] He went on to explain,

> Someone needed to step out of the chaos and do it. When we sat around and talked about who was in a position to do it, it made the most sense for me to do it just because of what I'd done on the issue before. . . . We also saw this as a potential issue that could be an "us versus them." We knew the public was on the side of the Prop 99s of the world and that Republicans for the most part were much more beholden to tobacco companies than Democrats, even though Democrats have had their fair share over the years. I knew that Philip Morris was looking to underwrite a huge piece of the Republican convention in San Diego. . . . So there were good political reasons for doing it also.[20]

Knepprath understood Katz's political motives: "We were going to concede to him as the author of the bill his ability to do what he wanted, but I think it was at that meeting that we really launched then the effort to do our grassroots stuff and to really build the campaign around his bill."[2]

THE COALITIONS FORM

Following the December 1995 meeting, ANR, AHA, and Glantz decided to move ahead without ALA and ACS, in the hopes that, once things started happening, the two other organizations would join them. Adams

invited Roman Bowser, AHA's executive vice president, to a meeting to
work out how ANR would run a grassroots campaign coordinated with
AHA's lobbying effort. AHA was to help finance this campaign by providing $25,000 to ANR. Under Bowser's leadership, the AHA had been
evolving from an organization that did not even have a lobbyist before
1988 to one that was willing to engage in a political fight. When asked
about this change, Bowser replied,

> I think that if we look back over time—the origin of Prop 99, the passage,
> the lawsuits—I think you see somewhat of an escalation of our activity and
> involvement each step of the way. The more I learned about it, the more in-
> terested I was in it. . . . When the lawsuits started, then we started getting a
> little bit concerned. I think that the real turning point for me was [when] Stan
> Glantz called our national executive vice-president and left him a voice mail
> message saying that "we've really got some problems out here with Prop 99"
> and . . . he passed the message to me. . . . I knew who he [Glantz] was. I
> wasn't real thrilled about meeting him because I'd read some unflattering
> remarks he made about the Heart Association. Anyway, I called him back. I
> asked him if there was anything I could do to help him, what he wanted, and
> that was the turning point, that telephone conversation, because he spent
> quite a bit of time with me basically educating me on what was really going
> on behind the scenes with Prop 99. Also, I did not realize until then that we
> were in serious danger of losing the whole thing. . . . [but] I was still bound
> and determined to have the American Heart Association stay with the Ameri-
> can Cancer Society and the American Lung Association.[23]

When the meeting started, Bowser announced that the ACS had just told
him that it would put $120,000 into an effort to save Proposition 99
on the condition that ACS run the campaign. ANR and Glantz reacted
skeptically, as did Adams. They were concerned that ACS, as the least
combative of the voluntary health agencies, would simply adopt earlier
failed strategies, and Glantz urged Bowser to move ahead with the original plan to work with ANR. Bowser, although doubtful about ACS, felt
that he simply could not ignore his colleagues at ACS and ALA. The meeting ended without agreement on how to proceed.

The next several weeks were devoted to extended discussions among
ANR, AHA, and Glantz on how to deal with ACS. By mid-January,
Glantz felt that saving Proposition 99 was impossible.[7] ACS and ALA
were unwilling to confront the CMA and the governor, and AHA was
unwilling to move without them. The governor had released an unacceptable budget, but the health groups did nothing more than issue a
press release. On Friday afternoon, Glantz told Carol that he was recog-

nizing reality and giving up. Carol replied that the only reason ANR was involved was because of pressure from Glantz and that without Glantz, ANR would drop out, too. (She had joked that she knew Glantz would write the history of Proposition 99 and she did not want ANR blamed for letting it die.) Glantz called Adams and Bowser as a courtesy. Adams asked Glantz to keep an open mind over the long Martin Luther King Holiday weekend.

The following Tuesday, Adams called Glantz and Carol and said that AHA had decided to break with ACS and ALA and asked them to reconsider working with AHA. AHA intended to confront the CMA and the governor and mount a major campaign to reengage the public in the future of Proposition 99. Carol was particularly surprised. Following the December meeting, ANR had decided not to get involved in the Proposition 99 reauthorization fight. Rather than simply saying no to AHA at that time, Carol had laid down a set of four conditions that AHA would have to accept about the campaign that she was sure would scare them off:

> One, that it'll really be hard hitting. And that means taking on Pete Wilson and the CMA. Two, that I can find a grassroots coordinator who I really trust, because otherwise I can't do this. Three, they were going to have to pay us. And, four, we're not going to be in a coalition with Cancer and Lung, given their position on not wanting to bash the governor and the CMA. . . . It was clear that they had different strategies in mind. So they chose us and you could have blown me away. I thought I was off the hook. . . . So there we were. Stuck running a campaign![3]

When asked about the change at AHA, Mary Adams said,

> We were not going to sit back on our heels and watch yet another year go by and dismal failure. Cancer and Lung put together this group called . . . "Keep the Promise to Our Kids, the Coalition to Restore 99." They were going along on a similar path but in a much less rapid way and a much less contentious way. . . . They were simply . . . not going to play an "in your face" game. . . . And my thought had been from the get-go that we had played nice in the past and it didn't work; that we had to take the gloves off and play the game differently, period.[5]

AHA committed $50,000 for a grassroots lobbying campaign and hired a Republican lobbyist. Up until that point, the health voluntaries were closely allied with the Democratic Party; now the Republicans controlled the Assembly. AHA, ANR, and Glantz began a paid advertising campaign to publicize the failure of the governor and the Legislature to fol-

low the will of the voters. They also started to work to force the CMA to
stop supporting the tobacco industry.

Meanwhile ACS, joined by ALA, had been pursuing their noncon-
frontational reauthorization strategy. Beerline explained, "We're going
to be nonpartisan, positive, try to take the high road and create win-win
situations. . . . Heart decided that the campaign that we were putting together was not aggressive enough and that they wanted to have a more
aggressive campaign but still remain a member of the coalition. And, of
course, they were talking by then with ANR. And we basically told Heart
that they couldn't have it both ways. . . . And ANR, of course, has their
own style, the way they do things."[8] Beerline went to on to say that if
AHA went off to work with ANR in ANR's style, then AHA could not
be part of the old coalition.

While not willing to be confrontational, ACS was planning to change
its tactics from the past. The organization planned to devote staff to coordinating a grassroots campaign and to hire a professional public relations firm to help attract media attention to Proposition 99 and arrange
meetings with editorial boards.

THE "HALL OF SHAME" ADVERTISEMENT

The core of the ANR/AHA strategy was to bring the issue of Proposition 99 back before the public, with the expectation that an informed
and engaged electorate would force the politicians to implement Proposition 99 the way the voters intended. The media had come to view
Proposition 99 as just one more fight over money in Sacramento. So the
first step in accomplishing this goal was getting the media interested in
the issue by publishing a very strong advertisement in the *Sacramento
Bee* attacking Governor Wilson and CMA lobbyist Steve Thompson for
their roles in the Proposition 99 diversions. This advertisement, which
appeared on January 30, 1996, featured photographs of Governor Wilson and Steve Thompson as the mock nominees for the "Tobacco Industry Hall of Shame" (figure 16).

The advertisement attracted Thompson's attention. Nancy Miller of
the law firm Hyde, Miller & Owen wrote Bowser, objecting that "your
political advertisement is personally and professionally damaging to
Mr. Thompson. He would like a retraction of the damaging and inac-
curate statements in an ad of equal size placed in the *Sacramento Bee* as
soon as possible. He is requesting approval of the language of such an

Nominated* for the

TOBACCO INDUSTRY
HALL OF FAME

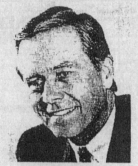

Pete Wilson
Governor

Refuses to fully fund California's tobacco education and research programs, defying court rulings and the mandate of the voters who passed Prop. 99.

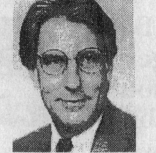

Steve Thompson
California Medical Association

Tobacco industry cheered when he led CMA's raid on tobacco education dollars. Former top aide to Willie Brown (largest recipient of tobacco $$ in the history of the California legislature).

If you believe these

Tobacco Industry Heroes

Belong in a **HALL OF SHAME** instead:

Call:

Governor's office: (916) 445-2841
Tell him to enforce the law we passed.

California Medical Association: (415) 882-5100
Tell them Steve Thompson made them a pawn of the tobacco industry.

* Nominated by the American Heart Association and
Americans for Nonsmokers' Rights, who paid for this ad.

Figure 16. "Hall of Shame" newspaper advertisement. Americans for Nonsmokers' Rights and the American Heart Association ran the advertisement in the *Sacramento Bee* on January 30, 1996, to indicate that the rules of the game on Proposition 99 had changed. (Courtesy of Americans for Nonsmokers' Rights) ad." [24] Steve Thompson followed this letter with one on CMA letterhead to Bowser that read:

> The issue of whether the Child Health [and] Disability Prevention program should be funded in part with Prop. 99 health education funds goes back to initial implementation of the initiative. While members of the initial Prop. 99 coalition disagreed on this issue, a compromise was reached to fund CHDP from health education to ensure enactment and maintain a common front against the tobacco industry whose major objective was to eliminate the television advertising program. This initial agreement occurred two years prior to my joining CMA. As a legislative staff person at the time, I supported the agreement because the threat to the advertising program was very real. . . .
>
> As tobacco tax revenues declined as a result of the many successful efforts following the enactment of Proposition 99 . . . indeed, including efforts of the Heart Association . . . competition for fewer dollars became intense, and what was once considered a compromise became an "illegal raid" on the tobacco education account. . . .
>
> Through legal counsel, I requested (in addition to Dr. Lewin's request), that you apologize for your untrue advertisement. As the attachments indicate, you have no intention of doing so. In fact, while litigation was never mentioned in Ms. Miller's letter to you, you threatened to counter sue ("slap-suit") if I chose to pursue the issue legally. Outside of fulfilling an enormous emotional need . . . which will stick in my craw for a long time to come. . . . I don't believe litigation will result in civilizing this debate. I believe you've done your cause an enormous disservice and hope you reflect on the value and ethics of your current tactics.[25]

Thompson also defended Governor Wilson, who, in his view, "was also unfairly smeared in your ad." [25]

Adams was sure that her new offensive was going to get her organization sued, although Bowser shrugged off the Thompson letter as bluster. Carol and Glantz passed the threatening letter on to the *San Francisco Chronicle* and it made news:

> Darts, not hearts, are flying this Valentine's Day between the American Heart Association and organized medicine: The nonprofit group claims that California doctors have run off with Governor Wilson and the tobacco industry.
>
> The latest spat—nasty even by Sacramento standards—began two weeks ago when the California office of the American Heart Association signed a newspaper advertisement "nominating" Wilson and the California Medical Association lobbyist Steve Thompson to the "Tobacco Industry Hall of Fame." . . .
>
> Wilson was not amused by the ad. And Thompson—one of the most prominent figures in the state capital—had his personal lawyer fire off a demand for a retraction.

Dr. Jack Lewin, executive director of the California Medical Association, called the name-calling "unconscionable" and "slanderous" in a letter to the heart association and threatened legal action if more advertisements appear.

"The heart association will print no retraction," said Mary Adams, chief lobbyist for the California charity.

Adams said that the association will forge ahead with a publicity campaign that challenges doctors' roles in the battle over anti-smoking programs. "This is a diversion from the American Heart Association's way of doing business, but that just underscores the importance we attach to this," said Adams. "It's time to get this issue out in the open." [26]

The media was finally paying attention to Proposition 99 again.

The fact that AHA had allied itself with the "radicals" at ANR also interested the media. Steve Scott of the *California Journal* observed,

> The Heart Association's participation was crucial to the credibility of those ads. ANR is a wonderful organization. They do a lot of good stuff but they are viewed by the Sacramento press, which winds up covering this, as kind of the radicals. They're the ones who are beating the drums. When the Heart Association came on, then all of a sudden you had this group that is perceived as "centrist," one of the moderates. So one of the moderates had gone over to the other side and all of a sudden you had a situation where the voluntaries couldn't claim unanimity. Lung and Cancer couldn't say, "Oh well, ANR— they're just out there on the fringes." [4]

Thompson also apparently mobilized support from other medical groups. The California chapter of the American College of Emergency Physicians, the California Association of Obstetricians and Gynecologists, the California Society of Plastic Surgeons, and the California Society of Anesthesiologists all responded to the "Hall of Shame" advertisement by writing an open letter to the California senators and Assembly members to lampoon the same "hit list" of projects that they had lampooned in 1994 during the hearings on AB 816. The letter from the specialist groups made it sound as though the same old fight about money was about to surface again.

CMA lobbyist Elizabeth McNeil was unhappy with the advertisement, not only because it attacked the CMA but also because she felt it would make Wilson more intransigent:

> The first ad was pretty devastating as far as moving anything politically, and we thought that shut the door completely to doing anything. . . . I think that turned off a lot of people, not only in the Capitol but around here. I think it was a very stupid move politically. I think it hurt his kids, hurt his family, and he's been someone who has always fought for kids' programs and health pro-

grams. . . . But it just dug the governor in. The governor called up Steve and
said, "Forget it, I'm not going to compromise on this and all conversations
are off, basically."[27]

The AHA and ANR shrugged off these criticisms. They purposely had
designed the ad to get people's attention, believing that it was better than
being ignored. Isenberg thought the 1996 advertising campaign had
value, and he also confirmed that it enraged Thompson: "Thompson
was beside himself. God, he was so mad. My wife took . . . the one with
Steve in it. She altered it a little bit and said, 'Steve Thompson, drug
dealer' [laughter]. Anyway, Steve didn't think that was very funny. Well,
it's like everything else in politics, it escalates the battle. It certainly irritated Wilson, agitated the California Medical Association. Did it have
some impact? Might have had some impact, together with the second
lawsuit."[22]

THE WELLNESS GRANT

In March the California Wellness Foundation, which had financed the
voter education campaign about Proposition 188, gave the ANR/AHA
media strategy a huge shot in the arm: a $250,000 grant to run a series
of advertisements on the status of the Proposition 99 Health Education
and Research programs and their importance. The campaign was not
designed to lobby for any particular piece of legislation, but rather to
educate and involve the public in the debate over the future of Proposition 99.[28]

    The Hall of Shame ad had attracted the attention of Herb Gunther,
director of the Public Media Center in San Francisco, which had run the
nonpartisan advertising campaign on Proposition 188 with a grant from
the Wellness Foundation a year earlier (see chapter 11). Gunther had
been interested in helping restore the integrity of Proposition 99 but had
not met any credible players with whom to work. The fact that the AHA
had adopted such an aggressive approach impressed Gunther, and he arranged a meeting between Glantz and Wellness Foundation president
Gary Yates to discuss Proposition 99. Glantz later described the meeting
in an interview:

> Gary basically said, "I know what you want. You want some money to run
> ads about Prop 99 and I had thought it over and decided not to do it." I had
> pitched the idea to him at the meeting after an adequate amount of wine, and
> my whole idea of engaging the public. They had just come off this victory in
> [Proposition] 188 and really shown a whole new way foundations could play

a positive role in public health. I basically said we wanted to do something like the 188 campaign and that the Heart Association was showing some guts. And it turns out that Wellness had been kind of watching. Tobacco isn't one of their priority areas, but they'd been watching Prop 99, wanting to do something to help and not seeing any place to put the money, because they looked at it as the same old same-olds, making the same old mistakes.

And they had noticed the [Hall of Shame] ad, too. And they had seen the article about the threats from the CMA, too, and were impressed by that. And were impressed that the Heart Association was willing to do it. ANR had a very good reputation with them for some other projects they'd been involved with.

And in the end Yates said, "Okay, I'm interested in doing this." And he looked at Gunther and he said, "How much money is this going to take?" And Herb said, "A hundred thousand dollars." And then Yates looked at me. I mean, that was more money than I had thought we had needed at the beginning. And then Yates looked at me and he says, "You know, you don't take on the CMA and the governor and lose. How much do you need to win? Can you win for a hundred thousand dollars?" And I said, "I'm pretty sure." And he said, "I don't want to be pretty sure. I want to be sure. How much do you need to be sure?" And I thought for a minute, took a deep breath, and said, "A quarter of a million dollars." And he looked at me and he said, this was about nine-thirty on a Thursday night, and he says, "I want a grant on my desk by five o'clock Tuesday morning for $250,000. I want ANR Foundation to be the fiscal agent. And you work it out with them and Heart and the Public Media Center." So we had one hysterical weekend of putting together this proposal.[7]

The resulting grant to ANRF paid for a series of advertisements to be developed by the Public Media Center in concert with Glantz, ANR, and AHA. The ads were to appear in major California newspapers and discuss issues surrounding Proposition 99. In addition, there were funds for public opinion polling and grassroots education. Gunther knew the hard-hitting advertisements would be out of character for the voluntary health agencies: "Our side invariably thinks the only way you win is by being nice, and the voluntaries are into that. I mean certainly around tobacco issues, it's been about, 'Oh, you know, I hope my back isn't hurting the heel of your shoe, Governor. We really appreciate your standing on us in this way. Let us know what else we can do to make you even more comfortable.' And that's the approach the voluntaries have had."[29]

Carol invited ACS and ALA to a meeting at the Public Media Center to discuss the strategy and encourage their participation. Beerline, however, had very little interest in Gunther's approach:

At the ad agency that was going to run their campaign, we had a major meeting. And all the players were there and we spent a lot of time talking about

our differences on how we wanted to run the campaign and basically what we
agreed upon at that point in time [was] that there was no way that we could
come together on this. So ANR and Heart would wage their campaign, we
would wage ours, we would keep each other informed. They felt very comfortable about the type of campaign that they had in mind and we dubbed it
the "black hat." . . . We said, "Okay, but we're not going to do it and we can
see that this might present some political problems in Sacramento and we're
going to have to distance ourselves from you." . . . But there was just no other
way that we could reconcile it because of the extreme difference in the way
that we were planning to run our campaigns.[8]

While ACS and ALA tried to work within the existing power structure
(which included the CMA), AHA, ANRF, Glantz, and Gunther started
trying to change it. Their first goal was neutralizing the CMA.

THE CMA HOUSE OF DELEGATES MEETING

AHA and ANRF believed that the CMA's pro-tobacco position originated with its political leadership and did not enjoy particularly broad
support among its physician members. To force the issue, they ran a full-
page ad in the California edition of the *New York Times* on February 29,
1996, during the CMA's annual House of Delegates meeting. The advertisement was an "open letter" signed by former surgeon general C. Everett Koop and other physicians and scientists telling the CMA, "It is
time to change" (figure 17). The advertisement helped stimulate a major
floor fight over CMA's position on Proposition 99. Roger Kennedy, a
physician from Santa Clara County who also served as chair of his local
tobacco control coalition, was involved in the floor fight and later recalled, "It really became clear that we were not going to win based on
the resolution, which was a very definite statement that the CMA should
change its position . . . but I think that we got what we could. In retrospect, I'm sorry I didn't push harder. . . . I think that going down to flam-
ing defeat in the face of the public may have accomplished more in the
long run. . . . There's no question that the leadership of the CMA was

Figure 17 (*opposite*).   Newspaper advertisement designed to change the
CMA's pro-tobacco position. The American Heart Association and the American Nonsmokers' Rights Foundation ran this advertisement in March 1996
during the CMA's annual House of Delegates meeting to stimulate discussion
of the CMA's stance on tobacco issues. It helped precipitate a vigorous floor
debate that marked the beginning of changes in CMA policy. (Courtesy of
American Nonsmokers' Rights Foundation)

An Open Letter to the California Medical Association

"The CMA believes that it is not in the best interest of physicians to battle the tobacco industry..."
CMA Medical Executives' Memo, June 13, 1988.

——— IT IS TIME TO CHANGE ———

In 1988 the people of California enacted Proposition 99, which increased the tax on tobacco and allocated at least 25 cents of every dollar raised to anti-tobacco education and research. Just as the voters had hoped, the resulting campaign has prevented the smoking of billions of packs of cigarettes.

It is not surprising, given this success, that the tobacco industry has done everything in its power to kill Proposition 99. What is surprising, however, is the fact that the California Medical Association has become the "cover" for the tobacco industry's attack on California's anti-smoking campaign.

The motive, articulated by the CMA's lobbyists and public relations staff, sounds noble – that poor women and children need medical care. This claim ignores the fact that 70 cents of every dollar Proposition 99 raises *can and has been legally used to fund medical services*, over $3 billion to date. We do not believe that the money the voters mandated for education and research should also wind up being spent on medical services.

The relentless pressure from the CMA, combined with the tobacco industry and its political allies, including Governor Pete Wilson, has all but destroyed the anti-tobacco education program and shut down the research program.

The result of the CMA's actions, whether intended or not, has been an increase in smoking in California, particularly among children. We view this as a clear violation of the first principle of medicine, "do no harm."

In its defense, the CMA has argued that the state budget crisis allows diversion of money mandated by the voters for anti-tobacco education and research. The courts have rejected this argument and ruled repeatedly that the use of Proposition 99 education and research money to provide medical services is illegal.

Governor Wilson, the defendant in these cases, is appealing. In the meantime, over $120 million that the people and the courts said must be used to prevent tobacco use sits in the state treasury as smokers die and children start to smoke. The CMA and Californians for Smoker's Rights are the only two organizations to file *amicus curiae* briefs in support of the Governor. We find it appalling that the Governor is wasting taxpayer money on these appeals and that the CMA is wasting physicians' money supporting Wilson's efforts to dismantle one of the most successful public health interventions in the world.

We believe that current official CMA policy does not reflect the true will of a majority of California physicians, or even the membership of the CMA.

There are members of the CMA planning to try and change this policy at the March 2-5, 1996, meeting of the House of Delegates. They want the CMA to fight against the tobacco industry and see that Proposition 99 is implemented as the voters intended. We applaud their efforts and urge you to support them; it is time for the CMA to break ranks with Governor Wilson and the tobacco industry and support Proposition 99 as the voters mandated.

C. Everett Koop, *Former U.S. Surgeon General*	John W. Farquhar, MD
Gregory W. Albers, MD	R.E. Fulton, MD
Jacob Bastacky, MD	Gordon L. Fung, MD, MPH
Dennis W. Biggs, Jr, MD	Stanton A. Glantz, PhD
Lester Breslow, MD, MPH	Robert C.W. Jones, Jr
Ralph Brindis, MD, MPH	Ronald M. Krauss, MD
Bruce H. Brundage, MD	Joel M. Moskowitz, PhD
Patricia A. Buffler, PhD	Bryce L. Reeve, MD, MPH
William G. Cahan, MD	Howard A. Rockman, MD
Robert Clark, MD	Stanley A. Rubin, MD
Patrice L. Des Pois, MD	John Slade, MD
Victor S. Dorodny, MD, MPH	Sidney C. Smith, Jr, MD
W. Allan Edmiston, MD	Gregory W. Thomas, MD, MPH
Eldon E. Ellis, MD	David B. Tillman, MD, MPH
Coyness L. Ennix, Jr, MD	Michael J. Wong, MD

This ad is endorsed by the American Heart Association and was paid for by the American Nonsmokers' Rights Foundation. For more information, write: ANRF, 2530 San Pablo Ave., Suite J, Berkeley, CA, 94702.

Public Media Center

not going to take a firm position that they would absolutely oppose any reallocation of funds." [30] ALA was working through its own doctors who were CMA members to get a resolution supporting full funding. According to Najera, "We took this to the public to make it a public debate at the House of Delegates. We literally organized a public debate for what I would say was the first time on the floor of the board, of the House of Delegates for CMA." [2]

The eventual CMA resolution was less than the public health advocates wanted. On March 3, 1996, the CMA House of Delegates voted to support full funding of Proposition 99's Health Education and Research programs if the governor and Legislature were willing to fund the "challenged programs" from the state General Fund. [31] If the governor and Legislature refused to use the General Fund, the CMA would continue to accept Proposition 99 funds for these programs, despite the court rulings. The CMA refused to withdraw its friend of the court briefs in support of the governor's position on AB 816 and SB 493. But in April 1996 the CMA did release a statement announcing its opposition to the governor's proposed budget concerning the use of the Health Education and Research Accounts to fund medical services. [32] Lewin saw the House of Delegates vote as representing a "fairly dramatic" change:

> I think that the change was because I'm a new leader and I was able to go directly to the doctors in the CMA and ask them what they wanted, what they believed in. And it was very clear that they were quite willing to support education and research as well as indigent health care and that they hadn't been asked the question in that way, that they didn't think you should undermine education for indigent health care. But they didn't think you should cut indigent health care to enhance education. Their strategy was that all of these things were too important and that the state had enough resources to do all three of these things and do them well. [10]

The CMA joined the ACS/ALA's Coalition to Restore Proposition 99, a decision that had the effect of isolating the governor. According to CMA lobbyist Elizabeth McNeil, the CMA action not only isolated the governor but also "showed them [the administration] and all these other groups, we're going work for something else and that isolated them, which made it difficult for them. In some ways made it more difficult for us to bring them around because they were a little upset with us about that." [27] The CMA's changed position made it less likely that the governor and tobacco industry could use medical necessity as the excuse for gutting the Proposition 99 Health Education and Research programs.

THE PHILIP MORRIS MEMO

One of Wilson's major responses to the criticism that he was pro-tobacco had always been that he took no direct campaign contributions from the tobacco industry. This claim ignored the fact that the tobacco industry was a major source of money for the California Republican Party— $165,727 in the 1995–1996 election cycle[16]—and that Wilson was the political leader of California Republicans. In any event, Wilson's defense hit a major snag when ANR obtained a March 4, 1990, internal memo between two Philip Morris lobbyists in Washington reassuring company executives that Wilson's act of returning some campaign contributions from the company did not mean that he was anti-tobacco. The Philip Morris lobbyists reported:

> Wilson is only sending about 16K of the 100K he collected. This 16K only includes checks he received either from a tobacco company or anyone working for a tobacco company, i.e., Hamish Maxwell [CEO and chairman of the Philip Morris Executive Committee], Mrs. Ehud [wife of Ehud Houminer, CEO of Philip Morris USA], Bill Murray [former president of Philip Morris].
>
> Apparently, he has also done this with other "controversial" industries such as lumber, chemicals, and others. The decision to do this was Wilson's alone, and in response to a wave of negative campaigning in California that not only attacks the candidates, but those who give to them as well.
>
> *You will be pleased to know that Pete called Hamish to explain that he was doing this to protect Hamish as well as himself. You will also be pleased to know that Pete is still "pro-tobacco."*[33] [emphasis added]

Wilson first saw the memo when he was being interviewed on camera by correspondent Peter Jennings for an ABC news special on tobacco. Wilson did not immediately say the memo was a lie, which limited what his staff could say later. (To the disappointment of many California tobacco control advocates, the exchange was not included in the final broadcast.) The memo, and the fact that the $84,000 retained by Wilson came from a variety of advertising agencies, law firms, and others who worked for the tobacco industry, received wide media coverage.[34–37]

ANRF and AHA also featured the memo in their first full-page advertisement attacking Wilson for diverting Proposition 99 anti-tobacco money into medical services, which ran on April 16 in the *New York Times,* and later in the *Sacramento Bee* and *Los Angeles Times* (figure 18). The advertisement reprinted the original memo and asked the question "Is this why Governor Pete Wilson is gutting Proposition 99 anti-tobacco education and research programs?" The ad also posed this

Is this why Governor Pete Wilson is gutting Proposition 99 anti-tobacco education & research programs?

In 1988, despite tens of millions of dollars spent by the tobacco companies opposing it, Proposition 99 was approved by California voters, raising cigarette taxes and creating anti-tobacco programs that have dramatically reduced the number of smokers and prevented thousands of cases of cancer and heart disease. Thanks to Prop. 99, smoking in California has declined by 2 billion packs —a drop of nearly $3 billion in tobacco sales.

Alarmed by Prop. 99's success, tobacco companies have turned to their backroom political allies in Sacramento to wage a behind-the-scenes campaign to gut the initiative's anti-smoking education and research programs. Political spending in California by the tobacco companies has increased by tenfold. They've hired a small army of slick lobbyists and political operatives. And they've deluged state politicians with cash contributions.

IS WILSON SERVING THE PUBLIC OR THE TOBACCO COMPANIES?

It's no surprise that the tobacco industry is sabotaging this program. But to have Governor Pete Wilson, who is described by Philip Morris as "pro-tobacco," undermining these programs is as cynical as it is calculated. Governor Wilson continues to divert funds mandated by voters for anti-tobacco education programs to pay for medical services. The audacity of the action is matched by its illegality.

This governor, in concert with some politicians whose entire careers have been spent slashing children's programs from the state budget, would now have you believe they stand on the side of poor, helpless children.

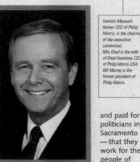

"Buffy" and "Jim" are most likely Kathleen M. "Buffy" Linehan, who works overseas for Philip Morris; James W. Dyer, Philip Morris lobbyist, currently staff director for the House Appropriations Committee. The two worked in the same office in 1990.

Hamish Maxwell, former CEO of Philip Morris, is the chairman of the executive committee; Mrs. Ehud is the wife of Ehud Houminer, CEO of Philip Morris USA; Bill Murray is the former president of Philip Morris.

In fact, Prop. 99 already allows 70% of its revenues specifically for indigent medical services —with over $3 billion available to pay doctors for treating poor children. In brazen defiance of state voters, Governor Wilson has illegally defunded anti-tobacco education and research programs by using the earmarked revenue for other purposes.

What the Governor and his tobacco patrons have done to Prop. 99 is a perfect example of everything that's wrong with our political system. It's time to get mad. It's time to fight back. It's time to remind Governor Wilson — and all the bought

and paid for politicians in Sacramento — that they work for the people of California. Not the tobacco companies. It's time to remind them who's the boss. Tell the Governor to stop playing games with Prop. 99 and start obeying the voters. Use the coupons below. Thank you.

Proposition 99:

- Passed by California voters in 1988
- Raised cigarette taxes by 25 cents
- Established the Tobacco Tax Surtax Fund
- Generates about $500 million a year
- Cut smoking by 2 billion packs and is considered the best anti-smoking program in the world
- Earmarks 25 percent of the Tobacco Tax Surtax Fund for anti-smoking education and research programs
- Allocates 45 percent for indigent healthcare
- Allocates 5 percent for the environment
- Allocates 25 percent by the legislature for any of the four mandated programs
- $3 billion in Prop. 99 funds are legally available for indigent health services without Governor Wilson's illegal diversion of the 25 percent allocated for the anti-smoking fund
- Governor Wilson has lost three times in court over illegal diversions of tobacco tax money, costing taxpayers over $500,000 in legal fees
- Researchers estimate Californians smoked 584 million more packs of cigarettes as a result of the Governor's efforts to sabotage Prop. 99 anti-smoking programs
- Tobacco companies have increased political spending in California by ten fold...now spending money faster in Sacramento than in Washington D.C.
- In a leaked tobacco industry memo, Governor Wilson is described as "pro-tobacco"
- With the help of the California Medical Association, Gov. Wilson has raided the 25 percent set aside for anti-tobacco education and research programs to give doctors more money to provide medical services for poor children—on top of the 70 percent already allowed for that purpose.

AMERICAN HEART ASSOCIATION

AMERICAN NONSMOKERS' RIGHTS FOUNDATION

Tell Pete Wilson to Put It Back.

American Nonsmokers' Rights Foundation
2530 San Pablo Ave., Suite J
Berkeley, CA 94702

NAME

ADDRESS

I support your efforts to protect the nation's most successful tobacco control campaign. Don't let Governor Wilson and the tobacco industry destroy Prop 99. Please send me more information on how I can help protect the anti-tobacco education campaigns I voted for.

Governor Pete Wilson
State Capitol
Sacramento, CA 95814

NAME

ADDRESS

You are supposed to uphold laws, not undermine them. The anti-tobacco education and research campaigns paid for by a tobacco tax I voted for in 1988 have saved thousands of lives in California. Stop playing games with Prop 99. Put the funding back. I'll be watching.

question: "It's time to ask the Governor who he really works for: The people of California or the tobacco companies?"

The tension between the ANRF/AHA and the ACS/ALA's Coalition to Restore Prop 99 was growing because the Coalition kept pressuring ANRF and AHA to tone down the attacks on Wilson. On April 29, after the advertisement featuring the Philip Morris memo ran, Coalition co-chairs Beerline and Martin wrote to the presidents of ANR and AHA calling on them to work to restore Proposition 99 "in a more positive way utilizing its media campaign to inform and educate the public on the real issues regarding the restoration of Prop. 99 funds."[38] ACS and ALA still hoped that the Legislature and the governor could be convinced to support the program with "a plethora of data and new information that will prove convincing and effective in restoring these important funds."[38]

They distributed their letter to the governor, the Legislature, and the media. According to Martin, they felt that they had to write the letter to "everybody" to say that they had nothing to do with the advertisements:

> Basically we said, "We share the same goal, there's no doubt about that, but your tactics and our tactics are not the same. We will pursue a positive campaign and we are notifying everybody that we have nothing whatsoever to do with those ads." And we hand-delivered that to the governor's office and we made a lot of phone calls saying, "Look, we don't have any control over the ads, there's nothing we can do about them. This is being done by these two groups and these two groups alone, period. We're out of this." And actually we finally did get that message across. I think that if we had not separated ourselves from those ads, we would have been dead politically at the Capitol.[39]

Carol found the letter highly offensive: "The tone was very patronizing, the whole 'we're glad you share our goals.' Not 'we're glad we have the same goals,' not 'we recognize that your goals are the same as ours.' 'We're glad you share our goals. You're welcome to share our goals.' We're welcome to join their coalition. We're welcome to sit at their table. Of course, we're not really welcome."[3] The whole point of the ANRF/AHA campaign was to avoid sitting at tables.

Figure 18 (*opposite*). Newspaper advertisement attacking Governor Pete Wilson for his pro-tobacco policies. The American Heart Association and the American Nonsmokers' Rights Foundation ran this advertisement in California's major newspapers to educate the public and media about what had happened to Proposition 99 and to focus attention on Governor Pete Wilson's role in dismantling the Tobacco Control Program. (Courtesy of American Nonsmokers' Rights Foundation)

THE GOVERNOR'S MAY REVISION

Meanwhile, as the disagreements among the parties in the field were playing out, competing bills were being introduced in the Legislature on how
to implement Proposition 99. The Senate Health Committee considered
two bills on April 17, the day after the media stories broke about the
memo calling Wilson "pro-tobacco," and both were passed out of committee, including one sponsored by Senator Diane Watson (D-Los Angeles) requiring full funding. The Assembly Health Committee passed a
full-funding bill sponsored by Assembly Member Katz on April 23 by a
12-1 vote. (After the hearing, several other members signed on to the
bill, resulting in a 15-1 vote in favor of the bill.) McNeil believed press
coverage of the issue the day before in the *Los Angeles Times* played an
important role in convincing the chair to let the bill out of committee.
The *Times* reported that the chair of the Assembly Health Committee,
Bret Granlund (R-Yucaipa), who had been quoted as saying, "I'm a free
enterprise, no-tax smoker," had taken at least $44,500 in tobacco in-
dustry campaign contributions.[40] According to McNeil,

> There was heavy-duty, behind-the-scenes lobbying with the CMA and the
> chairman of that committee to get that bill moved out. Ten minutes before the
> bill was heard, I was out in the hallway with the Assemblymen Katz and Brett
> Granlund, the chair. . . . he was getting some bad press in the *L.A. Times* at
> the time, which really helped. And I just said, "Well, look, this is going to go
> through the budget process and you're going to look terrible for not allowing
> this issue to move through the process and holding it up, and it's got a long
> ways to go and you're going to be criticized and seen as pro-tobacco, and
> there's no reason to do that." . . . So he agreed to let it out of committee. He
> had to signal that to the rest of his caucus to get it out because otherwise that
> bill was not going to come out.[27]

Under such scrutiny, the Assembly Health Committee was unwilling to
vote publicly against Proposition 99's Health Education and Research
programs. The bill later, however, stalled in the Assembly Appropriations Committee and died without a vote.

The Assembly Appropriations Committee passed the governor's proposal contained in his May revision of the budget. (The May revision is
considered the governor's "real" budget because it is adjusted to reflect
new economic data.) In the May revision, Wilson proposed releasing
$147 million in reserve Proposition 99 funds, including $33 million in
the Health Education Account and $41 million in the Research Account,

with the rest for medical services. The funds were available due to higher-than-expected revenues (because tobacco use was no longer falling, partially as a result of cuts in the anti-tobacco program) and underspending in several Proposition 99 medical programs, including ones illegally funded out of the Health Education Account. The additional $74 million in spending on Health Education and Research was to be a one-time expenditure. The governor was still not willing to allocate all of the Proposition 99 money as specified in the initiative. All of the new monies were to target youth, which was justified by the release of data showing that in 1995 adult smoking prevalence had dropped from 17.3 percent to 16.7 percent while youth smoking prevalence had risen again, this time from 10.9 percent to 11.9 percent.[41]

REACTION TO THE GOVERNOR'S NEW BUDGET

The reaction to the governor's proposal was mixed. AHA and ANRF responded with a new full-page advertisement headlined "The tobacco industry knows that the best way to get kids hooked on cigarettes is to say they're for 'Adults Only.' Why is Pete Wilson using tax dollars to help them?" The advertisement took issue with the governor's plan to focus on youth and argued that strategies that focused only on youth played into the tobacco industry's efforts to hook young smokers. The tobacco industry, according to internal memos, tries to attract young smokers by presenting the cigarette as "one of the initiations into the adult world" and as "part of the illicit pleasure category of products and services."[42] Smoking is linked to the illicit pleasure category through alcohol consumption and sex.

Not surprisingly, the Coalition to Restore Prop 99 took a more measured approach: "We are encouraged the Governor has recognized the importance of funding tobacco education, prevention, and research and believe he has taken a critical first step. However, we have very serious concerns about his proposed programmatic changes which may not be consistent with Proposition 99."[43] In a separate memo to ALA directors and staff, Caitlin Kirk, director of communications at ALA, and Najera commented that "although the proposal is a positive step, we have serious concerns and many questions about the details. We are quite concerned about the overall effectiveness of a tobacco control program that would require all funds to be spent on youth-focused education and research projects."[44] Knepprath explained,

Our coalition was very unified against the revise. We put out a "reject the revise" fact sheet to the Legislature and flogged that around. And I think that helped CMA maybe soften its position on that. . . . I think their posture on it was "Let's be more positive about it and try to work out our differences." We were saying, "Uh-uh, this is bad on its face. Go back to square one." We were able to, I think, through our combined efforts to convince [Senator Mike] Thompson and the budget committee that there needed to be a different approach to using the supplemental funds.[2]

While differing in how aggressive they were willing to be, the AHA/ ANRF and ACS/ALA camps were converging on their policy goals. The CMA, while a member of the ACS/ALA coalition, was also acting independently and had probably helped negotiate the governor's position in the May budget revision.[9] The CMA was not waiting for the Coalition as a group to act before going to the governor.

The objections of the health groups were getting the media's attention. On June 3 the *San Francisco Chronicle* carried as its lead editorial "Smelling the Smoke of Governor's Plan," which criticized the governor's May revised proposal:

Governor Wilson recently proposed a compromise that would shift $147 million of previously diverted Prop. 99 funds to tobacco education programs, but that would still fall short of the 20-percent level approved by voters. The Governor's plan also limits the education spending to programs aimed at teenagers, instead of a broader approach. Also, his proposal is a one-year deal, leaving tobacco education funding vulnerable to vagaries of future budget conditions. . . . The Katz and Watson bills reassert the state's long-term commitment to fight smoking. California voters delivered the mandate—and the money—eight years ago. This effort must not be undermined by Wilson and other friends of tobacco in Sacramento.[45]

On that same day, TEROC met and DHS director Kim Belshé came to the meeting to defend the governor's proposal. Jennie Cook, chair of TEROC, along with other committee members, echoed the public health groups' concern about focusing so exclusively on youth. The program, according to Cook, worked best when it included youth, communities, and adults all together. According to Belshé, the decision on how to spend the dollars was based on smoking rates. For the previous two years there had been an increase in the rates of smoking for youth. But what also emerged at the meeting was that for the second half of 1995 adult rates were also increasing. For the first six months of 1995, the percentage of adults that smoked was 15.5 percent but in the second six months this figure went up to 17.9 percent. Reporting the overall figure of 16.7 percent for the year disguised the uptick in adult smoking.[46] Several major newspapers reported on the apparent effort to disguise the upturn in the adult smoking rate, creating more bad publicity for the administration.[47,48]

In the Capitol, Senate Budget and Fiscal Review Committee staffer Diane Van Maren was working with Senator Mike Thompson to develop their own budget proposal:

> I did multiple renditions of various options with the intent of doing a two-thirds vote because that's what Senator Thompson wanted, maintaining indigent health care as best we could, providing an increase particularly for the media campaign, which Mike thinks is particularly excellent. And there has been very good analysis of that to show that it is excellent. To provide an increase to the competitive grants area locally and then also provide good funding to the schools. From a political context of course the governor did not want to provide much funding to the schools because "Oh, that's Delaine Eastin, and that's a Democrat and that's the Superintendent of Schools," so he didn't want to do that. . . . A lot of it came from the concern that came forth regarding the increase in adolescent smoking. We need to know more about what the schools are doing and we provided additional funding, $2 million, to do an evaluation in that area this year, but at the same time we also felt that it was important to provide the schools with more funding for a couple of reasons. One, they have a captive audience obviously. Two, because of the increase in adolescent smoking and chewing tobacco and related tobacco products, that was where we needed to get a firmer message across that smoking isn't cool no matter what the movies show and all the rest of it.
> . . . And then restoring the Research Account. And we also went along with the governor on his $5 million for the rural health grants, and we also went along with the governor on the $2 million for the evaluation of school program, and we also . . . provided General Fund monies to backfill for indigent health care.[21]

The state constitution requires a two-thirds vote in both houses of the Legislature to pass a budget bill. By deciding that the Proposition 99 revenues would be appropriated with a "two-thirds bill" rather than one that required a four-fifths vote, Thompson was signaling that there would not be any new diversion of Proposition 99 money.

On June 5 the Budget Conference Committee, comprising members of both houses, began meeting to complete the state budget, including decisions on what would happen with the Proposition 99 funding. The Senate was working with Senator Thompson's proposal, and the Assembly was presenting the governor's revised budget. On June 10 the *San Francisco Examiner* ran as its lead editorial "A Plan Goes Up in

Smoke: The Governor and Legislators Must Restore Mandated Funding
to Prop. 99 Anti-Smoking Programs Aimed at Youthful Addiction." The
editorial encouraged the Legislature to give the Health Education and
Research Accounts full funding.[49] On June 12 the Budget Conference
Committee agreed, on a 6-0 vote, that Proposition 99 reauthorization
would be drafted as a two-thirds bill, which meant that the initiative's
funding percentages would not be violated for the first time since the
voters passed Proposition 99.

The health groups were making progress.

ATTEMPTED RESTRICTIONS ON THE MEDIA CAMPAIGN

Full funding of the Health Education and Research Accounts was only
one problem that tobacco control advocates faced. As illustrated by the
Governor's May budget revision, tobacco control now had to deal with
efforts by the tobacco industry's political allies to withhold money from
effective programs and instead fund ineffective ones. The governor had
already tried to focus the campaign on youth. Now Speaker Curt Pringle
(R-Garden Grove) proposed that the media campaign be prohibited
from attacking the tobacco industry and limited to publicizing the health
effects of smoking. He wanted the advertisements to "be based solely on
the health implications of tobacco use and on the health implications of
refraining from tobacco use."[50] Echoing tobacco industry rhetoric, he argued that taxpayer dollars should not be used to attack a legal industry.

Reflecting another common tobacco industry strategy for reducing
the effectiveness of anti-smoking advertising, Pringle wanted the ads
to focus on children between the ages of six and fourteen, a strategy,
Adams said, that "dooms the entire campaign to fail."[51] These restrictions would have forced DHS to stop using effective messages that had
changed the social environment and helped reduce smoking in favor of
ones that public health professionals had long known to be ineffective.[52]
Pringle also wanted $5 million set aside for cessation.

Senators Thompson and Lockyer and Assembly Member Katz were
strongly opposed to media account restrictions, although they were willing to include the cessation language as a compromise with Speaker
Pringle in order to protect the media campaign.[21] Though it was not realized at the time, this $5 million was money currently appropriated for
the media campaign that the governor had not spent and which would
have been carried over to the next year in the media account. Thus, the
cessation compromise was effectively a cut in the media campaign.

In addition, following the lead of his predecessor, Willie Brown, Speaker Pringle also tried to insert language in the authorization for the Research Account that would block it from funding research of a "partisan political nature." [53] (ANRF and AHA protested this incursion of politics into the Research Account debate by running an advertisement, which included side-by-side photos of Pringle and Brown, who despised each other.) According to Katz, "Pringle and the governor were very, very serious about attacking Stan [Glantz] and the research, writing into Prop 99 or the budget that the ads couldn't attack the tobacco companies." [20]

Pringle was widely criticized for his stance. The editorial in the *Sacramento Bee* on June 28 was representative: "Tobacco industry executives plainly don't enjoy turning on the television and seeing ads telling Californians that the industry profits at the expense of their health. They don't like it when researchers unmask their marketing and political strategies. It's not hard to understand why they want the Legislature to undermine those elements of Proposition 99. What's harder to explain, and impossible to justify, is the speaker's willingness to do their work." [54] Pringle's language putting limits on what the media account could be used for was eventually dropped.

THE RESEARCH ACCOUNT

Significant changes also occurred in 1996 in the way the Research Account was to be spent. Up to that time, the University of California had been left wide discretion in selecting which research projects to fund using the peer review process. On one side, the public health advocates had been critical of the University of California for not focusing the research effort more directly on tobacco in the form of applied research. On the other side, the governor and Pringle were trying to impose more political control on the content of the research program. In the May budget Governor Wilson had proposed that TEROC be required to hold hearings and approve projects for funding. Since the majority of TEROC's members are appointed by the governor, this would increase his control over the program.

The public health groups vigorously objected to giving TEROC control over individual research projects, as well as to Pringle's language designed to stop "partisan political" research, as infringements on academic freedom. Rather than demanding that the Pringle language be dropped, however, the university attempted to finesse the point. The university convinced the governor to agree to a procedure whereby TEROC would hold a hearing and make recommendations to the Department of Finance on the university's "expenditure plan," which was a general plan for how the money was to be spent, rather than act on specific projects. The university argued that it had to submit expenditure plans to the Department of Finance anyway, so this was not a significant change. As in prior years, the university was reluctant to make any waves regarding Proposition 99 if it meant offending the governor.

Public health advocates were furious with the university for proposing this compromise because they thought it might be possible to get rid of the language altogether. According to Martin, "The [university's] budget people were trying to work a deal without understanding the issues. I was just floored. . . . I read this and I said to Cathrine [Castoreno, the UC lobbyist], 'Don't they know these people aren't their friends?' So we were shocked, because I don't believe that was necessary. . . . UC should never have caved in on that."[39]

On July 1 the University of California's vice president for health affairs, Cornelius Hopper, attempted to clarify the university's interpretation of the language. "A research program expenditure plan," he wrote, was understood to be "a general expenditure plan identifying the range of targeted research areas. As we have made clear to all parties, we do not intend to submit for review each grant proposal we wish to fund."[55] The letter went on to say that the university "interprets the phrase, 'research or other activities of a partisan political nature,' to mean activities pertinent to political parties. As a matter of policy, the University of California does not engage in such activities and the TRDRP [Tobacco Related Disease Research Program, which administers the Research Account] would not fund research that does so." The letter specifically affirmed that research related to public policies for tobacco control would be funded and that the university had no control over the uses to which its research was put by others.[55] Hopper also phoned Glantz and assured him that the university did not consider his work to be of a "partisan political nature" and that he would be free to compete for funding from the Research Account. (Glantz, whose research was by then supported by the National Cancer Institute and the American Cancer Society, did not apply for funding from the Research Account that year.)

According to Castoreno, the university was trying to accommodate the political process while holding firm on the issue of academic freedom: "We put out a letter to clarify our understanding of the language which very specifically is to share an overall plan about the areas we're intending to fund and how much money we're prepared to contribute to each of those areas, but definitely not to allow any external party to second-guess the actual projects we fund. And within that, we plan to fund public policy research." [56] Both the Legislature and the Wilson administration consented to Hopper's interpretation of the Research Account.

While the public battle had been over the imposition of political control over the research program, the big change in the final budget language actually represented an important victory for the public health groups regarding the priorities for the research program. The relevant passage read as follows:

> Of the funds appropriated by this item, $60,422,000 is to be allocated for *research regarding tobacco use, with an emphasis on youth and young adults, including, but not limited to, the effects of active and passive smoking, primary prevention of tobacco use, nicotine addiction and its treatment, effects of second hand smoke and public health issues surrounding tobacco use.* These funds may not be used to support research or other activities of a partisan political nature, and shall be allocated primarily for applied research. In addition, prior to its use of this $60,422,000, the university shall submit a research program expenditure plan to the Department of Finance for approval. The Tobacco Education [and] Research Oversight Committee shall conduct public hearings on the proposed expenditure plan and make recommendations to the Director of Finance regarding approval of the plan. [57] [emphasis added]

The university was directed to develop a program of research with much more direct relevance to tobacco. While Pringle's language remained, it had no practical effect. TEROC held its hearing and approved the expenditure plan later that year, as did the Department of Finance. The university was free to use the peer review process to select specific projects for funding, and the new program had a stronger tobacco focus. The following year, the requirement for the TEROC hearing and the Department of Finance's approval of the expenditure plan was dropped.

THE FINAL BUDGET NEGOTIATION

At a June 19 meeting of the Budget Conference Committee, chaired by Senator Mike Thompson, a spending plan for Proposition 99 was passed that allocated the full 20 percent to the Health Education Account and 5 percent to the Research Account. Of the $131 million allocated to Health Education, $5 million was to go to support cessation programs,

$25 million to the media program, $43 million to schools, $31 million to competitive grants, and $27 million to LLAs. The Research Account was given $60 million.[58]

On June 20 ANRF and AHA released the results of the public opinion poll they had commissioned from the Field Institute to determine the extent of public support for Proposition 99. The results indicated overwhelming support among both Democrats and Republicans for Proposition 99 as it was passed by the voters—80.1 percent of voters supported the Proposition 99 revenue allocations. In addition, 55.3 percent of voters said they would be less likely to vote for a candidate who took campaign contributions from the tobacco industry, and 56.4 percent thought that the industry had a "great deal" of influence over those who accepted industry money.[59]

On July 8 the Assembly and Senate approved the budget, which included the Proposition 99 programs. A related bill, AB 3487, authorized the programs by permanently removing the sunset provision and leaving the program appropriations to be determined through the yearly budget process. The governor signed the budget on July 15.

The only downside of the final decision was that the funds were appropriated for only one year. Program authorization alone, however, became a moot issue with the removal of the sunset language. Miller was unhappy to have Proposition 99 in the budget bill because, ironically, this made it more susceptible to back-room deals out of the public eye:

> . . . decisions in the budget aren't made like in a public hearing and you don't get to testify. Nobody does. It's done by the pols in the back room, and that's where they're going to assign the money. . . . And I think for a year or two we're stuck with that. One of the reasons they didn't extend us for more than a year is because they want it in the budget. And I think that CMA wants it there as well as Mike Thompson and others, because that puts it under their control. It takes it away from Diane Watson and Tom Hayden, Richard Katz. . . . The commitment to [Proposition] 99 is real thin in the Legislature still, despite everything we've done.[9]

McNeil, however, saw having the program in the budget as the only real alternative: "That was our preference to do this in the budget, because we thought that was the only way we were going to get the governor to go along. . . . if you had it in the budget, it's part of a bigger deal and there are lots of other issues and the governor doesn't have to put his signature on a Prop 99 bill. . . . It's not a single Prop 99 bill where he has to say, 'I caved in.'"[27] In any event, the 1996–1997 budget marked the first time that the Legislature had passed a bill consistent with Proposition 99. The Health Education Account received its full 20 percent of revenues and the Research Account its full 5 percent. There were no unacceptable restrictions on the expenditure of Health Education Account funds, and the Research Account expenditures were refocused in ways that the public health groups had advocated.

In the end, Wilson acquiesced to full funding of the Health Education and Research Accounts. Isenberg described Wilson's personal style in these terms: "He may be a Marine and Marines may be trained for assault, but Pete Wilson when mad digs his foxhole deeper and never budges. He's a very stubborn guy."[22] When asked why Wilson eventually shifted his stance on Proposition 99 funding in 1996, Isenberg replied, "Because everybody badgered him. The administration badgered him. 'You're losing the lawsuit, stop this.' . . . And you know, after a while, even Pete Wilson wears down when his advisors come [to him with] 'You're not winning this fight, now let's get out of here.' It's only whatever it is, $20 million, $30 million, $40 million."[22]

In addition, the tobacco industry itself had become more of an issue and the industry's partisan support for the Republicans had turned into a liability. The Philip Morris memo identifying Wilson as "pro-tobacco" also made it more difficult for Wilson to defend his actions as good public policy. As Miller explained, "The industry left him in a bad spot politically by shifting their donations so dramatically to the Republicans. It did two things. One, it alienated the Democrats and, two, it provided some convincing evidence to the press that there was indeed some substance to our claim that the diversion wasn't about a budget shortfall. It was about stopping [Proposition] 99. And the third one is related to that and that was the discovery of the Philip Morris memo regarding Wilson and his being a friend. . . . What it did for the reporters was give credibility to our argument."[9] The governor also had to face the reality that there would be no four-fifths vote in 1996, so he could not even attempt to alter the percentages of tax revenues going to the different accounts. In short, for Wilson, there was little good news coming from the Legislature on Proposition 99. With the public watching, with no Democratic support, and with no recession to provide cover, he was left with little choice but to support the full-funding effort. The only other cover he had had—the CMA—had also switched sides. By returning to the public arena and taking a principled position of demanding that the will of the voters be respected, the public health advocates had succeeded.

ENGAGING THE MEDIA

Public opinion both influences and is influenced by events, but public opinion is activated only when those events are reported in the mass media; even then, the way opinion leans is often dependent on how events are interpreted in the media.[60] Thus, it was essential that the media perceive Proposition 99 as an important issue and frame the issue as "following the will of the voter."

The media had not paid significant attention to the Proposition 99 programs between the 1989 passage of AB 75 and 1994. Scott of the *California Journal* had assumed that although programmatic initiatives were disputed, the money was going into the voter-approved categories:

> I have to say that it wasn't until the Lung Association and the Cancer Society suddenly started complaining about the diversions that I started noticing it at all, and more people started noticing it. Because the assumption had always been, and I'm guilty of this as much as anyone, but a lot of times what we look at as journalists to sort of guide us in determining what's a real issue and what's not a real issue is the attitude of the constituent groups. . . . They were never thrilled about them [the diversions], but they never raised them as an issue. I mean they never raised them as an issue to the level that they were seeking media on it. So the assumption was that if nobody's making any noise about this, then it's just not that big a deal.[4]

Scott differentiates between raising an issue and raising it "to the level they were seeking media on it." One of the by-products of running only an insider campaign is that the press is unlikely to be informed about the problems and issues. Without the press, it is harder to rally the kind of public opinion required to influence policy.

Some of the media coverage of Proposition 99 was in news reports, and some of it was paid for by the principals. The key players credited the increased media interest in the Proposition 99 funding effort with being important, although they differed over why it occurred. ACS and ALA saw their public relations firm as key, while ANR and AHA saw their advertising campaign as important; others thought that tobacco had just become a hotter media story generally because President Bill Clinton was making tobacco an issue in national politics. It was, in fact, a combination of all these factors.

ACS and ALA had hired the public relations firm Sturges, Zegas, and Metzger. Bobbie Metzger, who was married to Willie Brown's former chief of staff, carried weight with both the Legislature and the press. According to Beerline,

Probably one of the better decisions that we made was to hire this organization. They're extremely well connected politically in Sacramento. They have an excellent reputation, and they have access to the media that staggered me. . . . They basically took over the media part of this campaign from that point on, from April through July. And we had press conferences, press briefings. They set us up with all of our editorial board visits, numerous radio, TV interviews. . . . After the word got out that we had hired Metzger, [people commented,] "Well, the Coalition must be serious this time if they hired Metzger et al." So apparently they didn't think much of the prior efforts, that we were just going symbolically through the motions, but by having Metzger on board, apparently that sent an entirely different message to the legislators.[8]

The Metzger firm arranged for Martin and Beerline to have meetings with all the major editorial boards.

Isenberg, when asked about the media attention, attributed it mainly to advertising and the successful framing of the issue: "They advertised. They have learned the issue, which for them Prop 99 is just another way of saying campaign contributions. Tobacco campaign contributions. It becomes an opportunity to write the story; it's a fight. You can always get a good quote, call Stanley [Stanton Glantz] for a quote, call up whoever you want for a quote. Wilson's people are always outraged. And so it's a good fight, it's a constant fight, and the press media loves fights. That's how they explain issues."[22] Julia Carol agreed:

The first thing that got their attention was the break between the coalitions, and that actually helped get media attention. It said something is happening differently. The Heart Association breaking with Cancer and Lung caused a big uproar. That first ad that we sent out, the reverberations have not yet stopped from that ad on many levels. . . . That ad shocked the pants off of everybody. . . . And then the Philip Morris memo and our subsequent ad campaign. The fact that ABC was working on the story generates interest within the media. You know everybody wants to beat them to the punch. . . . There's peer pressure in journalism as to who is reporting on what. I also think the voluntaries [principally ACS and ALA] did a good job of getting editorials written. They did do editorial board visits and you know they were a part, particularly Lung, was a part of the grassroots sort of getting attention in the field. I think the troops were more mobilized because they were more excited because something was happening for a change. . . . I mean everyone needed to be woken up. One big giant wakeup.[3]

Opinions about the series of ANRF/AHA advertisements varied from those that found them counterproductive to those that deemed them to have had a considerable positive effect on the effort to stop the diversions. Scott thought they had "a tremendous effect." He went on to say,

> Even though they [ACS and ALA] "distanced" themselves from it, it provided ammunition for the voluntaries who were working within the system to really force the issue. . . . I think that even though they felt as though they were sort of being subtly attacked and that they had been trying to work this deal out with the Medical Association, they felt as though it undermined them. They didn't want to piss the Medical Association off, but on some level I think they felt as though, "Well, you'd better deal with us because you don't know what those lunatics are going to do." . . . So it gave them clout with the Medical Association that they might not have otherwise had. On a broader perspective, I think it put the Medical Association's Sacramento lobbyists on the hot seat because the whole, I mean, one of those ads was, "Why is the California Medical Association supporting Pete Wilson? Why is the California Medical Association supporting something that the tobacco industry supports?" [4]

Scott continued to discuss the effect of the advertising campaign on Wilson.

> All of a sudden Pete Wilson, if he sticks to the hard line on the tobacco tax diversions, . . . in the political context, you can't say that it's anything but doing the tobacco industry's bidding. Wilson, if he still aspires to any kind of life beyond the governorship, he can't allow that to be a rap against him because it's pretty clear that's an issue that is playing well with the electorate. So I just don't think there's any question but those ads had an impact. Again, one of the ways you measure that impact is how mad the people who were targeted got about them and they got mad. Wilson was breathing fire about them. [4]

On the other hand, a number of key players felt that the ads had been ineffective and perhaps even counterproductive. Among them was Lewin, who commented, "Their strategy this year was embarrassing Governor Wilson. Originally they thought by embarrassing the CMA, they could change the CMA. That was clearly one of their strategies. I would assume they think they won on that one. And they had nothing, it had nothing to do with that. If anything, that strengthened the resolve within CMA to do nothing." [10] Martin also thought that the ads had a negative effect:

> I think it had a very negative effect at the Capitol because one of the things you avoid is blaming one person for everything bad that's ever happened. It is a smash-in-your-face kind of ad campaign that I think is very counterproductive. The other problem we had was that people read the ad and because they knew the Lung Association and Cancer Society's position on Prop 99, they thought we had written and paid for the ad too. They didn't read the sponsors' names. So we got many negative calls, both Lung and Cancer got lots of calls, "What are you doing, why are you doing this?" . . . *This is not the way the game is played at the Capitol.* [39] [emphasis added]

Of course, that was the point of the ads. ANRF and AHA wanted to change the way the game was played.

THE END OF THE DIVERSIONS

The battle in 1996 was the last time that the governor or the Legislature tried to divert Proposition 99 money from the Health Education and Research Accounts into medical services. The 1997, 1998, and 1999 appropriations followed Proposition 99 and proceeded with little controversy (figure 19). This hands-off attitude is particularly interesting, given that the Court of Appeal eventually ruled in 1996 that SB 493, which expressly amended Proposition 99, might be legal and sent the issue back to the trial court for an evidentiary hearing. The Court of Appeal ruled that AB 816 was illegal because money from the Health Education and Research Accounts could not be used to fund medical services. In SB 493 the Legislature moved money out of the Health Education and Research Accounts into the medical service accounts and then appropriated the money. The Court of Appeal said that the plaintiffs had not put evidence into the record that demonstrated that this diversion of funds was "inconsistent with the purposes" of Proposition 99. This decision left the door open for further attempts at diversion, but the Legislature did not try.

The issue on SB 493 was that no evidence had been entered at the trial court level regarding the effects of the diversions on the Health Education and Research programs. If the existence of the programs had been jeopardized by the cuts, then the amendments were not consistent with the purposes of the initiative. On the other hand, if the programs were continuing to operate successfully, then the court was unsure that the diversions were, in fact, inconsistent with the purposes of the initiative. The Court of Appeal had no factual basis on which to make that decision. The voluntary health agencies and ANR appealed the SB 493 decision to the California Supreme Court, but the Supreme Court did not take the case, leaving the advocates with the decision whether to return to the trial court to introduce new evidence.

In the meantime, the $43 million that was being contested in court (see chapter 13) sat in reserve within the Health Education and Research Accounts. (The governor had spent the contested funds from AB 816 on anti-tobacco education and research after he lost the appeal, as well as about $22 million of the contested funds from SB 493.) In 1998, Glantz

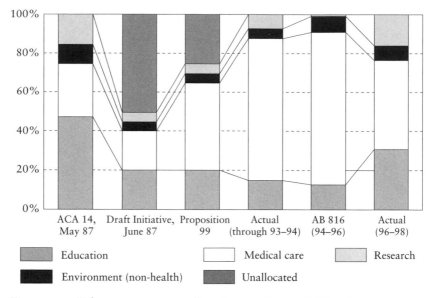

Figure 19. Tobacco tax revenue allocations, 1987–1998. The vigorous campaign mounted by health groups restored funding for the Proposition 99 anti-tobacco education and research programs starting with the 1996–1997 fiscal year.

suggested to Van Maren that the Legislature simply appropriate this money for anti-tobacco education and research; in exchange, the health groups would drop their lawsuits. Senator Thompson and the Legislature agreed, and these funds were appropriated, which would have ended this litigation and provided more money for anti-tobacco education and research. Rather than concur with this resolution, however, Wilson used his line-item veto to scuttle the deal because Lee Sanders had refused to drop the SAYNO lawsuit over the AB 75 and AB 99 diversions.[61]

CONCLUSION

Several factors contributed to the success of the health groups in 1996. While differing in tone and style, they all expanded the scope of the conflict beyond the Legislature and governor to include the general public. They also returned to the principled position of respecting the will of the voters rather than simply treating Proposition 99 as a fight over money. As a result, the media paid much closer attention to the Proposition 99 allocations than they had in the past.

Other things had changed. The California Medical Association was no longer pushing for diversions. The state's fiscal picture had improved. Repeated lawsuits had found the diversions illegal. The governor was linked to the tobacco industry in a year when such linkage was particularly embarrassing. The tobacco industry was an increasingly less desirable ally. The Legislature had changed from a Democratic body, heavily controlled by Willie Brown, a very strong ally of the tobacco industry, to one in which the Assembly was Republican and the Senate was Democratic. At the same time, the tobacco industry became increasingly partisan in its campaign contributions, which reduced the allegiance that Democrats felt toward the industry. The extent of the industry's clout in California policy making had changed dramatically since 1978 when Peter Hanauer and Paul Loveday launched Proposition 5.

For tobacco control advocates trying to defend citizen initiatives in legislatures, the challenge is to exercise vigilance and to use their greatest source of power—public opinion. When asked what tobacco control advocates did differently in 1996, Isenberg said, "They just screamed bloody murder. You know, the old oil, squeaky wheel analogy is not a bad one in all of this." [22]

Even with full funding, however, the tobacco education programs had to be implemented by public agencies, so the governor and his appointees were still in charge of most of the Health Education Account. After all, in its first analysis of how to reduce the effectiveness of the Proposition 99 media campaign back in April 1990, the Tobacco Institute had identified influencing the administration as a way to neutralize the program. [62] Thanks to the leadership of Ken Kizer (director of DHS in the Deukmejian administration) and Governor Deukmejian's willingness to take a hands-off position regarding the Proposition 99 programs, the industry had at first been unable to apply this strategy. But times and people changed, and the Wilson administration had already demonstrated a willingness to impose political restrictions on the scope and content of the anti-tobacco program. With full funding of the Health Education Account in hand, tobacco control advocates could turn their attention to program implementation.

It is possible to spend a large amount of money on an ineffective campaign, and the Wilson administration did precisely that.

CHAPTER 15

Political Interference in Program Management

In 1990 the tobacco industry had considered lobbying the Deukmejian administration to weaken the tobacco control program, particularly the media campaign, but it recognized that this strategy was unlikely to succeed.[1] The industry quickly recognized that Governor George Deukmejian had a hands-off approach to day-to-day program management and that Ken Kizer, director of the Department of Health Services (DHS), was committed to the anti-smoking program. Thus it was more productive to concentrate on working with the Legislature and others such as the conservative California Medical Association (CMA) and the liberal Western Center for Law and Poverty to divert anti-tobacco education and research funds into medical services. This situation changed as soon as Pete Wilson was inaugurated governor in 1991. According to Kizer, who stayed on at DHS until a successor was named, things changed immediately: "There were some comments from . . . [Wilson's] office that they were unhappy and would like to see any subsequent ads toned down, and wanted to review any of them."[2] As the administration slowly strangled the program, it lost its effectiveness.[3]

The battle over program content intensified over time, particularly after June 1996, when the Legislature stopped diverting money from the Health Education and Research Accounts into medical services. The health groups, which had become reasonably used to and proficient at fighting the tobacco industry directly and in the Legislature, had a much more difficult time engaging in administrative battles to insure that the Health Education money was spent effectively and not wasted on activities that the tobacco industry considered "acceptable."[4,5]

SQUASHING THE MEDIA CAMPAIGN

The media campaign had been a focal point for controversy ever since the tobacco industry tried to kill it off in 1989 in AB 75, Proposition 99's first implementing legislation (see chapter 5). In 1990 the industry recognized the power of paid counter-advertising and had conducted its own focus group testing of the California advertisements.[6–8] As the implementation of Proposition 99 continued, the media campaign continued to be controversial, with California tobacco control advocates working to maintain a no-holds-barred tone and the tobacco industry and its allies seeking to soften the tone and limit the scope of the campaign to targeting children and pregnant women or else to presenting health messages. Assembly Speaker Curt Pringle (R-Garden Grove) had even attempted to write these restrictions into law in 1996 (see chapter 14).

In 1990 the media campaign got off to a strong start. The first wave of advertisements, launched in April of that year under AB 75, included thirteen television spots and twelve radio spots, supplemented with three more television spots in February 1991. The campaign also included supporting billboards and print advertising. In addition to its aggressive tone, the DHS Tobacco Control Section (TCS) tied the advertising to the needs of the local programs. TCS convened a large Media Advisory Committee, consisting of various stakeholders and representatives of local and ethnic programs, to review emerging advertising concepts and provide feedback.

In January 1992 Governor Wilson tried to eliminate the media campaign by refusing to sign the new contract with the advertising agency, Livingston and Keye (previously keye/donna/perlstein; see chapter 10). The broadcasting of anti-smoking advertisements ended immediately, as did the development of new advertisements. Although the American Lung Association (ALA) successfully sued to force the administration to sign the contract in May 1992, the governor's action significantly disrupted the campaign. Although DHS began running the old advertisements again, no new media was available until February 1993. This delay meant that two years elapsed between waves of new material. Once the campaign restarted, Livingston and Keye released eleven television spots in February, supplemented with four more in November, and a total of seven radio spots. Despite the delay, the new advertisements maintained the tone of the earlier campaign, which focused on discrediting the tobacco industry and highlighting the dangers of secondhand smoke.

In the fiscal years 1994–1995 and 1995–1996, the Legislature continued to allocate money—nearly $12 million annually—to the media campaign. The allocation, however, did not insure that a quality program would result or even that the money would necessarily be spent. Instead of continuing the Deukmejian administration's policy of treating the development and approval of the advertising spots as a matter to be dealt with by public health professionals inside DHS and its advertising agency, the Wilson administration required the advertisements to be approved by the secretary of health and welfare, Sandra Smoley, and the Governor's Office. As a member of the Sacramento County Board of Supervisors in 1990, Smoley was one of only two votes against the Sacramento Clean Indoor Air Ordinance. The rate of production of new material fell dramatically. Only five television spots were released in September 1994 and four in September 1995. These television spots were supplemented by eleven radio spots. The administration then stopped all production. There were no new advertisements between September 1995 and March 20, 1997. In 1995–1996 the Wilson administration spent only $6.5 million of the $12.2 million appropriated by the Legislature for the media campaign. This $5 million in unspent funds was the $5 million that Speaker Pringle succeeded in allocating to smoking cessation efforts in 1996, effectively cutting the media campaign in half.

The efforts to squash the media campaign paid off for the tobacco industry. The weakening of the media campaign, in both content and intensity, was associated with an end to the drop in tobacco consumption in California (figure 20). The California Tobacco Survey, conducted in 1998 by John Pierce of the University of California, San Diego, under contract to DHS, demonstrated that smoking stopped falling in California in 1994, at the same time that the funding diversions accelerated and the media campaign and other programs were scaled back and toned down.[3,9] The loss of program effectiveness after 1994 meant that Californians smoked 840 million packs of cigarettes (worth about $1.2 billion to the tobacco industry) between 1994 and 1998 that would not have been smoked had the program remained as effective as it was between 1989 and 1994 (figure 21).

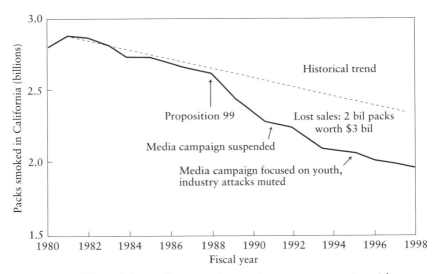

Figure 20.   Effect of the media campaign on cigarette consumption. After 1994, when Governor Wilson toned down the media campaign and focused on youth, the Tobacco Control Program lost its effectiveness. Even so, from passage in 1988 through 1998, the program prevented about 2 billion packs of cigarettes from being smoked (compared to the historical trend), worth $3 billion to the tobacco industry.

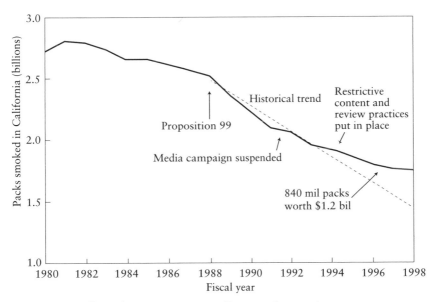

Figure 21.   Effect of restrictions on media campaign on cigarette consumption. Wilson Administration policies that scaled back and toned down the anti-tobacco education campaign slowed the decline in cigarette consumption. As a result, 840 million packs of cigarettes, worth $1.2 billion to the tobacco industry, were smoked that would not have been if the early trend had been maintained.

"NICOTINE SOUNDBITES"

The funding cuts and slowdowns in producing new media materials were only some of the problems faced by the media campaign. The controls placed on the content of the media campaign were even more harmful. In 1994 TCS, working with its new advertising agency, Asher/Gould, produced a thirty-second television advertisement, "Nicotine Soundbites" (figure 22), that used actual footage from the landmark April 14, 1994, congressional hearing conducted by Representative Henry Waxman (D-California) at which the chief executives of the major cigarette companies denied that nicotine was addictive. The advertisement began with an image of the executives standing with their right hands raised swearing to tell the truth. Four of the executives, William Campbell of Philip Morris, James Johnston of RJ Reynolds, Thomas Sandefur of Brown and Williamson, and Donald Johnston of American Tobacco, all deny, each in turn, that nicotine is addictive as their names and companies flash on the screen. The advertisement ends with the question "Do they think we're stupid?" Public health advocates loved the advertisement and the tobacco industry went berserk.

The advertisement was first aired on September 29, 1994. On October 6, lawyers for RJ Reynolds wrote DHS on behalf of the company's chief executive officer, James W. Johnston, claiming he was defamed and demanding an apology.[10] They also wrote to television station KABC in Hollywood, alleging that the advertisement was false and defamatory and demanding that the broadcasts end immediately.[11] They told Asher/Gould, "Your creation of an intentionally altered videotape is clearly outside the limits of legal or ethical behavior, and my client shall hold your agency, and everyone in this project, personally responsible."[12] The lawyers demanded that Asher/Gould "set aside and preserve every document . . . in your possession or custody and control relating to the development, production, and distribution of the offending commercial."[12] Finally, they demanded that DHS director S. Kimberly Belshé undertake "an immediate withdrawal of a television advertisement sponsored by your Department which contains a false and defamatory attack upon our client."[13]

By October 17, 1994, KABC and two other television stations had pulled the advertisement off the air. Bruce Silverman, the president of Asher/Gould, had offered to indemnify several stations, including the Los Angeles NBC affiliate, to keep the advertisements on the air. According

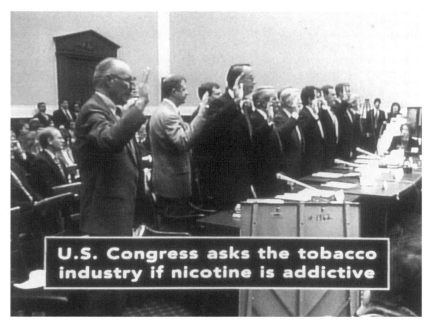

U.S. Congress asks the tobacco industry if nicotine is addictive

Figure 22. "Nicotine Soundbites" television advertisement. DHS created the thirty-second ad from footage of the Waxman hearing. The ad showed tobacco industry executives stating, under oath, that they did not believe nicotine was addictive. The Wilson administration prohibited the airing of the ad after the tobacco industry complained. (Courtesy California Department of Health Services)

to Silverman, "We don't see this as a horrible risk because we don't believe that KNBC or anyone, for that matter, including us, will really be sued by Johnston."[14] The threat to sue and the knuckling under by three stations to the threat, however, attracted broad media coverage.[15–19] The *Minneapolis Star Tribune* had this to say in an editorial of October 17: "Under the circumstances, a tobacco executive threatening to sue for libel should be funny—if his threat hadn't worked. Incredibly, the TV stations—in San Francisco, Oakland and Los Angeles—caved in to the pressure and took the commercial off the air. . . . Given all the jibes aimed at the tobacco industry, it's amazing its leaders would choose to fight this one. These ads simply underscored the oft-repeated fact that tobacco industry executives are expert prevaricators. Why should they be sensitive about that? After all, if you already make a profit from causing death, the charge of lying about it shouldn't be too hard to live with."[20]

Belshé publicly defended "Nicotine Soundbites" in a letter replying to Johnston's attorneys. She wrote,

> This is to inform you that the Department of Health Services will not withdraw or alter the advertisement in question. Further, we adamantly deny any allegation of defamation resulting from this advertisement. . . . The point made by the ad, we believe, is that while individual industry executives may be able to make certain statements which are literally true in a narrow legal context, these statements do nothing to give credibility to the overall industry position that tobacco is not a harmful product.
>
> Furthermore, I would like to take this opportunity to express my grave concerns regarding recent attempts which have been made to intervene in the airing of these ads by local television stations.[21]

"Nicotine Soundbites" remained on the air. But after DHS's public display of support, the administration quietly shelved it in early 1995.[22]

Beginning in 1995, the Wilson administration refused to air the spot, despite repeated requests to do so by public health advocates, including a formal request by the Tobacco Education and Research Oversight Committee (TEROC).[23] The administration's repeated excuse was a desire to avoid litigation (something it had no aversion to if the plaintiffs were the public health groups).[24] TEROC countered with a specific recommendation that it would endorse use of Health Education Account money to defend the advertisement in court, if necessary. Since "Nicotine Soundbites" was made up entirely of footage of the Waxman hearing, edited down to fit a thirty-second spot, and since truth is a defense, such litigation was extremely unlikely. Other states later aired the advertisement with no legal repercussions.

The content controls were not restricted to "Nicotine Soundbites." In September 1994 Sandra Smoley personally intervened to remove 190 billboards bearing the message "Secondhand Smoke Kills: Are You Choking on Tobacco Industry Lies?" (figure 23). Smoley ordered that the billboards be papered over at a cost exceeding $10,000, even though Belshé had approved them. When her role became public because of materials that Americans for Nonsmokers' Rights (ANR) had obtained from DHS under the California Public Records Act, Smoley defended her position to the American Cancer Society (ACS), ANR, and the American Heart Association (AHA), saying that she ordered the billboard pulled because *"it was found to be offensive for government to use taxpayer funds to call a private industry a liar"* (emphasis added).[24] Smoley, a registered nurse, did not approve of accusing the tobacco industry of lying, despite the fact that accelerating litigation against the tobacco industry was re-

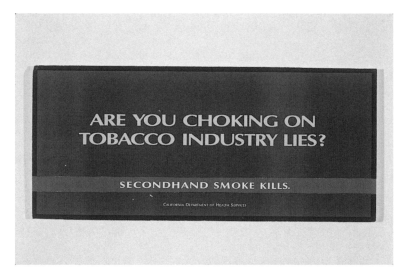

Figure 23. "Are You Choking on Tobacco Industry Lies?" billboard.
Sandra Smoley, California's secretary of health and welfare, ordered
DHS to paper over the billboards because she did not believe that it was
appropriate to accuse the tobacco industry of lying. (Courtesy California
Department of Health Services)

vealing, almost daily, new disclosures of the tobacco industry's lies to the
public about nicotine addiction, cancer, and marketing to kids over the
last half century.[25,26]

Smoley also killed the television advertisement "Insurance," which
pointed out that insurance companies owned by tobacco companies gave
nonsmoker discounts and then asked the question "What do the tobacco
guys know that they're not telling us?" She objected to an image of tobacco executives shredding documents. When the advertising agency offered to remove the few seconds of video showing the shredding, she still
refused to allow the advertisement to be aired. In response to complaints
by the public health groups about the administration's action, Smoley
blamed them for raising the issue: "Your organizations have given unwarranted emphasis to the decision not to air an ad known as 'Insurance.' . . . While the ad had much potential, and *could have been aired*
with further work, DHS dropped the ad immediately after your press
conference" (emphasis in original).[26] The state spent over $250,000 pro-
ducing "Insurance," only to leave the finished ad gathering dust on the
shelf because the public health groups had asked where it was.

IMPLEMENTING PRINGLE'S PRO-TOBACCO POLICIES

In June 1996 Speaker Pringle had tried to insert language into the budget that would have eliminated the media campaign's attacks on the tobacco industry, meeting a long-standing objective of the tobacco industry. While Pringle lost in the Legislature, the Wilson administration quietly used administrative procedures to accomplish the same thing.

DHS used contracting procedures in an effort to slow down the media campaign. At the time the 1996–1997 budget was signed, the contract to administer the media account was held by the advertising agency Asher/Gould, which had won it in May 1994. This contract contained an option for DHS to renew it for two years, beginning July 1, 1996. As early as June 1996, Asher/Gould had delivered storyboards (pen and ink versions of the proposed advertisements) to TCS for a new media campaign scheduled to begin that fall. Based on the past successes of the campaign, several of these proposed advertisements featured attacks on the tobacco industry.

Rather than simply exercising its option to extend Asher/Gould's contract for two years so that the agency could move ahead with the work, DHS issued a new Request for Proposals for the media campaign on August 2, 1996 (for the period from January 1, 1997, through December 31, 1999). This action set in motion a protracted process of submitting bids, judging proposals, and handling appeals for the agencies that were not selected. Some people in TCS, as well as in the public health community, were concerned that the entire process was designed as an attempt to replace Asher/Gould, since the administration distrusted the agency's president, Bruce Silverman, for consistently pressing for strong anti-industry advertisements. In the end, Asher/Gould won the new contract, but the process delayed the development of the planned advertisements. In a great show of circular logic, the time required for this process became one of the administration's excuses as it came under increasingly strong criticism from TEROC and public health organizations for delays in releasing new advertising.

One of these new advertisements was "Cattle," which showed cowboys—portrayed as Marlboro Man types—rounding up children as a metaphor for the tobacco industry's efforts to hook kids on cigarettes (figure 24). "Cattle" began with the words "This is how the Tobacco Industry wants you to see them" and was originally to feature one of the cowboys lassoing a kid and dragging him to where another cowboy was waiting with a branding iron labeled "Tobacco Industry." The final line was, "The Tobacco Industry. If you knew what they thought of you, you'd think twice." Another advertisement, "Thank You," a television advertisement that eventually became a radio spot, was a sarcastic "thank you" letter from the tobacco industry to kids in appreciation for their loyalty in spite of overwhelming evidence that tobacco kills. It began with the words "The Tobacco Industry would like to thank . . . " and ended with "Sincerely, the Tobacco Industry." These anti–tobacco industry advertisements soon hit a brick wall.

During the summer of 1996, it was reported that Mike Genest, the assistant deputy director for prevention services at DHS and someone who was widely viewed as the governor's political watchdog in the department, and Dr. James Stratton, the state health officer and DHS deputy director for prevention services, summoned Silverman to a closed-door meeting in Sacramento to discuss what would be acceptable and what would not be acceptable in the advertisements that were under development. When Silverman walked into the room, he found four terms written on a blackboard: "tobacco industry," "profit," "nicotine addiction," and "lies." The DHS managers reportedly stood up and drew a line through each of these terms; they were not to appear in any of the advertisements.

In July 1996 Genest said that everything that Asher/Gould had presented for youth was controversial and would need to be approved several layers up the chain of command.[27] He questioned the efficacy of attacking the tobacco industry, prompting Silverman to write Dileep Bal, head of the Cancer Control Branch (which includes TCS), that "the only effective method I know of to achieve that [a reduction in tobacco use] via advertising is with the 'Manipulation' strategy that we just tested."[28] In addition to expressing general concerns about attacking the industry, Genest wanted the phrase "Tobacco Industry" changed to "Big Tobacco."[27] Nothing was approved to go into production.

In addition to slowing the approval process, the Wilson administration made other changes designed to tone down and slow up the media campaign. Under previous policy, once an anti-tobacco advertisement was approved, TCS and the media contractor used their professional judgment in deciding when to run it. In August 1996, when Asher/Gould suggested again running "Industry Spokesmen," the very first Proposition 99 anti-tobacco advertisement (which had not been aired for several years), Genest announced a new policy: every advertisement was to be cleared *for each use*, even if it had been approved in the past.[29] The approval process included not only DHS management but also the

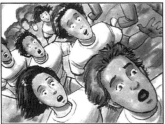

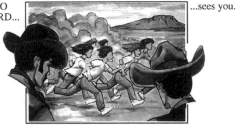

Figure 24. Original version of the television advertisement "Cattle." As originally proposed by Asher/Gould, the advertisement was a strong anti–tobacco industry message depicting kids being captured and branded by the industry. The handwritten note indicates that the DHS management ("12th floor") wanted references to the tobacco industry deleted, consistent with administration policy to avoid naming the tobacco industry.

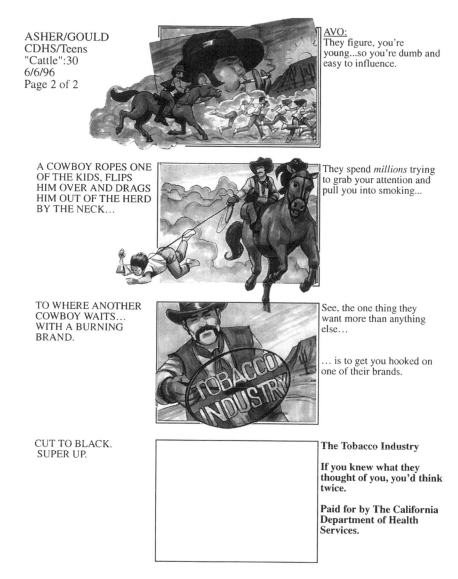

ASHER/GOULD
CDHS/Teens
"Cattle":30
6/6/96
Page 2 of 2

AVO:
They figure, you're young...so you're dumb and easy to influence.

A COWBOY ROPES ONE OF THE KIDS, FLIPS HIM OVER AND DRAGS HIM OUT OF THE HERD BY THE NECK...

They spend *millions* trying to grab your attention and pull you into smoking...

TO WHERE ANOTHER COWBOY WAITS... WITH A BURNING BRAND.

See, the one thing they want more than anything else...

... is to get you hooked on one of their brands.

CUT TO BLACK.
SUPER UP.

The Tobacco Industry

If you knew what they thought of you, you'd think twice.

Paid for by The California Department of Health Services.

Figure 24. *Continued.*

personal stamp of approval of Secretary Smoley. This new policy effectively shelved forty existing television and thirty radio advertisements that had been produced at a cost of millions of dollars to the taxpayers. It also ensured that advertisements such as "Industry Spokesmen," "Nicotine Soundbites," and others that the industry found so objectionable would not be put into the advertising rotation by TCS or the media contractor. Bal protested this new policy as "a fundamental change that I for one was unaware of until now." [30] Between the delay over the new spots and the need for reapproval of the old, there was clearly no intention of getting the media campaign up and running in a hurry.

The administration continued to impose tighter political controls on the media campaign. On September 16, 1996, Joe Munso, chief deputy director of the DHS Office of Public Affairs (OPA), the agency's public relations office, distributed a memo announcing that he would "review advertising concepts *before* they are focus group tested or shared with stakeholders/interested parties" (emphasis in original).[31] Thus, an official charged with protecting the administration's political and public relations positions would review proposed advertisements for political acceptability before any formal evaluation of the advertisements for quality or effectiveness as public health messages could take place. As these delays gradually ground the media campaign to a halt, with nothing but the old, "acceptable" advertisements being run, departmental staff began informing the administration that the advertisements were so overexposed that they had likely lost their effectiveness.[32]

Finally, Belshé wanted TCS to justify not only the attacks on the tobacco industry but also the entire strategy of "countering pro-tobacco influences in the community." This strategy, along with "reducing exposure to environmental tobacco smoke" and "reducing youth access to tobacco," was one of the three main themes in all of DHS's programming, including media, local programs, and the competitive grants. Robin Shimizu, a staff member at TCS who was helping with the media campaign, warned Dileep Bal that "these priorities were developed and renewed with the assistance of the tobacco control communities throughout California and do not simply belong to DHS/TCS. To back away from, or to have to justify the use of, any one of them, or to eliminate one of the priorities would be viewed harshly by everyone involved in tobacco control in the state as well as other states, unless there were a very strong rationale for doing so." [33] Bal forwarded Shimizu's comments to his boss, Don Lyman, head of the Chronic Injury and Disease Control Division, with a comment of his own: "'Countering pro-tobacco influences in the community' is the very signature piece of our efforts to date, as any of the cognoscenti within or without the state will attest to. To have that questioned in an issue memo you or I have not seen is beyond anything. Any fundamental shift of these proportions without community input will produce quite a mushroom-cloud, besides being ill-conceived. Caveat emptor." [34] Bal further offered to host "a full-scale consensus conference of the national cognoscenti" to discuss the issue, implying that those who were requesting the justification did not really want this level of public discussion of the issue. He also suggested that the "countering" strategy was being held to a higher standard of proof of its efficacy than other DHS interventions.[35] The strategy remained intact.

SHUTTING OUT THE PUBLIC HEALTH COMMUNITY

During the first years of the California anti-tobacco media campaign, both DHS and the advertising agency had actively involved members of the public health community, including TEROC, in the development of the advertising campaign with the aim of coordinating the media campaign with the community-based tobacco control activities and receiving expert advice on the content of the campaign.[36] Recognizing that efforts to slow down and weaken the media campaign would spark controversy within the public health community, the administration shut this group out of the review process.

As the legislatively constituted oversight committee for the Proposition 99 program, TEROC had a particular interest in the development and implementation of the advertising campaign. TCS had routinely, if informally, involved TEROC in the development of the advertising campaign by asking its members to review storyboards for advertisements that were under development. The administration quit involving TEROC in the review of the storyboards. The administration argued that TEROC was a "security risk" and that sharing the advertisements with TEROC would increase the likelihood that the tobacco industry would gain access to them. To this, Cook responded, "The TEROC is not an outside party; it is to be part of the process; and it is being deprived of the tools necessary to function." [37] One of the other TEROC members wryly observed that DHS apparently considered twelve-year-olds in a focus group less of a security risk than the TEROC members.[37]

At the December 10, 1996, meeting of TEROC, the committee discussed the delays in the media campaign and the new closed review process used for approving new media. Stratton announced that decision making about the media campaign had been removed from TCS. He also claimed that he had the final say over the content of the advertisements. No one believed him, but he was the first of a long line of officials who claimed to have the final say (in order to provide political cover for Smoley and the governor). TEROC formally requested to be allowed back into the process, specifically asking for the opportunity to see and comment on the storyboards for planned advertisements; Stratton refused.[38,39]

The veil of secrecy extended to the advertising firm as well. The new Asher/Gould contract issued on December 1, 1996, contained a new clause, nicknamed the "Silverman Clause," barring the advertising agency from discussing the media campaign with anyone without prior written approval from DHS management.[40]

The administration had a good reason for wanting to keep TEROC and the other members of the public health community out of the process. They had secretly weakened the June advertisements, just as public health advocates had feared.

By the December 1996 TEROC meeting, all the storyboards submitted by Asher/Gould in June had been modified to remove the prohibited words "the tobacco industry" and "addiction." "Cattle" now began with "This is how the guys who make cigarettes . . . ," and the final line was simply "If you knew what they thought of you, you'd think twice" (figure 25). The text of the advertisement "Thank You" had also been changed, from "The Tobacco Industry would like to thank . . . " to "Those of us who make cigarettes would like to thank you." The final line, "Sincerely, the Tobacco Industry," was still included in the December 5 presentation attended by TCS staff, Lynda Frost (deputy director of the Office of Public Affairs), Genest, and Stratton, but it was later deleted.[41]

Another new advertisement, "Rain," which featured cigarettes raining down on a playground, was based on the theme of hooking kids, but it never mentioned the tobacco industry by name. The opening line was "We have to sell cigarettes to your kids," and the final line was "How low will they go to make a profit?" Viewers were left with the impression that the advertisement was about retailers.[42]

Another proposed new advertisement, "Voicebox" (later known as "Debi"), was to attack the industry for lying about nicotine addiction. It featured a woman smoking through a tracheostomy opening, stating that the tobacco industry had lied to her about the addictive nature of its products. At the December meeting, the industry attack approach was deleted, and the advertisement instead promoted the state's "800" quit line. In the revised December version neither of the prohibited terms "addiction" or the "tobacco industry" was used. The advertisement instead featured a smoker who could not quit in spite of undergoing a tracheotomy, urging others to give quitting a try. An anti-industry advertisement had been converted into a cessation spot, one that implied quitting was impossible—a strange message from a public health department.

The effort to tone down the attacks on the tobacco industry flew in the face of the research on message effectiveness that Asher/Gould had conducted for TCS. In response to requests from administration officials for more and more justification for the anti-industry strategy, Asher/Gould hired an outside evaluator to study the question. In a November 1996 summary of its focus group research on different advertising messages and in a December 1996 memo to Colleen Stevens, head of the media campaign at TCS, Christine Steele, the Asher/Gould senior vice president responsible for the campaign, reported the results.[43,44] Five advertising strategies were tested on youths between the ages of twelve and eighteen in focus groups in Sacramento and Los Angeles. The messages tested were: (1) manipulation of kids by the tobacco industry, (2) the dangers of secondhand smoke, (3) the short-term health effects of smoking, (4) the risk of romantic rejection, and (5) the elimination of risks to the environment caused by smoking, with results including cleaner beaches, fewer trees destroyed to produce cigarettes, and fewer animals harmed by eating butts. Of the five, manipulation by the industry was the strongest message in the groups. According to Steele, "The body language of kids clearly revealed that this [anti-industry] strategy provided kids with an emotional wake up call. They sat up straight, they grimaced, they shook their heads, they became riled up and vocal—they at least became concerned about this formerly 'low interest' topic." [44] The administration was unmoved.

The ACS, which had been passive through the battles with the administration, started to take more proactive positions in 1996. One reason may have been that the administration was ignoring TEROC chair Cook, a longtime and high-level volunteer in ACS. Another reason may have been to recover from an embarrassment that occurred when the ACS's San Francisco unit awarded tobacco industry ally Willie Brown its "Humanitarian of the Year" award.[45–48]

On February 4, 1997, the presidents of the ACS, AHA, and ANR wrote Smoley to express their frustration with the "administration's ostensible defense of an industry responsible for the deaths of more than 42,000 Californians each year—the tobacco industry." [49] The three organizations protested the long delay in the production of new media

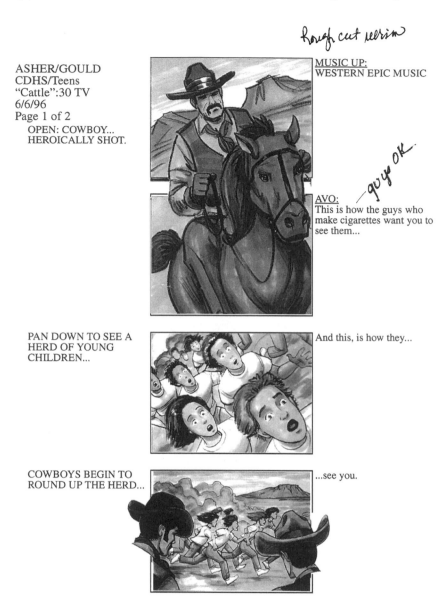

ASHER/GOULD
CDHS/Teens
"Cattle":30 TV
6/6/96
Page 1 of 2
    OPEN: COWBOY...
    HEROICALLY SHOT.

MUSIC UP:
WESTERN EPIC MUSIC

AVO:
This is how the guys who
make cigarettes want you to
see them...

PAN DOWN TO SEE A
HERD OF YOUNG
CHILDREN...

And this, is how they...

COWBOYS BEGIN TO
ROUND UP THE HERD...

...see you.

Figure 25.   The toned-down version of "Cattle." In accordance with Wilson administration policy, all references to the tobacco industry were deleted. In addition, the images were softened.

output and urged Smoley to release a campaign that featured the original campaign themes: "the tobacco industry lies," "nicotine is addictive," and "secondhand smoke kills." [49] Meanwhile, John Miller, chief of staff to Senator Diane Watson (D-Los Angeles), chair of the Senate Health

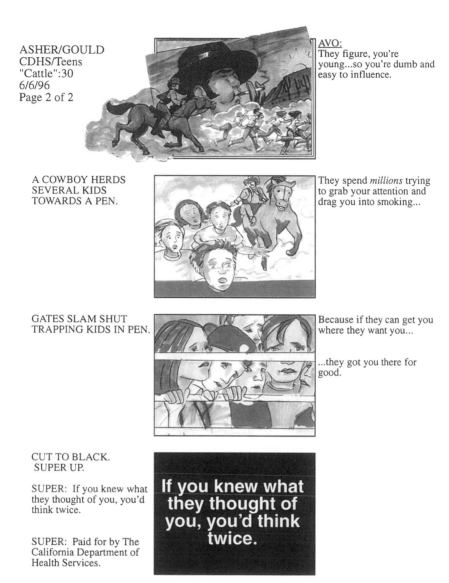

ASHER/GOULD
CDHS/Teens
"Cattle":30
6/6/96
Page 2 of 2

AVO:
They figure, you're
young...so you're dumb and
easy to influence.

A COWBOY HERDS
SEVERAL KIDS
TOWARDS A PEN.

They spend *millions* trying
to grab your attention and
drag you into smoking...

GATES SLAM SHUT
TRAPPING KIDS IN PEN.

Because if they can get you
where they want you...

...they got you there for
good.

CUT TO BLACK.
SUPER UP.

SUPER: If you knew what
they thought of you, you'd
think twice.

SUPER: Paid for by The
California Department of
Health Services.

If you knew what they thought of you, you'd think twice.

Figure 25. *Continued.*

Committee, was threatening to hold hearings on the way the media campaign was being conducted. It would take Smoley until March 7, over a month, to respond that nothing would change.[25] In response, AHA, ACS, and ANR took out a full-page advertisement in the West Coast edition of the *New York Times* featuring the infamous Philip Morris memo about Wilson and accusing the Wilson administration of refusing to release hard-hitting television spots and removing billboards to protect the tobacco industry.

On April 15, 1997, the ACS, AHA, and ANR presidents wrote the governor requesting a meeting to discuss their concerns about the performance of his secretary of health and welfare.[50] The letter went unanswered for a month. On May 16, the governor's deputy chief of staff and cabinet secretary wrote saying, "I am aware of your previous communications with the Health and Welfare Agency and the Department of Health Services. Both Secretary Smoley and Director Belshé have forthrightly represented the Governor's position to you."[51] Smoley, with Governor Wilson's explicit approval, was implementing Pringle's policy of refusing to attack the tobacco industry, even though the Legislature had rejected his language. The health groups accepted this rebuff quietly.

THE TEROC PURGE

Cook called an emergency meeting of TEROC for Monday, February 10, 1997, to follow up on Stratton's refusal to share information about the media campaign with TEROC and to decide what action TEROC should take in response. For Cook, as an ACS volunteer, it was hard to have to engage in political fights over the program. ACS had stayed out of the 1992 lawsuit over the media campaign filed by ALA, preferring to try to work things out with the governor. In the 1996 reauthorization fight, ACS had distanced itself from the aggressive strategies used by ANR and AHA. But Cook, as chair of TEROC, realized that the assault on the media campaign had to end. When asked about the changing ACS role, she explained,

> It's very hard, very hard. Within the Cancer Society, we have a lot of divisions that are doing tobacco programs and are fighting their legislators and fighting their governors to make sure the money is spent. But we have some that won't do it still. They will not get into the fray that way. They don't understand that. To them, it's just getting into the legal system and they don't think we should be in the legal system. And I think we have become better advocates for the patient and for the prospective patients because we are in the legal system now. We are willing to speak up and say these things just cannot occur.[52]

Cook's strong action in calling the emergency meeting could pose trouble for the administration by attracting public attention and energizing the ACS and other health groups, even though eight of TEROC's thirteen members are appointed by the governor (two are appointed by the speaker of the Assembly, two by the Senate Rules Committee, and one by the superintendent of public instruction).

On the Friday before the TEROC meeting, Stratton announced a major shakeup of TEROC. Three physicians on TEROC who had been strong advocates for the anti-tobacco education campaign were replaced with individuals closely allied with the Wilson administration. Breslow and Dr. Reed Tuckson, president of Drew University of Medicine and Science in Los Angeles, were told that they had been replaced in an action allegedly taken three months earlier by Speaker Pringle, a Republican, the day before the Democrats took over the Assembly. Neither Pringle nor DHS had given any previous indication of these changes, even though TEROC had met in December, after the date on which Pringle supposedly made the appointments; and the associated paperwork had ostensibly been "lost."[53] In addition, the governor removed Paul Torrens, a professor of public health at UCLA who had been another outspoken advocate for a strong program.

In the physicians' places, Pringle had allegedly appointed Hal Massey, a retired Rockwell Executive who had been active in ACS, and Doug Cavanaugh, the president of Ruby's Restaurants, an opponent of smoke-free restaurants and bars who was, according to Pringle, "familiar with the tobacco debate, balancing regulations with people's right to smoke."[53] Wilson replaced Torrens with Dr. George Rutherford, who had been the state health officer in the Wilson administration and responsible for the Proposition 99 program until he left to join the faculty at the University of California. Wilson also appointed Stratton to TEROC, making him a member of his own oversight committee.

The TEROC purge, combined with a dismantled media campaign, made news.[53–59] Well over a hundred people came to the TEROC meeting on the afternoon of February 10, compared with the ten to fifteen nonmembers who usually attended. Audience members included the heads of a number of county tobacco use prevention programs who emphasized the key role the media campaign played in their efforts. Without the "air cover" created by the media, the impact of their local programs was more limited. Steve Hansen, a member of the board of the California Medical Association, suggested Stratton was guilty of "public health malpractice."[39]

TEROC eventually agreed that Cook should write to Belshé, informing her of the committee's unanimous vote (even including Stratton's) to request a meeting to review the storyboards for the current and future media spots; Belshé rebuffed the request.[37,60]

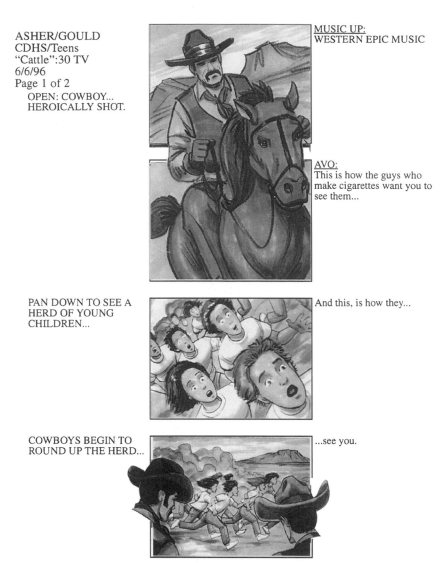

ASHER/GOULD
CDHS/Teens
"Cattle":30 TV
6/6/96
Page 1 of 2
   OPEN: COWBOY...
   HEROICALLY SHOT.

MUSIC UP:
WESTERN EPIC MUSIC

AVO:
This is how the guys who
make cigarettes want you to
see them...

PAN DOWN TO SEE A
HERD OF YOUNG
CHILDREN...

And this, is how they...

COWBOYS BEGIN TO
ROUND UP THE HERD...

...see you.

Figure 26.   "Cattle" as finally produced. In response to strong pressure from
public health advocates, the words "tobacco industry" were added into the
voiceover at the end of the advertisement.

THE STRENGTHENED ADVERTISEMENTS

In February 1997 the administration responded to pressure about the
advertisements by again revising the televised advertisements, although
this fact was not made public at the time. On February 28, 1997, Lynda

ASHER/GOULD
CDHS/Teens
"Cattle":30
Version 1 (TO BE RECORDED)
3/3/97
Page 2 of 2

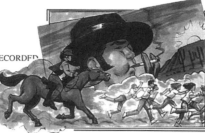

AVO:
They figure, you're
young...so you're dumb and
easy to influence.

A COWBOY HERDS
SEVERAL KIDS
TOWARDS A PEN.

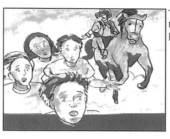

They spend *millions* trying
to grab your attention and
push you into smoking...

GATES SLAM SHUT
TRAPPING KIDS IN PEN.

Because once they get you
where they want you...

...they got you for good.

CUT TO BLACK.
SUPER UP.
SUPER: The Tobacco
Industry. If you knew
what they thought of you,
you'd think twice.

SUPER: Paid for by The
California Department of
Health Services.
funded by the Tobacco Tax
Initiative.

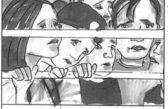

If you knew what they thought, you'd think twice.

AVO: The Tobacco
Industry. If you knew what
they thought of you, you'd
think twice.

PAID FOR BY THE
CALIFORNIA DEPARTMENT OF
HEALTH SERVICES.
FUNDED BY THE
TOBACCO TAX INITIATIVE

Figure 26. *Continued.*

Frost okayed the restoration of the phrase "the tobacco industry" in the
"Cattle" advertisement, changing the revised version, "If you knew what
they thought of you, you'd think twice," back to "The Tobacco Industry. If you knew what they thought of you, . . . " (figure 26). In "Rain,"
the voiceover comment at the end was changed to "The tobacco indus-

try. How low will they go to make a profit?" In addition, "Thank You," which had become a radio spot, now had the words "Tobacco Industry" both in the opening sentence and in the last line.

By the time Asher/Gould prepared the final storyboards on March 3, 1997, two versions of "Voicebox" were planned. In addition to the cessation advertisement, a version was recreated that emphasized addiction and the behavior of the tobacco industry. In it, the actor says, "They say nicotine is not addictive. How can they say that?"; the tag line at the end was "The tobacco industry denies that nicotine is addictive."

At the TEROC meeting on March 25, John Pierce, director of the California Tobacco Survey, presented the latest California smoking prevalence data, which showed that smoking rates for both youth and adults appeared to be going up. Overall, youth smoking, which had been as low as 8.7 percent in 1992, rose to 11.9 percent in 1995 and remained flat in 1996 at 11.6 percent. The annual Behavioral Risk Factors Survey conducted in house at DHS showed that adult smoking prevalence had increased from 16.7 percent to 18.6 percent between 1995 and 1996,[61] reversing a downward trend that had existed for nearly a decade.[24,62] The increase in smoking rates received wide media coverage.[62–64] Public health groups blamed the increase on the fact that the administration had not fully funded Proposition 99's anti-tobacco education programs and on its reluctance to attack the tobacco industry. Sean Walsh, the governor's press secretary, commented that he was frustrated because Wilson was being blamed for everything—"including [the comet] Hale-Bopp." [62] He referred to the public health groups' criticisms as "Chicken Little–like comments made by zealots in the anti-smoking community." [64]

TEROC finally saw the new advertisements at its March 25 meeting, after they were released to the public, and Cook indicated that the members' reactions were mixed.[37] The advertisements as released, nine months after Asher/Gould originally proposed them, were similar to those originally conceived by the advertising agency.

While the health groups did manage to get the 1997 advertisements strengthened, the administration's reluctance to go after the tobacco industry remained. On February 10, 1998, Christine Steele of Asher & Partners (the new name for Asher/Gould) was once again having to justify to Genest the strategy of countering tobacco industry influence, commenting that "this approach is important, relevant and, without question, necessary." [65]

THE 1998 HEARINGS

By 1998, the Legislature had become sufficiently concerned about the conduct of the media campaign that it held several oversight hearings to investigate the matter. Senator Mike Thompson (D-Santa Rosa) held three hearings of the Budget and Fiscal Review Committee. After two unsatisfactory appearances by DHS officials, Thompson demanded that the advertising agency appear before the committee. In preparation for the hearing, Stratton called Hal Asher of Asher & Partners to coach him about what they were to say at the hearing. According to a memo Asher wrote to his coworkers, "They [Stratton, on behalf of the administration] want us to say . . . with all clients we present a lot of ideas . . . some stay . . . some go. They want us to say . . . the state is *not stalling*. (He initiated this—not his exact words.) They rejected some ideas. Had input . . . and then accepted many of the new commercials. In other words . . . they help in the process . . . and this is like any client! . . . That the *state added value* to the campaign" (emphasis in original).[66] Stratton emphasized the need not to air dirty laundry in public and for everyone "to be on the same page." According to Asher, Stratton wanted them to say, "We are extremely excited about the new commercials that we are in the process of producing . . . and we think they will be the most effective yet."[66] By May, DHS had, in fact, killed virtually every idea that Asher & Partners had presented for countering tobacco industry influence.

Responding to the administration's stated concern that they would have to release materials to the tobacco industry if they showed them to TEROC, the Senate Budget and Fiscal Review Committee approved, in a bipartisan 5-0 vote, language to protect DHS in this regard. The language was designed "to ensure that the materials shared with the statutorily created group [TEROC] not constitute putting this into the public domain." The governor vetoed the language in the budget, although the new language corrected the nominal security problem that the administration was citing to lock TEROC out of the process.[67] Senator Watson's September 16 hearing of the Senate Health Committee featured extensive questioning of Stratton, who finally admitted publicly that Smoley forbade the use of certain words in the anti-tobacco advertisements, such as "lies" and "profits."

The full truth about the administration's efforts to weaken the media campaign finally came out at an October 16, 1998, Senate Judiciary

Committee hearing because Senator Adam Schiff (D-Pasadena) subpoenaed Asher & Partners to allow them to testify fully, despite the "gag clause" in their contract with DHS. In response to written questions, Asher & Partners wrote,

> Campaigns which exposed the tobacco industry's marketing *tactics* have been approved. Campaigns which take on the tobacco industry in a more universal manner have generally been disapproved for being "anti-business" and because they did not focus narrowly on the tobacco industry's "marketing tactics." All commercials which "personified" the tobacco industry were disapproved for "showing executives in a negative light." . . .
>
> In our best professional judgment, California . . . is not getting the most effective advertising campaign we can produce in the area of "counter advertising" for all of the reasons previously discussed.
>
> Bottom line: effectiveness could be improved if:
>
> 1. Creative decisions were based on which messages would be most impactful against consumers as opposed to politics.
>
> 2. All creative decisions were left to the Tobacco Control Section. They get the job done quicker than the multiple approval levels which exist in the administration. They also tend to focus more on a given message's effectiveness rather than its political implications.[68] [emphasis in original]

Asher & Partners also confirmed that, in 1997, "after intense pressure from tobacco control activists, the Administration finally allowed us to use the phrase 'the tobacco industry' and asked us to quickly redo all of our creative materials to reflect the reneging of this restriction."[68]

TRYING TO CONTROL TEROC

As TEROC became an advocate for the media campaign, the political appointees at DHS started to investigate how they could increase their control over this nominally independent oversight committee. In addition to replacing outspoken members, DHS also tried to exercise control over the meeting minutes, the Master Plan that TEROC was required to prepare for the Legislature, and the meeting agendas.

In 1997 Jennie Cook, chair of TEROC, became aware that the DHS administration had issued instructions for it to edit the TEROC minutes. Cook explained, "I mean, when they got to the point where they were reviewing the minutes before I ever saw them and taking stuff out, I really blew my stack. Those are our minutes, they're not the department's minutes, those are our minutes. I want everything in it."[52] The review process affected more than just the minutes. On March 4, 1997, Genest sent an e-mail to TCS specifying, "In no event, should TCS TEROC staff simply distribute an agenda or other materials to TEROC without first consulting with TCS management."[69] Bill Ruppert, the TCS member who staffed TEROC, wrote to Bal to inquire about the procedure for approving minutes:

> In the past, we FAXed the draft minutes to the chairperson of TEROC, made any corrections requested by the chair, and then mailed the final out to the members. . . .
>
> For the December 10 [1996] and February 10 [1997] TEROC meetings, there was [a] great deal of confusion and delay over approval of the minutes. *There were requests from the Deputy Director level and Division level for review of drafts even before these drafts went to the Chairperson.* It is unclear what the role of these levels was at the time, whether it was approval or not. The chairperson told me that she did not want anyone changing the minutes.[70] [emphasis added]

Bal forwarded the note on to Lyman, who responded, "The rule is, 'no surprises.' If the minutes are acerbic the front office wants to know BEFORE they appear in front of them from some other source." He claimed that otherwise the review was just for quality control purposes.[71]

The agenda for the June 17, 1997, meeting also caused controversy when Stratton demanded that Pierce be removed from the agenda, probably anticipating that Pierce would present results from the California Tobacco Survey showing that the program was being compromised by the funding diversions and the hindrances to the media campaign. According to Lyman, Stratton "does not want to see his face! . . . Tell them Pierce is in San Diego busilly [*sic*] working away to get data for September."[72] Lyman also said that Stratton wanted the report from the University of California to be longer and for the university to be put on the "hot seat." He also wanted the report from CDE to "talk longer and invite more questions on their productivity."[72] Cook was furious when Ruppert conveyed these suggested changes, especially the order that she "un-invite" Pierce.[73]

The political leadership at DHS was particularly worried that a presentation by Pierce at TEROC could put embarrassing results on the program's loss of effectiveness before the public. Stratton responded on May 30 that "with respect to Dr. Pierce, it has always been our policy to share data when it is ready for release. In the case of his contract, that means after he had conducted the analysis, put it in writing, and shared with the contract management and technical staff in TCS for approval and release. At the last TEROC meeting, this process was not followed.

I expect our usual procedures to be followed this time." [74] Pierce could come to the meeting, but only after DHS reviewed his presentation. Michael Johnson, the head of evaluation at TCS, wrote to Bal to assure him that he would get advance data from Pierce: "I will forward to you and up through the appropriate channels." [75] Lyman also noted, "We will 'read him the riot act' and place a 'heavy' on each side of him at TEROC to assure he does not open a new bag of unexpected tricks for them." [76]

The administration had succeeded in purging TEROC before the February 10 meeting, leaving no strong voices on the committee beyond Cook's. She was joined on May 19, however, by Professor Stanton Glantz of the University of California, San Francisco, when Senator Bill Lockyer (D-Hayward) appointed Glantz to TEROC. Given Glantz's strong opposition to the tobacco industry and politicians who supported industry interests, many observers were surprised to see Lockyer—author of the 1987 Napkin Deal, which gave the tobacco industry immunity from product liability in California—appoint Glantz to TEROC.[77] Lockyer's decision seemed to reflect the continuing shift in overall Democratic policy away from its staunch pro-tobacco position during Willie Brown's tenure as speaker. Glantz provided Cook with an important ally on the committee.

At the time Glantz joined TEROC, he found it in the process of finalizing its Master Plan for the next two years of the California Tobacco Control Program. He considered the recommendations diffuse and not clearly focused on program implementation, and he worked with Cook to strengthen and focus them. In July TEROC issued its new Master Plan, with the following recommendations for future program direction:

1. Vigorously expose tobacco industry tactics.

2. Press for smoke-free workplaces and homes.

3. Accelerate cessation of smoking in persons between the ages of 20 and 39.

4. Strengthen school-based tobacco use prevention education programs consistent with emerging research.

5. Implement more effective control of tobacco sales to minors.

6. Generate and adopt additional smoking prevention and cessation strategies that are relevant to the many racial and ethnic populations in California.

7. Link Proposition 99–financed research and evaluation efforts closely with Tobacco Control Program activities.

8. Increase the surtax on tobacco products by at least $1.00 per pack.

9. Oppose any settlement of tobacco litigation that benefits the to-bacco industry.

10. Coordinate Proposition 99–financed programs with other State and Federal tobacco control initiatives.[23]

Lyman described Stratton's reaction to the final draft: "The good Dr. Stratton is unhappy. . . . Stratton sees stuff in the recommendations that he still has trouble with and other TEROC members had trouble with too. He also remembers that this was to be referred to the writers to come back next time with another try at language. So, how come the rush-rush?"[78] TEROC had actually agreed to let Cook make corrections in accordance with feedback from members and then send the final version to the printer. DHS took its time printing the report and quietly released it during the doldrums of late August when most people were more interested in finishing up their summer vacation than debating tobacco control policy. While the University of California and CDE took steps to implement the TEROC Master Plan, DHS ignored them.

DELAYED IMPLEMENTATION OF THE SMOKE-FREE WORKPLACE LAW

When Governor Wilson signed California's smoke-free workplace law, AB 13, on July 21, 1994, it was scheduled to go into effect on January 1, 1995. Experience with similar laws passed at the local level had demonstrated the need for a period of several months of public education to achieve effective compliance. Despite several recommendations from TCS and other public health advocates, Smoley prohibited use of the advertising campaign to publicize California's then-new smoke-free workplace law.[79] At the time, Philip Morris was mounting its initiative campaign for Proposition 188 to overturn California's workplace smoking restrictions, and the tobacco industry was worried that the state would use the advertising campaign to educate people about AB 13 (see chapter 11).[80] Even after the health groups defeated Proposition 188, however, there was still no advertising to educate the public that virtually all workers had a right to a smoke-free workplace.

While the tobacco industry was unhappy about the smoke-free workplace law, it was apoplectic about the smoke-free bar provisions scheduled to go into effect on January 1, 1998. The industry made several unsuccessful attempts to get the law overturned in the Legislature, and by mid-1997 there was evidence that it would mount a major campaign to encourage people to ignore the law. This situation made an adequate period of public education, using the media campaign, particularly important. Indeed, TEROC specifically called for such a campaign in its 1997 Master Plan.[23]

In fact, TCS had started preparing for the January 1 implementation of the smoke-free bar law during the previous summer when it surveyed the local lead agencies to find out what information, materials, and approaches would be the best way to educate bar workers about the new law.[81] Philip Morris, through its public relations firm, Burson Marsteller, and its National Smokers Alliance, had been sending mailings to bar owners warning of severe economic ramifications if the smoke-free bar provisions of AB 13 were implemented.[82] Using Proposition 99 funds, TCS funded the ALA Contra Costa–Solano to manage a statewide program known as BREATH (which originally stood for Bar and Restaurant Employees Against Tobacco Hazards) to educate bar owners and employees about the law. BREATH created posters, handbooks, mailings, and a compendium of ideas that the LLAs could use to educate bar owners and dispel tobacco industry myths about the economic chaos that the law would allegedly trigger.

A 1996 DHS-commissioned Gallup poll found that more than three times as many bar patrons preferred a smoke-free bar as were happy with the current unregulated situation.[83] A 1997 poll by the nonpartisan Field Institute showed that 86 percent of bar patrons in California would stay in a bar the same amount of time or longer if it were smoke free, and 76 percent of California bar patrons were bothered by secondhand smoke in bars, restaurants, and other public places.[84] Even so, based on the experience of implementing the early smoke-free workplace laws, TCS wanted to educate both bar owners and employees, as well as patrons, about the new law well in advance of the effective date of January 1.

TCS asked its advertising agency, Asher & Partners, to present ideas and a time line for using the media campaign to fill this need in the spring of 1997 and expected to have radio spots and television ads running by June 1997. Despite the strong evidence that such an educational effort would help the law go into effect more smoothly, the administration put the media campaign on hold. DHS postponed the educational advertisements so as not to appear to lobby the Legislature to vote against the exemption.[85] ANR's Cynthia Hallett, who was working on implementing AB 13, rejected this argument: "Let's say they are trying to repeal the law that says you have to stop at a stop sign. Does that mean while this law is in debate, you don't have to stop at the stop sign? That the law will not be enforced because there is debate surrounding it?"[86] But the Wilson administration refused to prepare the public for the new law as long as the tobacco industry was trying to get it repealed. Smoley ignored the Master Plan and TCS and delayed approval of advertisements about the existing law, first proposed in May 1997, until October, a month after the legislative session ended. (Part of the delay was due to waiting for Smoley's return from a two-week vacation in China so that she could personally approve the advertisements.) It was not until late November of 1997 that DHS began running two advertisements promoting smoke-free bars—one on the radio and one on television.

PULLING THE ADVERTISEMENTS FOR SMOKE-FREE BARS

The controversy over advertisements about smoke-free bars extended beyond the state level. In the summer of 1997, in anticipation of the implementation of smoke-free bars, the Gold Country Coalition, based at ALA of Sacramento–Emigrant Trails (ALA-SET), created its own smoke-free bar radio advertisements as part of its approved work plan with TCS. The group knew that a public education campaign was going to be necessary for effective implementation of the law. No official enforcement mechanism is as effective as voluntary compliance and public demand.

Gold Country was also contractually obligated to do a "Save a Waitress" campaign, as project director Sue Smith explained: "In the contract it says clearly . . . if AB 13 bar phase-in seems to be in jeopardy, the region will create a campaign called "Save a Waitress." We created the campaign. . . . We sent scripts back and forth to TCS for approval, had one teleconference in which myself and two of my staff sat in with some TCS staff and people from Rogers [TCS's public relations firm], and they had a concern about a certain line that they thought might be potentially lobbying, so we dropped that line and went a different direction."[87] It was common knowledge that the tobacco industry was trying to get the law repealed and that DHS had long-standing regulations against "lobbying" with Proposition 99 money:

> Lobbying is communicating with a member or staff of a legislative body, a government official or employee who may participate in the formulation of the legislation, or the general public with the specific intention of promoting a yes or no vote on a particular piece of legislation. Such communication is considered lobbying only if its principal purpose is to influence legislation.

> Educating legislators, their staff, government employees, or the general public about your program or about tobacco-related issues in NOT lobbying.[88]

The planned text of the advertisement was reviewed on a teleconference with TCS on August 18. Some revisions were made, even though the advertisement did not appear to violate the lobbying rules. It did not include a call to action, address a particular piece of legislation, or express an opinion on a vote.

Gold Country's radio advertisement began airing on August 25, using the following script:

BARTENDER: Hi, I've been a bartender for a long time. When I worked in a smoky bar, it was like smoking a pack of cigarettes a day. Did you know that bar workers are the only employees not protected from secondhand smoke in the workplace?

SINGER: Hi. I'm David Mendenhall. Sometimes my throat is so sore from the poison in secondhand smoke that it hurts to sing with my band, Thicker Than Water. When all other workplaces went smoke free, I thought bars were next. Now it may not happen in January.

WAITRESS: I'm Laura Bass and I've been a cocktail waitress for years. When I feel sick and complain about cigarette and cigar smoke, some say to work someplace else. Where I work is not the issue. Staying healthy is.

BARTENDER: We've listened to your stories and sympathized with your problems. It's our job to serve you. Breathing secondhand smoke, though, should not be a condition of employment . . . even for those of us who work in bars.

SINGER: January 1st.

WAITRESS: Smoke-free bars for California.

BARTENDER: Sponsored by the Gold Country Tobacco Prevention Coalition through Proposition 99 funds.[89]

At the time, there was no pending legislation to modify AB 13. On August 28, 1997, the Assembly adopted language delaying smoke-free bars, which was sent to committee for a September 2 hearing. If no legislation passed by September 12, the deadline for the Legislature to act would pass.[90] Gold Country believed that the advertisement met the terms of the contract and the rules about lobbying; TCS did not.

On September 5, April Roeseler, chief of the Local Programs Unit at TCS, wrote Smith informing her that she had violated the contract rule prohibiting the use of TCS funds to support lobbying activities. Roeseler also informed Smith that "TCS is not to be billed for any costs related to producing or placing this radio ad."[91] Smith called Crocker Communications, Gold Country's media subcontractor, with instructions to pull the advertisement, but she was not happy with the decision. According to Smith, "I'm not a legal expert. But there's not a piece of the ad that meets any definition of lobbying."[87]

Because the company had already purchased the air time, Crocker asked Smith if she wanted to substitute an existing advertisement that had already cleared DHS review. She told them to do so, then went on a weekend bicycle trip. Crocker picked what was called the "Mahannah" advertisement, after the LLA director in Mono County. The text of the Mahannah advertisement consisted of the following:

MALE VOICE: Violent coughing, heavy breathing and hacking becoming softer.

FEMALE ANNOUNCER: We're doing so much to keep California's indoor public areas smoke-free. Now you can breathe easy in buildings, offices, restaurants and more. You should be proud of yourselves for taking such good care of each other. Now we need to work on the bars and nightclubs. Wouldn't you think?

(One single cough, male voice)

I thought so.

Smith came back to work on Monday to find a crisis. As she later recalled,

I'm off on a three-day bike trek and I come back and Jane [Hagedorn, executive director of the Sacramento ALA] comes running over and says she just got a call from DHS and that we were to report there in thirty minutes and to show how we had pulled this from the airwaves "or we pull your contract." Somebody apparently heard that ad on Monday, made a number of phone calls. That's why we got pulled in there. We were thinking we were getting pulled in for the "Save a Waitress." So we go to "Save a Waitress" and show the documentation from Crocker that says, "We pulled these advertisements." . . . However, these other advertisements are still running and that's when things got really worse. After that meeting a DHS representative (not from TCS) told me, "You're history."[87]

Both advertisements were pulled, but ALA-SET continued to be concerned about two aspects of the TCS letter. One was its broad definition of lobbying and the dangerous precedent it would set. The other was the request to revise the contract to remove the "Save a Waitress" piece. According to Smith, "That was considered by our local management team to be a cover-up by DHS and the Governor's Office. Compromises were made on both sides, but the one thing that the ALA-SET management refused to do would be to take it out of the contract. We were willing to concede the cost of the ad initially, but were not willing to 'make it go away.'"[87]

On November 25, 1997, ALA-SET decided to go with the status quo and accept a financial loss on the waitress ad, which meant that any expenses incurred after August 18 could not be billed.[92] Smith had this observation: "TCS was probably looking at the bigger picture. They were fearful that if we spoke out about this issue, the state would look at every piece of media that was ever distributed through Prop 99. I understood that fear. But I also think that politically, that we could have played some more trump cards that I didn't get to play. If I wasn't planning on staying around in this, I would have made a really big deal about this."[87]

On December 16, 1997, Smith received a final follow-up letter from Shimizu concerning "an inappropriate use of Proposition 99 funds in the production and placement of the radio ad, 'Save a Waitress.'"[93] Shimizu warned Smith about her action: "As you are aware, on August 18, 1997 staff at TCS advised you not to run the radio ad as you had drafted. However, you chose to produce and run a version of the radio ad without any further contact with TCS staff which resulted in the production of an ad deemed inappropriate for funding by Proposition 99. For the record, this is to notify you that if inappropriate advertisements are produced and placed in the future, your contract would be subject to termination."[93] Whether TCS was merely echoing orders from above and making the best of a bad situation or was independently asserting control over the field mattered little in terms of effect on the program. According to Smith, "I think it hurt all the regional efforts in terms of media. . . . I think what bothered me the most was the lack of support by a system that you've counted on being part of the solution with you."[87] Far from being insulated from the politics of the program, the field was heavily buffeted, and this buffeting extended to more than just local media programs. In Smith's view, this buffeting came as a surprise: "And I've heard different stories of who made the phone calls . . . about whether they were tobacco lobbyists or particular legislators, but there were two phone calls that were made. . . . That somebody can reach their fingers down into a localized media campaign that's created via contract by local people, and could make that go away. . . . And the intimidation was there at all times."[87]

THE CALIFORNIA TOBACCO SURVEY:
TCS "FIRES" JOHN PIERCE

From the inception of the Proposition 99 programs, the Legislature had funded a statewide prevalence survey, the California Tobacco Survey, to monitor the program's impact on smoking and to identify which ele-

ments of the program seemed to be most effective. The survey was conducted for DHS by the University of California, San Diego, and directed
by Professor John Pierce. Pierce and his colleagues had a record of finding politically unacceptable results beginning in 1991, when they reported that the media campaign contributed to a 17 percent drop in
smoking when Governor Wilson was trying to eliminate the campaign
on the grounds that it did not work. Nevertheless, on December 8,
1997, TCS wrote Pierce and his co-investigator, Elizabeth Gilpin, to inform them that TCS was amending their contract "in order to extend
the time period through June 30, 2000 and to augment the contract by
$3,052,332.... Essentially, the contract extension is for: the conduct of,
analyses of, and reporting on the 1999 California Tobacco Survey; the
conduct of, analyses of, and reporting on the longitudinal assessment of
adolescent smoking initiation study; and the completion of reports and
additional analysis of the 1996 California Tobacco Survey." [94]

Six months later, TCS reversed itself. On June 15, 1998, TCS wrote
the UCSD investigators to tell them that TCS "will not be renewing your
contract to conduct the 1999 California Tobacco Control Survey nor do
we plan to fund your proposed longitudinal study of adolescent smoking initiation." [95]

In the intervening months, Pierce and his coworkers had submitted a
draft report on the California Tobacco Survey concluding that, after
1994, the California Tobacco Control Program had lost its effectiveness.
TCS pressured the research group to make changes to the report. Over
time, the working relationship between Pierce's group and TCS deterio-
rated. After TCS abruptly notified Pierce that the contract would not be
renewed, Pierce observed:

> As I reflect on our experience with the State over the past year, I can only con-
> clude that the decision to terminate our contract was politically motivated.
> Our difficulties with the Department of Health Services staff began when we
> did two things:
>
>> a) Identified the coincidence between the halting of the decline in smoking
>> behavior and the diversion of money from the specific health education
>> accounts mandated by the Tobacco Tax Initiative.
>
>> b) Based on probabilities obtained from previous national and California
>> research, we projected that smoking rates in 15–17 year old adolescents
>> in California were likely to increase by 14% between 1996 and 1999. [96]

Pierce's report concluded that the initial success of the program, between
1989 and 1993, did not persist into the late period, 1994–1996. The

report suggested that a combination of reduced program funding, increased industry advertising and promotion expenditures, decreases in tobacco prices, and increased political activity contributed to the shift.[3]

DHS asserted that Pierce's contract was not canceled because of the work's quality but because Pierce was "too difficult to work with."[97] Members of DHS's own Evaluation Advisory Committee, who supported the quality of Pierce's work, also questioned the decision to terminate the contract but received no better explanation.[98,99] Mike Cummings, a cancer researcher from New York and chair of the Evaluation Advisory Committee, wrote Bal and Johnson on June 22, 1998:

> Finally, as co-chair of the Evaluation Advisory Task Force, I would like to express my deep dissatisfaction with the way the situation with Dr. Pierce was handled. First, it became apparent at the June Evaluation Advisory Task Force meeting that not all Task Force members were briefed on this situation and the concerns raised about Dr. Pierce's report. This situation was unfair both to Dr. Pierce and to our task force. Second, it is apparent that the decision to terminate Dr. Pierce's contract was made before the task force meeting for reasons unrelated to the scientific issues that were brought before the task force for discussion. It is an embarrassment that task force members first learned about the contract termination from Dr. Pierce and not from CDHS. The task force should have been notified of this decision before the meeting so that our time could have been used more productively to advise CDHS about future plans for the California Tobacco Survey. *Third, it appears that you were attempting to use our task force to raise concerns about the UCSD report in an effort to strengthen your case to terminate Dr. Pierce's contract.* Our task force members, who volunteer their time to your program, should never have been put in this position.[99] [emphasis added]

An editorial in the *San Diego Union-Tribune* captured the general outrage that greeted Pierce's firing:

> Earlier this month, a report by UCSD researchers came to light which concludes that California's anti-smoking campaign is coughing and wheezing for want of state support. This prompted the state agency that commissioned the report to start taking potshots at the messenger. Welcome to the world of power politics, where special interests generally prevail against the public interest. . . .
>
> What we have here is not a failure to communicate, but a refusal to capitulate. This report is scientifically sound while politically embarrassing to the folks in Sacramento looking to undermine the anti-smoking campaign. They and their tobacco buddies are doing whatever it takes, including attacking the integrity of respected scientists, to gut a program approved by the voters. And that is despicable.[97]

Cook, the chair of TEROC, however, refused to put the issue on the TEROC agenda when Glantz requested that she do so. She responded, "I have considered the various facts and assertions that have been made and have studied the responsibilities of TEROC, and have concluded that it is an internal administrative matter which the Committee should not get involved in."[100] Cook's decision to ignore Pierce's termination was all the more remarkable in light of an article by Pierce and his colleagues that appeared in the *Journal of the American Medical Association* the day before TEROC met; the article confirmed that the California Tobacco Control Program had declined in its effectiveness beginning in 1994.[3] These findings were widely publicized in the press on the morning of the TEROC meeting, but no one at the meeting mentioned the news coverage or Pierce's termination.[101–104] The courage to challenge the politicization of the media campaign did not extend to the evaluation process, even though TEROC's central purpose was to evaluate the campaign and report back to the Legislature on how to improve it.

CONCLUSION

At a project directors' meeting held in Palm Springs in June 1998, TCS staffer April Roeseler, in a speech to the directors, commented that TCS's unspoken motto was "we hire people who believe you can never have too much stress." That probably described the jobs of most project directors as well. For tobacco control advocates, Proposition 99 was to be their opportunity to put in place a model program, with its own funding source, that assured tobacco control advocates would be in the field as continuously as the tobacco industry. That the political process would not give them the freedom to produce that program was frustrating. One LLA director summed it up this way: "We had a pretty clear idea of what we need to do. . . . I think if the campaign had been allowed to work the way it was designed to work, I think we would be in pretty good shape. If we had a strong media campaign continuously and we had the counties and schools funded continuously, if everybody had been able to work the way it was supposed to, I think it would have been a lot more successful."[105] The successes in California were instead achieved only in the face of a hostile tobacco industry, an equally hostile political system, and a body of advocates at the state level who were often slow to act.

The long periods with no advertisements or no new advertisements in the media and the shift away from a hard-hitting campaign to softer,

youth-focused messages reduced the effectiveness of the California Tobacco Control Program.[3] The failure to implement a timely educational
campaign about California's smoke-free workplace law, particularly the
bar provisions, has made it more difficult to implement the law and, indirectly, supported tobacco industry efforts to neutralize the law.

For the campaign to succeed in the long run, it is necessary for the
nongovernmental organizations, especially the voluntary health agencies, to be willing to hold those charged with implementing the program
accountable. This is often difficult for them to do, since it requires acting against established political powers, not just the tobacco industry.
What is clear from the California experience, however, is that there are
as many opportunities for political interference with the anti-tobacco
education program through administrative actions as there are through
the legislative process. Strong action by outside groups is capable of influencing legislation and program content for the better. Lacking such
intervention, it is likely that in the long run the tobacco industry will
counter the program just as effectively through administrative controls
as by stealing the money.

CHAPTER 16

Lessons Learned

As the 1990s drew to a close, the landscape of tobacco control was worlds away from where it was when a few activists gathered in Berkeley with the odd idea that people should not have to breathe secondhand tobacco smoke. The voters of four states—California, Massachusetts, Arizona, and Oregon—had enacted large tobacco control programs funded through tobacco tax increases. The tobacco industry had been forced to promise to pay over $200 billion to states to settle lawsuits to recover the money smoking costs society in medical expenses, and many states were setting up tobacco control programs modeled on Proposition 99.

The California experience indicates that it is possible to reduce tobacco use rapidly through an aggressive anti-tobacco advertising campaign, combined with community-based programs that stress changes in the social norms around tobacco, so as to create a smoke-free society.[1] A successful program is not simply directed at keeping kids from smoking but at protecting nonsmokers from secondhand smoke and creating environments that facilitate smokers' decisions to cut down or quit. Most important, a successful campaign de-legitimizes tobacco use and the tobacco industry. When the California program followed these principles, the rate of decline in tobacco consumption tripled and the rate of decline in smoking prevalence increased significantly.[2-5] When the Wilson administration scaled back the program and shifted the focus to children, the progress slowed or stopped.[4-6]

Despite all the political problems, in its first eight years the California Tobacco Control Program prevented 2 billion packs of cigarettes (worth $3 billion to the tobacco industry) from being smoked. It also held teen smoking well below the rate that was occurring nationally. More important, the program saved lives. Because the risk of heart disease falls rapidly when someone quits smoking, during these eight years Proposition 99 prevented more than 14,000 heart attacks and strokes and saved over 2,500 lives.[7] It prevented over 10,800 low-birthweight births.[8] The $500 million in medical costs that were avoided from these causes of death alone amounted to more than the anti-smoking media and community programs cost. Proposition 99 also reduced deaths from lung and other cancers, asthma, sudden infant death, and other causes. These reductions are a stunning public health achievement.

The experience from California, however, shows that the tobacco industry does not give up easily. Indeed, the more effective the program, the more vigorously the tobacco industry and its allies will attack it. They fight to stop tobacco control programs from being enacted and, when that is not possible, they seek to subvert those programs by channeling them into unproductive areas, such as concentrating solely on children—the younger, the better.[9] (Indeed, the national settlement of state tobacco control litigation approved by most attorneys general in November 1998 limits anti-tobacco education to instruction provided to children; and forbids attack on the industry, despite the fact that anti-industry messages are an effective way to combat smoking.)[10] The tobacco industry is happy to see money disappear into the schools.

THE PLAYERS

One of the early California anti-smoking television advertisements, "A Couple More Good Years," captured the reality of battling the tobacco industry:

ANNOUNCER: The cigarette business in America is a dying business. But it is still very profitable. Obscenely profitable. So the tobacco companies are able to employ an army of spokespersons to deny the evidence and stall for time.

MALE TOBACCO INDUSTRY SPOKESPERSON: This is a very complex question. Statistics can't prove a causal relationship between smoking and disease. And there are Constitutional issues here.

FEMALE TOBACCO INDUSTRY SPOKESPERSON: We're accused of trying to get people to start smoking. We don't. We try to get people to switch. And, it's always been our policy that young people shouldn't smoke.

ANNOUNCER: The tobacco companies know the game is up. All they want is a couple more good years.[11]

The tobacco industry is highly motivated and unscrupulous. It has maintained its protected position in American and worldwide society by aggressively and single-mindedly defending its interests.[12] It acts professionally and strategically and thinks in the long term. It has an "army of spokespersons" and analysts and lawyers and public relations experts and lobbyists to protect its profits. The industry skillfully uses these resources to seek out allies within the political, cultural, and even medical communities.

Against this seemingly invincible army is a force made up primarily of well-meaning volunteers with limited experience and resources. While some of these people work in small activist organizations like Americans for Nonsmokers' Rights (ANR) and its predecessors, most are affiliated with the large voluntary health agencies: the American Lung Association (ALA), American Cancer Society (ACS), and American Heart Association (AHA). The large voluntary health agencies have tremendous public credibility and substantial resources, but historically they have been cautious and slow to act. Tobacco is but one priority for these agencies, and the tobacco industry is highly skilled at generating controversy about the political involvement of health groups to limit industry profits. Because the tobacco industry often works through intermediaries, these groups must be willing to confront not only the tobacco industry but also its partners and agents. Doing so is particularly difficult when the industry allies itself with powerful politicians or with groups, such as medical providers, who normally work with the voluntary health agencies. In many ways, the California story is about how the voluntary health agencies gradually developed the courage to enter the fray of hardball politics and do battle with not only the tobacco industry but also its allies.

The effort to pass Proposition 99 attracted a wide variety of players, including public health groups, environmental groups, and medical interests. The voluntary health agencies were willing to work with this mixed bag of partners in what they thought was a straightforward trade —support for the initiative in exchange for some of the money that the tobacco tax would generate. To attract the doctors and hospitals, the voluntary health agencies had dropped their claims on the new tax revenues from 47.5 percent to 20 percent for health education and from 15 percent to 5 percent for research. Naively believing that a deal was a deal, the health groups thought they could count on the medical players to support their goals once the initiative passed. Carolyn Martin, a volunteer with the ALA and the first chair of the Tobacco Education Oversight Committee, later summed up the hard lesson learned: "This was the first time money was set aside for tobacco education, and 'nice' non-profit voluntaries were not prepared for the vicious, powerball politics that money and tobacco create."[13]

The California Medical Association (CMA) was ready for the Proposition 99 legislative battle. The CMA was simultaneously working for and against Proposition 99, so it was well positioned regardless of the electoral outcome.[14] The CMA could claim credit for helping with the initiative campaign, thereby securing a seat at the bargaining table when the revenues were divided. The CMA could also claim credit for its efforts to subvert the initiative to avoid alienating the tobacco industry. By the time the tobacco industry was hatching its postelection strategy to counter the effects of Proposition 99, it was talking with the CMA about how to eliminate the Health Education Account money by moving it into medical care.[15,16] These needs trumped the CMA's concern for public health interventions to prevent and stop tobacco use. Within the legislative process, in fact, the medical groups had more in common with the tobacco industry than with the weaker public health groups.[17,18] They became even more dangerous when they were joined by the Western Center for Law and Poverty, a liberal group that advocated for health care programs for the poor. It took years for the health groups to accept this fact and recognize that the medical service providers needed to be watched and countered just as the tobacco industry did.

THE KEYS TO SUCCESS:
IDEAS, POWER, AND LEADERSHIP

Health policy entrepreneurs are most likely to be successful when they are solving a problem that the legislative leadership recognizes as important.[19] Unfortunately for tobacco control advocates in California in 1988, tobacco was not on the Legislature's agenda prior to Proposition 99. In fact, it was being kept off the agenda by powerful tobacco interests.

In contrast, health care for children was actively on the agenda, in particular the need for additional funding for the popular Child Health and Disability Prevention Program (CHDP). By funding CHDP with Proposition 99 Health Education Account money, the legislative leadership got money for CHDP, the CMA got money for doctors, and the tobacco industry kept money away from programs that reduced tobacco use.

To be successful in overcoming these legislative roadblocks and in securing implementing legislation that reflects public health priorities, tobacco control advocates had to exploit three factors: ideas (ways of framing the problem and creative approaches to solving it), power (generation of resources to translate ideas into action), and leadership (recognition of opportunity and commitment to challenge the status quo).[19] The public health advocates were weak in all three areas from 1989 until 1996, when advocates made a concerted effort to return to tobacco control's key power base—public awareness and involvement. The result in 1996 was funding for tobacco control programs in the way the voters had mandated.

After the funds were restored, however, the field of conflict simply shifted to the administration, where tobacco control advocates had to face the same problems all over again.

IDEAS: KNOWING WHAT YOU WANT

The way an issue gets framed often determines the solutions that will be pursued and who will be included in discussions of the issue.[20] So people make an effort to frame the issue so that their preferred solution becomes the chosen course of action.[21] Good tobacco legislation, from a public health standpoint, results when the tobacco use is framed as a public health issue and bad legislation results when it is instead framed as an issue of personal freedom.[22]

In the various California electoral campaigns, the tobacco industry tried to frame tobacco control as excessive government regulation, unfair taxation, or a violation of personal choice, while the public health groups tried to frame it as a health issue in which the tobacco industry was interfering with local decision making. In 1979, in analyzing the failure of Proposition 5, both proponent Paul Loveday and his opponents in the tobacco industry noted that the tobacco control side did not do a good job of staying on its issues.[23-25] By 1988, when they passed Proposition 99, public health groups had learned how to stick with their own messages and avoid discussing the industry's messages. By the time of Proposition 188 in 1994, tobacco control activists had done their polling and knew that calling Proposition 188 "the Philip Morris initiative" could kill it. They stayed on that message and won big.

While they had learned how to frame issues in electoral campaigns by
1988, the public health groups still had to learn the same lesson in legislative battles. They got off to a good start on framing the issue in the initial budget skirmishes in 1989. In January 1989, when Governor George
Deukmejian proposed the first Proposition 99 budget, he did not touch
the money in the Health Education and Research Accounts but used
money from the medical service accounts in a way that violated the intent of the initiative. The voluntary health agencies joined the CMA in
protesting this violation of the will of the voters. The voluntary health
agencies also used this argument to force the CMA and tobacco industry to back down on the Project 90 effort to divert funds out of anti-
tobacco education into medical services in the summer of 1989.

The health groups then made a key error at the end of June 1989 when
they agreed to use Health Education Account money to fund CHDP. By
doing so, they compromised their ability to frame the issue as "following
the will of the voters." Giving up some money for CHDP in exchange
for a decent bill, viewed from an insider perspective, was a reasonable
and appropriate action. As strategy, from an outsider's standpoint, it was
not. The health groups could no longer mobilize public support behind
the integrity of the initiative since they themselves had violated it. They
cleared the way for medical groups and others to frame the fight over
Proposition 99 revenues as sick children versus a silly anti-smoking campaign or as just another budget fight. In 1998, looking back on that first
year, Carolyn Martin recognized, "I think inexperience led to the first
CHDP diversions and we did abandon the moral high ground. We did
not understand or know how to use our newfound power." [13]

Even with the lawsuits in 1994 and 1995, when the courts ruled that
the diversions were illegal, the voluntary health agencies did not reframe
the issue as following the will of the voters. By not putting effort and resources into publicizing the victory, the health groups allowed Governor
Pete Wilson to frame the issue as one in which the courts encroached on
the Legislature's prerogative and disrupted medical care for the poor. By
resisting the compromises of 1994 and 1995, both in the Legislature and
in court, however, the health groups started to reclaim the issue of "following the will of the voter," which paved the way for the fight in 1996
to restore the Health Education and Research Accounts.

But getting the issue framed in a way that helps public health is only
part of the battle. Tobacco control advocates also need to know what
they want the money for. In 1989, when Proposition 99 passed, they were
not ready. Although the dangers of tobacco use were well defined, with

over 60,000 studies documenting the toll of tobacco use, in 1989 the methods for preventing tobacco use and for encouraging cessation were not as well defined.[26] The problem for the public health advocates was that, in the words of Cliff Allenby, Deukmejian's secretary of health and welfare, "They had no act."[27] Without an "act" in the form of a firm idea of what should be done with the money, the voluntaries were in a weak bargaining position.[28]

From the beginning, the CMA, Assembly Speaker Willie Brown (assisted by Steve Thompson), and the other health providers did "have an act." CHDP was in place and could readily be expanded. All it lacked was money. If part of the object was to prevent youth from starting to smoke, then all the health providers needed to do was to present a plausible argument that advice from a doctor was one route to achieving this goal. Looked at carefully, it was not really plausible that advising infants and toddlers not to smoke would be very effective. But no one challenged the plausibility of the program. The health groups deferred to the medical groups because they thought they had no choice.

Even in 1991, as it was becoming clear that the California Tobacco Control Program was working and tobacco use was dropping, the voluntary health agencies' lobbyists in Sacramento did not protect what the tobacco industry realized was a major strength of the tobacco control program: the local lead agencies. The lobbyists were willing to let the industry curb the local programs, apparently not realizing the degree to which cutting the local programs was an industry priority. Between reducing local funding outright, implementing Section 43 reductions, and diverting local money into Comprehensive Perinatal Outreach, Assembly Bill 99 served the tobacco industry's interests. The local programs were not fully restored until the fight of 1996 restored all funding to the California Tobacco Control Program.

From the start, the public health groups understood the value of the media campaign. While the lobbying effort was able to protect funding for the media campaign, including through such measures as the ALA lawsuit filed to protect the media campaign funds in 1992, the media campaign needed protection in addition to funding. The industry, if it could not kill the media campaign, wanted to limit its messages. By 1996–1997, the health groups were forced to learn how to pressure the administration for a high-quality media campaign.

By 1996, the tobacco control activists had an "act." They knew what they wanted; the issue was how to get it from the political process.

POWER: TURNING IDEAS INTO ACTION

To get their "act" through the political process, tobacco control activists needed political power, and the primary source of their power was public sentiment. To activate public sentiment, they had to keep the process as public as possible. Between 1989 and 1996, however, the health lobbyists did not exploit this resource. Until 1996, tobacco control advocates supported having the Proposition 99 programs designed by a conference committee, not by the policy committees of the Senate and Assembly. By sending the bill to a conference committee, tobacco control advocates lost the advantage of public debate and review. A conference committee is very much an insider forum in which the public is generally excluded from knowing what is going on or being given a chance to influence the process.[29] The public health groups have not been as successful at the inside game as the tobacco industry or the medical groups. Unlike the tobacco industry and medical groups, which are major sources of campaign contributions, public health groups do not make campaign contributions.[6,30–32] After the voluntary health agencies agreed to major cuts in AB 99 in 1991 in exchange for three years of program stability, the more powerful insider players simply ignored the deal. Even so, the voluntary health agencies continued to play the insider game, while not increasing resources for their lobbying efforts.

The agencies do, however, enjoy high name recognition and credibility with the public.[33] By contrast, the tobacco industry has very low public credibility. This difference in public standing means that outside strategies are likely to be the public health community's best means to achieve good tobacco policy, because the skills and resources of the voluntary health agencies tend to be amplified in public arenas while those of the tobacco industry are muted. But outsider strategies require a commitment of resources to a continuous public information effort. Equally important, they require a willingness to anger powerful politicians and interest groups by publicizing their misdeeds.

With nearly exclusive reliance on the insider strategy between 1989 and 1996, another problem for the public health groups was that the media and thus the public were kept uninformed and disengaged. To raise an issue in the insider circle is not the same as raising it with the media, which is an outsider strategy. The first major move outside the Capitol —when ALA filed a lawsuit in 1992 over the media funding—generated some publicity and protection for the media account budget. But when the later lawsuits over AB 816 successfully challenged the diversion of funds from Health Education and Research into health care, the voluntary health agencies did not use publicity about their victory to bring public pressure to bear on the governor or the Legislature. The legal victories, although clearly a successful use of outsider strategies, were not further amplified in the outsider forum. The court victory was instead viewed as a new piece of ammunition to bring into the insider game, not as a way to involve the public and get the media to frame the issue as "following the will of the voter."

In 1996 the tobacco control groups made a decision to engage the public and shift the focus away from Sacramento. Although AHA and ANR, on one hand, and ALA and ACS, on the other, engaged in different campaigns to restore the voter-approved funding levels to Proposition 99, there were some common themes in their approaches. Leaders in both coalitions sought to expand the scope of the conflict in 1996 to involve more than just the Legislature and the Sacramento insiders.[34] In particular, they worked to involve the media and the public more and to involve local level activists and agencies in the fight to restore the antitobacco programs. They committed time and money to the effort. Shifting the venue out of the Legislature into a more public arena meant that the debate over the future of Proposition 99 would occur in a venue in which the public health groups were more powerful and the tobacco industry and its medical allies were weaker. This more favorable venue contributed to the health groups' victory.

In the years following 1996, the Legislature continued to vote for full funding of the Proposition 99 Health Education and Research Accounts, even without a massive campaign to protect them. These votes were achieved even though the Court of Appeal had overturned the Superior Court's decision that SB 493 violated Proposition 99, leaving open the issue of whether or not the diversions were legal. Tobacco control activists had demonstrated that they could create the kind of public pressure it takes to leverage legislative behavior and, over time, impaired the ability of the tobacco industry to control the Legislature.

In 1998, after the smoke-free bar law went into effect, the Legislature withstood several attempts to overturn the ban, in spite of the tobacco industry's all-out attack on it. Tobacco control activists had, over the course of two decades, convinced the Legislature that people cared about tobacco control issues and had learned how to make it painful to ignore the public will on tobacco issues.

LEADERSHIP: SEIZING OPPORTUNITIES
AND CHALLENGING THE STATUS QUO

The ability to construct an "act" and to mobilize the power to implement it requires leadership that can both seize opportunities and challenge the status quo. Strong leadership means having people in place who are willing to pursue a tough and sometimes confrontational strategy. The voluntary health agencies are generally far less confrontational and much more willing to compromise than their advocacy group counterparts because the voluntary health agencies have multiple legislative issues and competing demands. Thus, historically the voluntary health agencies have rarely been effective advocates for tobacco control in the face of concerted opposition from the tobacco industry and its political allies.

The environmentalists continued their successes with Proposition 99 throughout its course. While the voluntary health agencies were having to justify their programs over child health programs, environmentalists successfully avoided having the issue framed as "mountain lions versus sick children" and kept more than their original allotment of 5 percent of the tax revenues. The fact that no one touched the environmentalists was a tribute to the environmental movement's combination of strong inside leadership and ability to use tough outsider strategies when needed.

Once Proposition 99 passed, rather than following the environmentalists' model and assuming a strong, unified, confrontational leadership posture to protect the anti-tobacco education and research programs, the health groups' lobbyists worked within the established power structure. They accepted the kind of legislative compromises that would have been expected within that system before Proposition 99 passed. They failed to capitalize on the power that they had just demonstrated by defeating the tobacco industry in the election.

During the fight over AB 75, the first implementing legislation, the reliance on the insider game by the voluntary agencies led to only modest compromises. With the election less than a year in the past, the Legislature was conscious of what the public wanted. Steve Scott, political editor of the *California Journal,* observed: "Their [the tobacco industry's] most important ally at the time was Speaker [Willie] Brown, but with the election still fresh in memory, even Brown's muscle couldn't pull enough votes for the industry to get its way in this battle. It was one of the first major losses suffered by the industry in the Legislature until that time." [35]

With the exception of the CHDP diversion, AB 75 was reasonably close to the voter mandate, and it is possible that those who were lobbying for the legislation believed it was due to the quality of their leadership. It is more likely that, as Scott observed, the Legislature was unwilling to thwart the public. But as the election faded in memory, the public health groups opted not to work to keep public sentiment activated and the media involved.

The voluntary health agencies' decision to compromise on AB 75 and allow funding of CHDP from the Health Education Account helped the CMA, CAHHS, and the tobacco industry and put the health groups in a difficult position. They began to protest the diversions in 1994. By 1995, Steve Thompson, who had become the CMA's chief lobbyist, could use the voluntary health agencies' previous actions to counter their emerging claim that the diversions were illegal; "Overall revenue," he said, "was diminished and what might have been, depending on one's point of view, a legal or illegal transaction initially has certainly become an illegal transaction today." [36] Having agreed to the diversions in the past, it was difficult for the health groups to claim the moral high ground about the illegality of those same diversions as money got tighter.

Thus, in 1994, in the face of their changed position and a tough budget year, the voluntary health agencies had a hard fight before them, again being fought with no more resources than they had before Proposition 99 passed. To complicate matters further, however, they were also trying to pass AB 13 in the midst of a rancorous debate within the health community over whether AB 13 was a good idea. At the same time, the tobacco industry qualified its own initiative, Proposition 188, for the ballot, which further drained resources and energy away from the Proposition 99 battles. Not surprisingly, 1994 was the worst year yet for Proposition 99 in the Legislature, with AB 816 diverting $301 million of the Health Education and Research revenues—34 percent of the money the voters had allocated to tobacco control—into medical programs.

If the absence of leadership from public health had been a problem in the first eight years of Proposition 99, the entry of strong leaders in 1996 was key to restoring the voter-mandated funding levels. In 1996, under the leadership of AHA executive vice president Roman Bowser, AHA joined ANR and Stanton Glantz and confronted the CMA in a successful effort to separate it from the tobacco industry. The ACS leadership became more involved in the legislative process instead of merely deferring to their lobbyists. The CMA leadership, too, took a more active role in setting policy on Proposition 99 rather than simply following its lobbyists' advice. Within the Legislature, the Democratic minority leader, Richard Katz (D-Panaroma City), a longtime supporter of tobacco control efforts, took a personal interest in Proposition 99, which changed the dynamic within the Legislature.

In addition to changing their behavior in Sacramento, the health groups involved their grassroots membership. All these actions shifted the control over the legislation away from the lobbyists and to the organizational leaders, who were more concerned with designing an effective tobacco control program than maintaining relationships within the Legislature.

CONCLUSION

Difficult as it may be for tobacco control advocates to demand accountability, tobacco control programs will not survive if the nongovernmental organizations that care about the program will not protect it. The preservation of the intent and spirit of these programs will not occur simply because an initiative is approved by the voters. This approval is a powerful force, but it must be used effectively by those who accept the responsibility for defending the public interest. Exercising oversight over the elected and appointed officials who had authority over the tobacco control program was even more challenging for the public health groups than getting the program enacted.

In the years immediately following an election or legislative action to create a tobacco control program, the effort to keep the will of the voters before the Legislature is not difficult, since both the press and the public are likely to be paying attention. But voter approval is likely to become less obvious and thus less powerful over time, and tobacco control advocates need to seek ways to keep the public informed and involved on the tobacco issue. If advocates instead retreat to playing only the insider political game, they will probably fail. They must be willing to withstand and embrace the controversy that the tobacco industry and its allies will generate.

The California story illustrates a few simple rules for beating the tobacco industry:

- The public is public health's best asset. Keep the fight public and the public engaged.

- The tobacco industry will try to work in the shadows and through intermediaries. Confront these groups and force them apart from the tobacco industry.

- The early implementing phases of tobacco control legislation are very important. Bad precedents, once set, are exceptionally hard to reverse. Avoid compromises early in the process.

- Do not be afraid of controversy; use it.

- Press for and defend high-quality programs. Beware of reasonable-sounding compromises in the anti-tobacco program (such as concentrating on kids or avoiding attacks on the tobacco industry), even when these suggestions come from "friends" in the health department.

- The battle does not end when a tobacco control initiative is passed.

- The battle does not end when the Legislature enacts implementing legislation, even if it is a good bill.

- The battle does not end when the health department or schools implement a good program.

- The battle never ends.

When the health groups are willing to take the risks and make the financial and other commitments necessary to confront the tobacco industry and its allies, the health groups can win despite the industry's superior economic resources. One only needs to visit a smoke-free bar in California to understand how dramatically reality has changed since a small group of activists met in Peter Hanauer's living room with the odd idea that people had a right to breathe clean indoor air.

They have shown over and over again that you can beat the tobacco industry.

Organizations, Programs, and People Involved in Tobacco Control in California

ORGANIZATIONS AND PROGRAMS

American Cancer Society (ACS)

American Heart Association (AHA)

American Lung Association (ALA)

Americans for Nonsmokers' Rights (ANR): A national nonprofit lobbying organization based in Berkeley, California, dedicated to protecting nonsmokers from secondhand smoke and keeping the tobacco industry out of the public policy-making process. American Nonsmokers' Rights Foundation (ANRF) is ANR's educational arm. ANR is the successor to Californians for Nonsmokers' Rights (CNR).

California Association of Hospitals and Health Systems (CAHHS): An organization that represents the interests of hospitals and health systems in the California Legislature.

California Department of Education (CDE): The state agency responsible for school-based Proposition 99 programs. It reports to the Superintendent of Public Instruction, an elected position that is independent of the governor.

California Medical Association (CMA)

Child Health and Disability Prevention (CHDP): The program established by California to meet requirements for the federal Early and Periodic Screening, Detection, and Treatment Program. It was the major program to which Proposition 99's Health Education money was diverted between 1989 and 1996.

Coalition for a Healthy California: The coalition of advocates who worked together to pass Proposition 99 and oppose Proposition 188. Its leadership came from the American Lung Association and the American Cancer Society.

Comprehensive Perinatal Outreach (CPO): A California program designed to insure that pregnant women receive prenatal care. It does not offer services itself but links women to services that can help them. CPO received money from Proposition 99's Health Education Account from 1991 through 1996.

Department of Health Services (DHS): The state agency responsible for all Proposition 99 programs except the school-based ones. It is part of the State Health and Welfare Agency, and its director is appointed by the governor. The Tobacco Control Section (TCS) was part of DHS.

Local Lead Agency (LLA): The umbrella name given to the county and city health departments charged with implementing Proposition 99 at the local level. There are sixty-one LLAs—fifty-eight county health departments and three city health departments.

Tobacco Control Section (TCS): The section of the Department of Health Services (DHS) that was responsible for administering Proposition 99 programs.

Tobacco Education and Research Oversight Committee (TEROC): The committee appointed to oversee the Proposition 99 Health Education and Research programs. In 1989 it was called the Tobacco Education Oversight Committee (TEOC) and only oversaw the Health Education programs. Its mission was broadened in 1994.

Western Center for Law and Poverty: A Sacramento-based advocacy organization concerned with health care for the poor.

PEOPLE

Adams, Mary: Lobbyist for the AHA; had been a lobbyist for the ACS (as Mary Dunn) when Proposition 99 passed.

Bal, Dileep: Head of the DHS Cancer Control Branch, which includes TCS.

Belshé, Kimberly: Southern California spokesperson for tobacco industry against Proposition 99, 1988; Director of DHS, 1993–1998.

Bowser, Roman: Executive vice president of the AHA.

Brown, Willie: Speaker of the California Assembly until 1995.

Carol, Julia: Executive Director of ANR.

Connelly, Lloyd: Member of the California State Assembly; helped organize Proposition 99.

Cook, Jennie: ACS volunteer and second chair of TEROC.

Coye, Molly Joel: Director of DHS, 1991–1993.

Deukmejian, George: Governor of California, 1983–1991.

Glantz, Stanton: Early tobacco control advocate; professor of medicine at the University of California, San Francisco; treasurer and president of ANR, 1980–1986.

Hanauer, Peter: Early tobacco control advocate; treasurer of the campaigns for Propositions 5 and 10; first president of ANR; member of the ANR board.

Hite, Betsy: ACS employee who worked on passage of Proposition 99; later a spokesperson for DHS.

Isenberg, Phil: Member of the California State Assembly; carried the first three pieces of Proposition 99 implementing legislation.

Kizer, Ken: Director of DHS when Proposition 99 passed.

Martin, Carolyn: ALA volunteer and first chair of TEOC.

Mekemson, Curt: Started Proposition 99 while working for ALA Sacramento–Emigrant Trails.

Merksamer, Steve: Former chief of staff to George Deukmejian; his law firm does lobbying for the tobacco industry.

Michael, Jay: CMA's chief lobbyist until 1992.

Miller, John: Aide to Senator Diane Watson; worked on the Proposition 99 implementing legislation.

Najera, Tony: ALA's chief lobbyist; led the lobbying effort on the Proposition 99 implementing legislation.

Nethery, W. James: ACS president; chair of Coalition for a Healthy California when Proposition 99 passed; worked on the first piece of implementing legislation.

Nicholl, Jack: Campaign manager for the Yes on Proposition 99 and No on Proposition 188 campaigns.

Nielsen, Vigo: Attorney for the tobacco industry.

Schilla, Peter: Chief lobbyist for the Western Center for Law and Poverty.

Smoley, Sandra: Member, Sacramento County Board of Supervisors; later Secretary of the Health and Welfare Agency under Wilson.

Thompson, Steve: Aide to Willie Brown; head of the Assembly Office of Research; chief CMA lobbyist after 1992.

Wilson, Pete: Governor of California, 1991–1999.

Important California Tobacco Control Events

April 1977	Berkeley passes an indoor air ordinance.
November 1978	Proposition 5 (statewide initiative covering clean indoor air issues) is defeated.
November 1980	Proposition 10 (statewide initiative covering clean indoor air issues) is defeated.
December 1980	Californians for Nonsmokers' Rights forms to pass local clean indoor air ordinances.
November 1983	Proposition P (San Francisco referendum) is defeated; smoke-free workplace law remains on the books.
November 1988	Proposition 99 (statewide initiative) passes.
October 1989	Deukmejian signs AB 75 (Health Education Account) and SB 1613 (Research Account), the first pieces of implementing legislation for Proposition 99.
April 1990	First California media campaign is launched.
June 1990	Lodi becomes the first city with restaurants 100% smoke free.
August 1990	San Luis Obispo becomes the first city with smoke-free bars.
May 1991	Molly Joel Coye replaces Ken Kizer as director of DHS.
July 1991	AB 99 passes, authorizing the Health Education Account until 1994.
January 1992	Governor Wilson attempts to shut down the media campaign.
April 1992	ALA sues to restore the media campaign.
June 1992	Sacramento voters pass Measure G, mandating smoke-free worksites, including restaurants.

December 1993   Governor Wilson vetoes bill reauthorizing the Research Account.

March 1994   ANR and Just Say No to Tobacco Dough file suit against diversions in AB 75 and AB 99.

July 1994   AB 13 passes, requiring 100% smoke-free workplaces on January 1, 1995; bars are given until January 1, 1997, to be smoke free (Legislature later extends date for bars to January 1, 1998).

July 1994   AB 816 passes, authorizing expenditures in the Health Education and Research Accounts until 1996 and increasing diversion of money from these accounts to medical services.

August 1994   ANR files suit against AB 816.

September 1994   ALA and ACS file suit against AB 816.

November 1994   Philip Morris initiative, Proposition 188, is defeated.

December 1994   Superior Court finds AB 816 illegal.

January 1995   Workplaces are required to be smoke free under AB 13.

July 1995   SB 493, authorizing expenditures in the Health Education and Research Accounts until 1996, passes. SB 493 sought to solve legal problems with AB 816.

July 1995   ANR and ALA, ACS, and AHA file suits against SB 493.

September 1995   Court issues a preliminary injunction against SB 493.

July 1996   Budget passes with full funding restored to the Health Education and Research Accounts.

January 1998   California bars become smoke free.

July 1998   Appellate Court rules unanimously that local ordinances are not preempted by either state or federal law.

References

CHAPTER 1

1. Pringle P. *Cornered: Big tobacco at the bar of justice.* New York: Henry Holt, 1998.

2. Glantz S, Slade J, Bero L, Hanauer P, Barnes L. *The cigarette papers.* Berkeley: University of California Press, 1996.

3. Glantz SA, Barnes DE, Bero L, Hanauer P, Slade J. Looking through a keyhole at the tobacco industry: The Brown and Williamson documents. *JAMA* 1995;274:219–224.

4. Hanauer P, Slade J, Barnes DE, Bero L, Glantz SA. Lawyer control of internal scientific research to avoid products liability lawsuits: The Brown and Williamson documents. *JAMA* 1995;274:234–240.

5. Bero L, Barnes DE, Hanauer P, Slade J, Glantz SA. Lawyer control of the tobacco industry's external research program: The Brown and Williamson documents. *JAMA* 1995;274:241–247.

6. Barnes DE, Hanauer P, Slade J, Bero LA, Glantz SA. Environmental tobacco smoke: The Brown and Williamson documents. *JAMA* 1995;274:248–253.

7. Slade J, Bero L, Hanauer P, Barnes DE, Glantz SA. Nicotine and addiction: The Brown and Williamson documents. *JAMA* 1995;274:225–233.

8. Glantz SA. Changes in cigarette consumption, prices, and tobacco industry revenues associated with California's Proposition 99. *Tobacco Control* 1993;2:311–314.

9. Begay ME, Traynor M, Glantz SA. The tobacco industry, state politics, and tobacco education in California. *Am J Pub Health* 1993;83(9):1214–1221.

10. Begay ME, Glantz SA. Tobacco industry campaign contributions are affecting tobacco control policymaking in California. *JAMA* 1994;272(15):1176–1182.

11. Monardi F, Glantz SA. Are tobacco industry campaign contributions influencing state legislative behavior? *Am J Pub Health* 1998;88(6):918–923.

12. Pierce JP, Gilpin EA, Emery SL, White M, Rosbrook B, Berry C. Has the California Tobacco Control Program reduced smoking? *JAMA* 1998;280(10): 893–899.

13. Koh HK. An analysis of the successful 1992 Massachusetts tobacco tax initiative. *Tobacco Control* 1996;5(3):220–225.

14. Heiser PF, Begay ME. The campaign to raise the tobacco tax in Massachusetts. *Am J Pub Health* 1997;87(6):968–973.

15. Aguinaga S, Glantz S. *Tobacco control in Arizona, 1973–1997.* San Francisco: Institute for Health Policy Studies, School of Medicine, University of California at San Francisco, 1997 October. (http://www.library.ucsf.edu/tobacco/az/)

16. Bialous SA, Glantz SA. Arizona's tobacco control initiative illustrates the need for continuing oversight by tobacco control advocates. *Tobacco Control* 1999;8:141–151.

17. Goldman LK, Glantz SA. *Tobacco industry political expenditures and tobacco policy making in Oregon: 1985–1997.* San Francisco: Institute for Health Policy Studies, School of Medicine, University of California at San Francisco, 1998 June. (http://www.library.ucsf.edu/tobacco/or/)

18. Wolinsky H, Brune T. *The serpent on the staff.* New York: G. P. Putnam's Sons, 1994.

19. Sharfstein J. 1996 congressional campaign priorities of the AMA: Tackling tobacco or limiting malpractice awards? *Am J Pub Health* 1998;88:1233–1236.

20. Pierce JP, Gilpin EA, Emery SL, Farkas AJ, Zhu SH, Choi WS, Berry CC, Distefan JM, White MM, Soroko S, Navarro A. *Tobacco control in California: Who's winning the war?* San Diego: University of California at San Diego, June 30, 1998.

21. Pierce JP, Evans N, Farkas AJ, Cavin SW, Berry C, Kramer M, Kealey S, Rosbrook B, Choi W, Kaplan RM. *Tobacco use in California: An evaluation of the Tobacco Control Program, 1989–1993.* La Jolla: University of California, San Diego, 1994.

22. Pierce JP. Evaluating Proposition 99 in California. Speech: American Heart Association, Nineteenth Science Writers Forum, January 12–15, 1992.

23. Glantz S. Achieving a smokefree society. *Circulation* 1987;76:746–752.

24. Sallis JF, Owen N. Ecological models. In: Glanz K, Lewis FM, Rimer BK, eds. *Health behavior and health education.* San Francisco: Jossey-Bass, 1997. pp. 403–424.

CHAPTER 2

1. [Review of scientific and public policy events relevant to smoking; incomplete document] Brown and Williamson Document 2114.02. March 15, 1973.

2. Roper Organization. *A study of public attitudes towards cigarette smok-*

ing and the tobacco industry. Prepared for the Tobacco Institute. Washington, DC: Roper Organization, 1978 May.

3. Kluger R. *Ashes to ashes: America's hundred-year cigarette war, the public health, and the unabashed triumph of Philip Morris.* New York: Vintage Books, 1996.

4. Hanauer P. Interview with Edith Balbach. June 4, 1998.

5. Hyink BL, Provost DH. *Politics and government in California.* New York: Longman, 1998.

6. Pepples E. Campaign report—Proposition 5, California 1978. January 11, 1979. Brown and Williamson Document 2302.05.

7. Stockdale J. Memo to Edward A. Grefe. August 25, 1977. Bates No. 2024372962/2966.

8. Taylor P. *The smoke ring.* New York, NY: Pantheon Books, 1984.

9. Pepples E. Letter to J. Swaab re: California Proposition 5. February 15, 1978. Brown and Williamson Document 2302.01.

10. Shartsis AJ. Letter to Ramsey Elliott. October 28, 1978.

11. Economic Research Associates. Memorandum report: Estimated costs for government occupied buildings to comply with the proposed "Clean Indoor Air Act." April 25, 1978. Americans for Nonsmokers' Rights Records, MSS 94-29, Archives and Special Collections, Library and Center for Knowledge Management, University of California, San Francisco.

12. Economic Research Associates. Memorandum report: Estimated cost for effective enforcement and prosecution of the "Clean Indoor Act." May 9, 1978. Americans for Nonsmokers' Rights Records, MSS 94-29, Archives and Special Collections, Library and Center for Knowledge Management, University of California, San Francisco.

13. Loveday P. Speech. Minneapolis, February 3, 1979. Bates No. 2024372711/2741.

14. V. Lance Tarrance & Associates. Memorandum to John D. Kelly and Stuart Spencer re: summary analysis of California Separate Sections Study. February 25, 1980. Bates No. 1005067831/7842.

15. Scott S. Memo to "Distribution." June 10, 1980.

16. Kennery D. Election 80: Campaigns compete for access to airwaves. *PSA Magazine* 1980 July;32ff.

17. Gilmour J, Bergland D, Flournoy H. Letter to Mr. Greenwood. August 15, 1980.

18. Soble RL. Opposition leaders claim proposition is deceptive. *Los Angeles Times* 1980 September 7;H3.

19. Bartlett R. Smoking-law foes start petition to snuff it out. *San Francisco Chronicle* 1983 June 15.

20. Hanauer P. Proposition P: Anatomy of a nonsmokers' rights ordinance. *New York State Journal of Medicine* 1985;85(7):369–374.

21. Ainsworth G. Memorandum to E. A. Horrigan, Jr., G. H. Long, and C. A. Tucker re: San Francisco campaign. July 16, 1983. Bates No. 50212 3473/3474.

22. Nelson Padberg Consulting. Campaign update: No on Proposition P:

San Franciscans Against Government Intrusion. September 8, 1983. Bates No. 2024078573/8652.

23. Nelson Padberg Consulting. Preliminary campaign plan. 1983 July. Bates No. 50212 3475/3481.

24. Johnston D. Anti-smoking foes claim names for S.F. referendum. *San Francisco Examiner* 1983 June 28;A1.

25. Hsu E. Smoking law backers organize S.F. group. *San Francisco Chronicle* 1983 August 18.

26. Nelson Padberg Consulting. Post election report. 1984 January. Bates No. 50065 0179/0189.

27. Tarrance VLJ. Research memorandum to Robert Nelson, John D. Kelly, M. Hurst Marshall, W. E. Ainsworth, James Cherry, Esq., K. V. R. Dey, Jr., Ernest Pepples, Esq., Stanley S. Scott, re: San Francisco Proposition P tracking. November 3, 1983. Bates No. 50388 7726/7728.

28. Ainsworth G. Memo to E. A. Horrigan, Jr., re: San Francisco campaign. November 4, 1983. Bates No. 50065 0286.

29. Tobacco Institute, State Activities Division. *California: A multifaceted plan to address the negative environment.* Washington, DC: Tobacco Institute, January 11, 1991. Bates No. 2023012755/2944.

30. USDHHS. *Reducing the health consequences of smoking: Twenty-five years of progress.* Rockville, MD: US Department of Health and Human Services, Public Health Service, Centers for Disease Control, Center for Chronic Disease Prevention and Health Promotion, Office on Smoking and Health, 1989. DHHS Publication No. (CDC) 89-8411.

31. Pritchard R. Tobacco industry speaks with one voice, once again. *United States Candy and Tobacco Journal* 1986 July 17–August 6;86.

CHAPTER 3

1. Mekemson C. Interview with Michael Traynor. November 18, 1992.

2. Mekemson C. Letter to Tony Najera re: ALA participation in cigarette tax initiative. October 8, 1986.

3. Connelly L. Interview with Michael Traynor. March 11, 1993.

4. Najera T, Mekemson C. Some initial thoughts on a cigarette tax initiative. October 14, 1986.

5. Connelly LG. Letter to Betsy Tram-Hite. November 20, 1986.

6. Hite B. Interview with Michael Traynor. February 26, 1993.

7. A-K Associates, Kinney P. Status and campaign plan for tobacco tax initiative. September 24, 1987. Bates No. 50660 9215/9232.

8. Hanauer P. Interview with Edith Balbach. June 4, 1998.

9. Carol J. Interview with Edith Balbach. August 8 and September 5, 1996.

10. Carol J. Comments on manuscript. 1998 October.

11. Mekemson C. Letter to Lloyd [Connelly], Jerry [Meral], Tony [Najera], Daryl [Young], Charles [Mawson]. Follow-up thoughts after meeting with Lloyd Connelly on October 22, 1986, re: cigarette tax initiative. October 27, 1986.

12. Begay ME, Glantz SA. Tobacco industry campaign contributions are

affecting tobacco control policymaking in California. *JAMA* 1994;272(15): 1176–1182.

13. Begay ME, Glantz SA. *Political expenditures by the tobacco industry in California state politics from 1976 to 1991.* San Francisco: Institute for Health Policy Studies, School of Medicine, University of California, San Francisco, 1991 September.

14. Sylvester K. The tobacco industry will walk a mile to stop an anti-smoking law. *Governing States Localities: Congressional Quarterly* 1989 May;34–40.

15. Paddock RC. Proposed 25-cent boost in cigarette tax rejected. *Los Angeles Times* 1987 May 19;3.

16. Green S, Chance A, Richardson J, Rodriguez R, Smith K. *California political almanac 1993–1994.* Sacramento: California Journal Press, 1993.

17. Rund CF, Henne JC. *The attitudes and opinions of California voters toward a cigarette tax increase.* San Francisco: Charlton Research Company, 1987 February.

18. Mekemson C. Letter to Betsy Tram re: some initial thoughts on the raw poll results as they relate to the proposed cigarette tax legislation. February 10, 1987.

19. V. Lance Tarrance & Associates. *California Constitutional Amendment Survey: A confidential report prepared for the Tobacco Institute.* Houston: Tarrance Hill Newport & Ryan, 1987 March. Bates No. 50661 0043/0062.

20. Hinerfeld DS. How political ads subtract. *Washington Monthly* 1990 May;12.

21. Hite B, Mekemson C. Californians overwhelmingly support tobacco tax increase. News release, April 21, 1987.

22. Howe T, Hite B, Mekemson C, Shannon T. Tobacco heir supports cigarette tax increase in California at informal hearing. News release, April 24, 1987.

23. Field M. *Californians favor more restrictions on smoking in public places, would approve big boost in cigarette tax.* San Francisco: California Poll, May 18, 1987.

24. Hite B. Letter to the Honorable Johan Klehs. May 12, 1987.

25. Najera T, Mekemson C. Letter to ALAC Board of Directors, ALAC Legislative Staff Workgroup, CTS Executive Committee, CTS Government Affairs, Affiliate Coordinators of Legislative Affairs, Affiliate Network Coordinators, Affiliate Presidents, Other Interested parties, re: ACA 14 and AB 2408—increase cigarette taxes. May 4, 1987.

26. Ainsworth G. Memo to G. H. Long and P. C. Bergson. April 9, 1987. Bates No. 50661 0209/0210.

27. Wiegand S. Cigarette tax proposal dies in Assembly. *San Francisco Chronicle* 1987 May 19.

28. Begay ME, Traynor M, Glantz SA. Extinguishing Proposition 99: Political expenditures by the tobacco industry in California politics in 1991–1992. San Francisco: Institute for Health Policy Studies, School of Medicine, University of California, San Francisco, 1992 September.

29. Glastris P. Frank Fat's napkin: How the trial lawyers (and the doctors) sold out to the tobacco companies. *Washington Monthly* 1987 December; 19–25.

30. Richardson J. *Willie Brown*. Berkeley: University of California Press, 1996.

31. Kennedy R. Interview with Edith Balbach. April 1, 1997.

CHAPTER 4

1. Mekemson C. Letter to Lloyd [Connelly], Tony [Najera], and Betsy [Hite], re: Tim's [Howe] draft of the initiative. May 13, 1987.

2. Mekemson C. Letter to Tony [Najera] and Betsy [Hite]. May 9, 1987.

3. Hite B. Interview with Michael Traynor. February 26, 1993.

4. Kiser D. Interview with Michael Traynor. January 13, 1994.

5. A-K Associates, Kinney P. *Status and campaign plan for tobacco tax initiative*. Sacramento: A-K Associates, Inc., September 24, 1987. Bates No. 50660 9215/9232.

6. Nicholl J. Interview with Michael Traynor. January 19, 1993.

7. Glantz SA. Interview with Edith Balbach. September 26, 1996.

8. Fairbank Bregman & Maullin. Executive summary report on a California statewide poll. San Francisco, September 10, 1987. Bates No. 50660 9272/9389.

9. V. Lance Tarrance & Associates. *California Constitutional Amendment Survey: A confidential report prepared for the Tobacco Institute*. Houston: Tarrance Hill Newport & Ryan, 1987 March. Bates No. 50661 0043/0062.

10. Green S, Chance A, Richardson J, Rodriguez R, Smith K. *California political almanac 1993–1994*. Sacramento: California Journal Press, 1993.

11. Price CM. Initiative campaigns: Afloat on a sea of cash. *California Journal* 1988 November;481–486.

12. Martin C. Comments on manuscript. 1998 October.

13. Coalition for a Healthy California. Executive Committee minutes. October 26, 1987.

14. Michael J. Interview with Michael Traynor. April 20, 1993.

15. Hitchcock D. Interview with Mike Traynor. December 8, 1992.

16. Wiegand S. Medical groups push tobacco tax increase. *San Francisco Chronicle* 1987 December 15.

17. Sample HA. Petition drive launched for 25-cent hike in cigarette tax. *Sacramento Bee* 1987 December 17.

18. Nicholl J. Letter to Executive Committee re: January financial situation. January 7, 1988.

19. Carol J. Interview with Edith Balbach. August 8 and September 5, 1996.

20. Nicholl J. Letter to Executive Committee. February 8, 1988.

21. Nicholl J. Letter to Executive Committee re: signature gathering update and financial position. March 24, 1988.

22. Californians Against Unfair Tax Increases. A petition to oppose the tobacco tax initiative. 1988.

23. Nethery WJ. Interview with Michael Traynor. May 11, 1994.

24. Michael J. Tobacco tax initiative. March 29, 1988.

25. Wright M. Tobacco tax signature totals by category. Bolinas, CA, 1988.

26. Farina J. Cigarette-tax initiative drive drawing very healthy response. *San Diego Tribune* 1988 May 3;A3.

27. United Press International. Cigarette tax, school aid head for ballot. *San Francisco Chronicle* 1988 May 3.

28. Rund CF, O'Donnell K. *The attitudes and opinions of California voters toward a cigarette tax increase.* San Francisco: Charlton Research, Inc., 1988 April.

29. Raimundo J. Interview with Michael Traynor. March 10, 1993.

30. Harris S. Factions fire up battle over tax hike for tobacco. *Los Angeles Times* 1988 July 7;3.

31. Marr M. *Proposition 99—The California tobacco tax initiative: A case study.* Berkeley, CA: Western Consortium for Public Health, 1990 April.

32. Green S. 4-year-old helps start tobacco-tax drive. *Sacramento Bee* 1988 July 7;A3.

33. Pfeiffer MT. Letter to Officers/Executive Committee re: authorization of $25,000 allocation to Coalition for a Healthy California. July 11, 1988.

34. Bowser RJ. Letter to W. James Nethery. September 27, 1988.

35. Marelius J. Tobacco tax initiative supporters claim "legal harassment." *San Diego Union* 1988 July 28;A5.

36. Field M. *Initial sentiment in favor of Prop. 95 (Housing and Nutritional Assistance), Prop. 97 (Cal-OSHA), Prop. 98 (School Funding), and Prop. 99 (Cigarette and Tobacco Tax).* San Francisco: California Poll, August 10, 1988.

37. Rund C, O'Donnell K. Letter to Jack Nicholl re: California poll data. August 11, 1988.

38. Robinson B. Backers of Props. 99, 103 still getting free TV time. *San Jose Mercury News* 1988 October 2.

39. Linderman CS. Campaign California Executive Committee meeting fairness doctrine—tobacco tax report. July 28, 1988.

40. Price C. Playing for time: Campaigns massage the "fairness doctrine." *California Journal* 1989 June;251–253.

41. Jessell HA. Antismoking coalition seeks return of fairness doctrine. *Broadcasting & Cable Magazine* 1994 August 22.

42. V. Lance Tarrance & Associates. *Prop 99 campaign study #3587.* Houston, August 4, 1987.

43. Adams M. Comments on manuscript. November 1998.

44. Langness D. Interview with Michael Traynor. January 19, 1993.

45. Mozingo RL. Memo to Dolph W. von Arx, W. G. Campion Mitchell, Gene Ainsworth, re: California tax initiative meeting—July 6, 1988. July 7, 1988. Bates No. 50765 9931.

46. California Medical Association. Executive memo re: tobacco tax initiative. June 13, 1988.

47. Hinerfeld DS. How political ads subtract. *Washington Monthly* 1990 May.

48. Holm P, Rund C. Letter to Jack Nicholl re: September survey results on Prop 99. September 15, 1988.

49. Field M. *Decline in voter approval margin of Prop. 99, cigarette tax increase initiative.* San Francisco: California Poll, September 22, 1988.

50. Reich K. Ads against tax hike on cigarettes challenged. *Los Angeles Times* 1988 September 9;3.

51. Reich K. TV initiative ads hype their own brand of truth. *Los Angeles Times* 1988 September 2.

52. Green S. Police chief rejects tobacco tax–crime link. *Sacramento Bee* 1988 September 23;A5.

53. Stein MA. Deception seen in anti-cigarette tax ads. *Los Angeles Times* 1988 September 28.

54. Flynn P. Campaign against cigarette tax increase called "sleazy." *San Diego Union* 1988 September 28;E1.

55. Scott J. Smoking costs state's taxpayers billions a year, report indicates. *Los Angeles Times* 1988 November 3.

56. Green S. State study finds smoking claimed 31,289 lives in '85. *Sacramento Bee* 1988 September 3.

57. Coalition for a Healthy California. Recipient Committee campaign statement. Sacramento, Office of the Secretary of State of the State of California, January 1–June 30, 1987–1989.

58. Californians Against Unfair Tax Increases. Recipient Committee campaign statement. Sacramento, Office of the Secretary of State of the State of California, January 1–June 30, 1987–1989.

59. Stein MA. Those who backed cigarette tax face tougher job: Seeing that it's spent right. *Los Angeles Times* 1988 November 10.

60. McNally R. Memo to David Townsend. November 28, 1988. Bates No. 50765 8838/9842.

61. Hanauer P. Interview with Edith Balbach. June 4, 1998.

CHAPTER 5

1. Waters G. Petition for Review. Sacramento: Supreme Court of the State of California, January 23, 1997.

2. Stein MA. Those who backed cigarette tax face tougher job: Seeing that it's spent right. *Los Angeles Times* 1988 November 10.

3. Winebrenner JT. Memo to P. J. Hoult re: California tax increase. November 21, 1988. Bates No. 50677 9941/.

4. Herson MB. Memo to Mr. Ralph Angiuoli re: California marketing program. January 12, 1989. Bates No. 507740 3093/3094.

5. Degener P. Memo to Distribution re: California retail promotion 12/88–1/89. November 18, 1988. Bates No. 2044195177/5180.

6. Connelly LG. Letter to Ernest J. Dronenburg, Jr. November 15, 1988.

7. Hager P. Justices declare tobacco tax constitutional. *Los Angeles Times* 1991 April 2;A3.

8. Kuzins M. Letter to Corey Brown. February 10, 1989.

9. Miller J. Interview with Stanton A. Glantz. July 12, 1998.

10. Miller J. Memo to Senator [Watson]. September 1988.

11. American Lung Association of California. *Proposition 99 implementation recommendations: Policy statement*. Sacramento, December 3, 1988.

12. Najera T. Memo to ALAC, Prop 99 oversight. December 13, 1988.

13. American Heart Association. *Recommendations for implementation of Proposition 99: Policy statement*. December 22, 1988.

14. Thompson S. Interview with Michael Traynor. June 30, 1995.

15. Miller J, Najera T, Adams M. Interview with Michael Traynor. June 20, 1995.

16. Begay ME, Glantz SA. *Political expenditures by the tobacco industry in California state politics from 1976 to 1991.* San Francisco: Institute for Health Policy Studies, School of Medicine, University of California, San Francisco, 1991 September.

17. Jacobson PD, Wasserman J, Raube K. The politics of anti-smoking legislation. *J Health Policy, Politics, and Law* 1993;18(4):787–819.

18. Kluger R. *Ashes to ashes: America's hundred-year cigarette war, the public health, and the unabashed triumph of Philip Morris.* New York: Vintage Books, 1996.

19. Richardson J. *Willie Brown.* Berkeley: University of California Press, 1996.

20. Monardi FM, Balbach ED, Aquinaga S, Glantz SA. *Shifting allegiances: Tobacco industry political expenditures in California January 1995–March 1996.* San Francisco: Institute for Health Policy Studies, School of Medicine, University of California, San Francisco, 1996 April.

21. CMA's new chief lobbying calls MDs to action. *California Physician* 1992 April;22.

22. Najera T, Miller J. Interview with Michael Begay. July 22, 1994.

23. Oliver TR, Paul-Shaheen P. Translating ideas into actions: Entrepreneurial leadership in state health care reforms. *J Health Policy, Politics, and Law* 1997;22(3):721–788.

24. Kingdon JW. *Agendas, alternatives, and public policies.* 2d ed. New York: Harper Collins, 1995.

25. State of California, Legislative Analyst's Office. *Analysis of the 1989–1990 budget bill.* Sacramento, 1989 February.

26. Carol J. Interview with Edith Balbach. August 8 and September 5, 1996.

27. Nicholl J. Memorandum to Executive Committee. December 8, 1988.

28. American Cancer Society. Proposition 99 Follow-up meeting—meeting notes. Oakland, December 15, 1988.

29. Martin C. Comments on manuscript. 1998 October.

30. Coalition for a Healthy California. Tobacco tax coalition unveils "Program for a Healthy California." Press release, January 5, 1989.

31. Elsner RH. Letter to W. James Nethery. January 4, 1989.

32. Kizer K. Interview with Michael Traynor. June 15, 1995.

33. Hafey JM. Letter to James Nethery. May 4, 1989.

34. Nethery WJ. Interview with Michael Traynor. May 11, 1994.

35. Coalition for a Healthy California. Minutes. May 15, 1989.

36. Williams G. Letter to W. James Netherly [*sic*]. May 15, 1989.

37. Marr M. *Proposition 99: The California tobacco tax initiative: A case study.* Berkeley, CA: Western Consortium for Public Health, 1990 April.

38. Langness D. Interview with Michael Traynor. January 19, 1993.

39. Cook J. Interview with Edith Balbach. March 19, 1998.

40. Hite B, Brown C. Tobacco tax initiative sponsors criticize governor's budget. Press release, January 10, 1989.

41. California Medical Association. News. Press release, January 10, 1989.

42. The Big Raid [editorial]. *Los Angeles Times* 1989 January 24; II.2.

43. Gregory B. Letter to Lloyd G. Connelly. February 24, 1989.

44. Scott S. Interview with Edith Balbach. September 18, 1996.

45. RJ Reynolds Tobacco. California short and long-range plans. 1989. Bates No. 50760 3756/3760.

46. Tobacco Institute, State Activities Division. *Project California proposal.* Washington, DC, February 21, 1989. Bates No. 2025848159/48192.

47. Nielsen, Merksamer. Memorandum to Executive Committee re: California state budget. December 15, 1988. Bates No. 50763 7136/7160.

CHAPTER 6

1. Martin C. Memorandum to E. A. (Tony) Oppenheimer, M.D., Spencer Koerner, M.D., Erna Barnickol, George Williams, re: Coalition for a Healthy California—February 3, 1989, meeting. February 5, 1989.

2. Najera A. Memo to George Williams and Carolyn Martin re: Prop 99—meetings—for the record. February 16, 1989.

3. Nethery J, Martin C. Letter to William Honig. March 10, 1989.

4. Second draft—Proposition 99 Health Education account. Sacramento: California State Legislature, February 7, 1989.

5. American Lung Association of California. *Public policy brief—Senate Bill 1099 (Watson)—Tobacco Use Prevention Act.* Sacramento, 1989 (February?).

6. Najera T. Memo to Dr. James Nethery, George Williams, Carolyn Martin. April 14, 1989.

7. Nielsen, Merksamer. Memorandum to Executive Committee re: California state budget. December 15, 1988. Bates No. 50763 7136/7160.

8. Gregory B. Letter to Lloyd G. Connelly. May 4, 1989.

9. Begay ME, Glantz SA. *Political expenditures by the tobacco industry in California state politics from 1976 to 1991.* San Francisco, Institute for Health Policy Studies, School of Medicine, University of California, San Francisco, 1991 September.

10. Goggin ML. *Policy design and the politics of implementation.* Knoxville: University of Tennessee Press, 1987.

11. Isenberg P. Interview with Edith Balbach. April 9, 1997.

12. Miller J, Najera T, Adams M. Interview with Michael Traynor. June 20, 1995.

13. Miller J. Comments on manuscript. January 31, 1999.

14. American Lung Association of California. Action Alert 1-89. Sacramento, July 7, 1989.

15. Cumming GH. Deposition of Gordon H. Cumming, Superior Court of the State of California, County of Sacramento, October 12, 1994. Case No. 379257.

16. Martin C. Comments on manuscript. 1998 October.

17. Miller J. Memorandum to Senator Diane Watson. June 26, 1989.

18. Muraoka S. Minutes—Coalition for a Healthy California. June 30, 1989.

19. Williams J, Isenberg P. *Case study on Proposition 99 (the cigarette tax).* Sacramento: California State University, Sacramento, November 20, 1995.

20. Tobacco Institute, State Activities Division. *Project California proposal.* Washington, DC, February 21, 1989. Bates No. 2025848159/48192.

21. Walters D. A smoky fight over initiative. *Sacramento Bee* 1989 June 29.

22. Walters D. A lousy way to make policy. *Sacramento Bee* 1989 June 15.

23. Knap C. "Unholy" pair: Tobacco, medical lobbies draw frowns. *Santa Maria Times* 1989 July 20.

24. Williams GR. Memo to E. A. Oppenheimer et al. May 17, 1989.

25. Connelly LG. Letter to Richard P. Simpson. May 24, 1989.

26. Cate G. Memo to Catherine Hanson. May 23, 1989.

27. Light J. Tobacco. June 27, 1989.

28. Michael JD. Memo to CMA Executive Committee. May 12, 1989.

29. Plested WG. Letter to the Honorable Robert Presley. July 14, 1989.

30. Cate GF. Letter to Members of the Conference Committee on AB 75. July 12, 1989.

31. California Medical Association. Minutes of the 738th meeting of the Council. July 21, 1989.

32. Takayasu M. Voluntary health organizations assail CMA's attempts to violate provisions of Proposition 99. Press release, July 31, 1989.

33. Ellis V. Doctors hit on anti-smoking program. *Los Angeles Times* 1989 August 1;3.

34. Lucas G. Flap over cigaret tax. *San Francisco Chronicle* 1989 August 1;A8.

35. Irwin L, Beerline D. Letter to colleagues. August 17, 1989.

36. Michael JD. Letter to Joe B. Tye. August 29, 1989.

37. Dunn M. Memo to Ron Hagen. August 24, 1989.

38. Marr M. *Proposition 99: The California tobacco tax initiative: A case study.* Berkeley, CA: Western Consortium for Public Health, 1990 April.

39. Scott S. Interview with Edith Balbach. September 18, 1996.

40. Lucas G. Tobacco lobbyists attack Prop. 99 plan. *San Francisco Chronicle* 1989 September 13;A7.

41. Chance A. Tobacco industry fights anti-smoking ads. *Sacramento Bee* 1989 September 13;A3.

42. Bronzan B, Isenberg P, Keene B, Rosenthal H. Memorandum to members of the Legislature. September 13, 1989.

43. Shuit DP. Conferees vote to fund no-smoking ad campaign. *Los Angeles Times* 1989 September 14;3.

44. Adams M. Comments on manuscript. 1998 November.

45. Walters D. The Capitol's sausage grind. *Sacramento Bee* 1989 September 15.

46. Thompson S. Interview with Michael Traynor. June 30, 1995.

47. University of California. Draft Prop 99 Research Account: Preliminary statement of principles. January 20, 1989.

48. Hopper CL. Memo to members of the Coalition for a Healthy California. March 7, 1989.

49. Scott S. Smoking out tobacco's influence. *California Journal* 1997 April; 14–18.

50. Allenby C. Interview with Michael Traynor. June 16, 1995.

51. Bal DG, Kizer KW, Felten PG, Mozar HN, Niemeyer D. Reducing tobacco consumption in California: Development of a statewide anti-tobacco use campaign. *JAMA* 1990;264(12):1570–1574.

CHAPTER 7

1. State of California, California State Legislature. Assembly Bill 75. Sacramento, October 2, 1989.
2. Tobacco Control Section, California Department of Health Services. *National Cancer Institute Planning Model*. Sacramento, 1989 December.
3. Hawkins J, Jenson J, Catalano RJ. Delinquency and drug abuse: Implications for social services. *Social Science Review* 1988 June;258–284.
4. Hawkins J, Catalano R, Kaggerty K. Risk and protective factors are interdependent. *Western Center News* 1993 September.
5. California Department of Education. Not Schools Alone. Sacramento, California Department of Education, 1991.
6. Cook J. Interview with Edith Balbach. March 19, 1998.
7. Kizer K. Interview with Michael Traynor. June 15, 1995.
8. Lee P. Keye/Donna to do anti-smoking ads for state. *Los Angeles Times* 1990 January 27;D2.
9. Scorching attack on cigarette firms. *Los Angeles Times* 1990 April 10;1A.
10. Keye P. What don't we know, and when haven't we known it? Speech given at Health Communications Day, Johns Hopkins University, Baltimore, October 13, 1993.
11. Scott S. Smoking out tobacco's influence. *Californian Journal* 1997 April:14–18.
12. California Department of Health Services. First the smoke. Now, the mirrors. Newspaper advertisement, *Sacramento Bee* 1990 April 11.
13. Johnson B. Anti-smoke torch flickers. *Advertising Age* 1990 April 16;1.
14. Roan S. State to launch anti-smoking ad campaign. *Los Angeles Times* 1990 April 10;A1.
15. Garfield B. California's anti-smoking ad fans flames of racial paranoia. *Advertising Age* 1990 April 16;70.
16. Lucas G. Deukmejian cool to blitz on smoking. *San Francisco Chronicle* 1990 April 11;1.
17. Malmgren KL. Memorandum to Samuel D. Chilcote, Jr. April 18, 1990. Bates No. TIMN 298437/298420W.
18. Gallup Organization, Stanford University, University of Southern California. *Final report. Independent evaluation of the California Tobacco Control Prevention and Education Program: Wave 1 data, 1996–1997*. 1999 February.
19. Tobacco Control Section, California Department of Health Services. Local lead agencies. Sacramento, 1989.
20. LLA Director 4. Interview with Edith Balbach. 1997.
21. LLA Director 3. Interview with Edith Balbach. 1998.
22. Hallett C. Interview with Edith Balbach. March 27, 1998.
23. LLA Director 6. Interview with Edith Balbach. 1998.

24. LLA Director 1. Interview with Edith Balbach. 1998.

25. Nielsen, Merksamer. Memorandum to Executive Committee re: California state budget. December 15, 1988. Bates No. 50763 7136/7160.

26. Glantz SA. Preventing tobacco use—the youth access trap. *Am J Pub Health* 1996;86(2):156–158.

27. LLA Director 9. Interview with Edith Balbach. 1998.

28. LLA Director 5. Interview with Edith Balbach. 1998.

29. Hanauer P. Interview with Edith Balbach. June 4, 1998.

30. LLA Director 2. Interview with Edith Balbach. 1998.

31. Williamson J. Statewide Projects Meeting minutes. May 7, 1993.

32. Honig B. Interview with Edith Balbach. January 4, 1994.

33. Yeates K. Interview with Edith Balbach. November 22, 1994.

34. TUPE Coordinator 1. Interview with Edith Balbach. Spring 1998.

35. TUPE Coordinator 2. Interview with Edith Balbach. Spring 1998.

36. Wolfe G. Interview with Edith Balbach. December 7, 1994.

37. Martin C. Interview with Edith Balbach. November 21, 1994.

38. Isenberg P. Interview with Edith Balbach. April 9, 1997.

39. TUPE Coordinator 3. Interview with Edith Balbach. Spring 1998.

40. Tobacco Control Section, California Department of Health Services. *Comprehensive tobacco control guidelines for local lead agencies.* Sacramento, September 11, 1990.

41. Balbach ED. *Interagency Collaboration in the Delivery of the California Tobacco Education Program* [Ph.D.]. Berkeley: University of California at Berkeley, 1994.

42. Moskowitz J. Interview with Edith Balbach. December 6, 1994.

CHAPTER 8

1. Roan S. State to launch anti-smoking ad campaign. *Los Angeles Times* 1990 April 10;A1.

2. Malmgren KL. Memorandum to Samuel D. Chilcote, Jr. April 18, 1990. Bates No. TIMN 298437/298420W.

3. Osmon HE. Memo to W. E. Ainsworth and R. L. Mozingo. April 12, 1990. Bates No. 50760 3741/3742.

4. Chilcote SDJ. Memorandum to the members of the Executive Committee. April 11, 1990. Bates No. TIMN 423498/423504.

5. KRC Research. Memo to Stanley Temko, Covington & Burling, re: California quantitative research. New York: KRC Research & Consulting. May 3, 1990. Bates No. TIMN 355366/355370.

6. KRC Research. *Qualitative research report: Reaction to California's Proposition 99 and its 1990 anti-smoking media campaign.* New York: KRC Research & Consulting, 1990 May. Bates No. TIMN 334989/335167.

7. Woodson WN. Memo to Samuel D. Chilcote, Jr., re: California advertising situation. May 14, 1990. Bates No. TIMN 355359/355360.

8. Tobacco Institute (?). California anti-tobacco advertising program. November 1, 1990. Bates No. 50779 3734/3735.

9. Slavitt JJ. Memo to Pat Tricorache re: TI youth initiative. February 12, 1991. Bates No. 2500082629.

10. Slavitt JJ. Memo to William I. Campbell. March 1991. Bates No. 2500082631/2634.

11. Harris TC. Memorandum to T. N. Hyde re: Planning meeting on impending "Prop 99" efforts. December 20, 1991. Bates No. 51199 9020.

12. Woodson W. Memorandum to Marty Gleason. May 13, 1991. Bates No. TIMN 378297.

13. Stratton, Reiter, Dupree & Durante. *Report to R. J. Reynolds Tobacco on the Tobacco Control Plan, State of California.* Denver, June 14, 1991. Bates No. 51319 3999/4061.

14. Hyde T. Memo to Tommy Griscom, Tom Ogburn, Roger Mozingo, Jim O'Mally, and Mark Smith, re: Stratton & Reiter's California research project. April 4, 1991. Bates No. 50777 7860/7863.

15. DiFranza JR, Godshall WT. Tobacco industry efforts hindering enforcement of the ban on tobacco sales to minors: Actions speak louder than words. *Tobacco Control* 1996;5(2):127–131.

16. DiFranza JR, Savageau JA, Aisquith BF. Youth access to tobacco: The effects of age, gender, vending machine locks, and "It's the Law" programs. *Am J Pub Health* 1996;86(2):221–224.

17. DeBon M, Klesges RC. Adolescents' perceptions about smoking prevention strategies: A comparison of the programmes of the American Lung Association and the Tobacco Institute. *Tobacco Control* 1996;5(1):19–25.

18. Tobacco Institute. Order form for "Helping Youth." Washington, DC, 1993, Bates No. TIMN 447189/447215.

CHAPTER 9

1. George Gallup. Cancer Society given highest ratings in test of special interest groups. Press release, April 16, 1989.

2. V. Lance Tarrance & Associates. *Kern County smoking study.* Houston, 1982 September.

3. Stumbo B. Where there's smoke. *Los Angeles Times Magazine* 1986 August 24:11–15.

4. Tobacco Institute, State Activities Division. *California: A multifaceted plan to address the negative environment.* Washington, DC. January 11, 1991. Bates No. 2023012755/2944.

5. Ifergan S-J, Milligan M. Tobacco Institute acknowledges role in fight against B.H. no-smoke law. *Beverly Hills Courier* 1987 April 24;3,10.

6. Arnold R. Judge rejects challenge to Beverly Hills smoking ban. *Los Angeles Times* 1987 April 3.

7. Hager P. High court declines to review smoking ban in Beverly Hills. *Los Angeles Times* 1987 May 21.

8. Ferris J. Smoke screen clouds Tobacco Industry action. *Contra Costa Times* 1991 June 23.

9. RJ Reynolds. In the news. *Choice* 1987;1(6):4.

10. Philip Morris USA. The lessons of Beverly Hills. *Philip Morris Magazine* 1991 Winter;6(1):22.

11. Philip Morris. *Smoker* 1988 July/August;1(6).

12. Fogel B. Testimony before the New York City Council. June 6, 1994.

13. US Environmental Protection Agency. *Respiratory health effects of passive smoking: Lung cancer and other disorders.* Washington, DC, 1992. USEPA Document No. EPA/600/6-90/006F.

14. Stoddard S. Interview with Bruce Samuels. April 10, 1991.

15. Samuels B, Glantz SA. *Tobacco control activities and the tobacco industry's response in California communities, 1990–1991.* San Francisco: Institute for Health Policy Studies, School of Medicine, University of California, San Francisco. 1991 August.

16. Drummond M. Council OKs smoking ban. *Lodi News Sentinel* 1990 June 7.

17. Stamos B. Interview with Bruce Samuels. November 14, 1990.

18. Turner B. Interview with Bruce Samuels. December 5, 1990.

19. LICAC. Campaign disclosure statement. July 1–December 31, 1990.

20. Ross P. Interview with Bruce Samuels. November 14, 1990.

21. Ross P, St. Yves E. Interview with Bruce Samuels. November 2, 1990.

22. TUFF. Ballot Measure Committee statements. July 1–December 31, 1990.

23. Dados A. Interview with Bruce Samuels. November 2, 1990.

24. RJ Reynolds. Independent Expenditure and Major Donor Committee campaign statement. July 1–December 31, 1990.

25. Carol J. Comments on manuscript. October 1998.

26. Levin M. Blowing smoke: Who's behind the building doctor. *The Nation* 1993 August 9–16;168–171.

27. Mintz M. Smokescreen / How the Tobacco Institute, its PR agents at Fleishman-Hillard and its lawyers at Covington & Burling helped turn a small-time Fairfax businessman into an international authority on indoor air quality and cigarette smoke. *Washington Post Magazine* 1996 March 24;12–30.

28. Begay ME, Traynor MP, Glantz SA. *The twilight of Proposition 99: Reauthorization of tobacco education programs and tobacco industry expenditures in 1993.* San Francisco: Institute for Health Policy Studies, School of Medicine, University of California, San Francisco, 1994 March.

29. Dempster D. Bad news for smokers in capital. *Sacramento Bee* 1990 September 12;A1.

30. Sacramentans for Fair Business Policy. General Purpose Recipient Committee statements. January 1–December 21, 1990.

31. Samuels B, Glantz S. The politics of local tobacco control. *JAMA* 1991; 266(15):2110–2117.

32. Davilla R. Smoking ban put on hold. *Sacramento Bee* 1990 November 1.

33. Eagan T. Memorandum to George Mimshew. September 20, 1990. Bates No. 50764 0402/0405.

34. Smith M. Memorandum to Tom Ogburn re: California update. April 17, 1991. Bates No. 50770 3343–3344.

35. Woodruff T, Rosbrook B, Pierce J, Glantz S. Lower levels of cigarette consumption found in smoke-free workplaces in California. *Archives of Internal Medicine* 1993(153):1485–1493.

36. Glantz S. Back to basics: Getting smoke-free workplaces back on track. Editorial. *Tobacco Control* 1997;6:164–166.

37. McAdam RS. Memorandum to Kurt L. Malmgren. November 27, 1991. Bates Number TIMN 0022833/839.

38. Glantz SA, Smith LRA. The effect of ordinances requiring smoke-free restaurants on restaurant sales. *Am J Pub Health* 1994;84:1081–1085.

39. Glantz SA, Smith LRA. The effect of ordinances requiring smoke-free restaurants and bars on revenues: A follow-up. *Am J Pub Health* 1997;87:1687–1693.

40. Glantz SA, Smith L. Erratum for "The effect of ordinances requiring smoke-free restaurants and bars on revenues: A follow-up." *Am J Pub Health* 1998;88:1122.

41. Glantz SA. Smokefree restaurant ordinances don't affect restaurant business. Period. *J Pub Health Management & Practice* 1999;5:vi–ix.

42. Laufer D. E-mail to Tina Walls re: San Fran. and CA. November 1, 1993. Bates No. 2045891104.

43. Glantz SA, Smith LRA. Erratum for "The effect of ordinances requiring smoke-free restaurants on restaurant sales." *Am. J. Pub. Health* 1997;87:1729–1730.

44. Price Waterhouse. *Potential economic effects of a smoking ban in the state of California.* N.p., 1993 May.

45. Tobacco Institute. 1992 referenda assessment. January 24, 1992. Bates No. ATX03 0311555.

46. Traynor MP, Begay ME, Glantz SA. New tobacco industry strategy to prevent local tobacco control. *JAMA* 1993;270(4):479–486.

47. Morris RC. Memorandum to Kent Rhodes re: Proactive opportunity, Placer County, California. April 25, 1991. Bates No. TIMN 184603/184620.

48. J. Moore Methods. *Sacramento County smoking ordinance.* Sacramento: Citizens for Healthier Sacramento/Yes on G, 1992 January.

49. Here comes the smoke. *Business Journal* 1992 April 13.

50. Malmgren KL. Memorandum to Samuel D. Chilcote, Jr., re: Expanded Local Program. November 30, 1992. Bates No. 51333 1953/1965.

51. Philip Morris Tobacco. Overview of state ASSIST programs. N.d. Bates No. 2021253353.

52. Aguinaga S, Glantz SA. The use of public records acts to interfere with tobacco control. *Tobacco Control* 1995;1995(4):222–230.

53. Helm MB. Letter to California Department of Health Services. April 4, 1991.

54. Newman FS. Memo re: California anti-smoking advertising. June 8, 1990. Bates No. 2022986403-6456.

55. Stratton, Reiter, Dupree & Durante. *Report to R. J. Reynolds Tobacco on the Tobacco Control Plan, State of California.* Denver, June 14, 1991. Bates No. 51319 3999/4061.

56. Pierce JP. Evaluating Proposition 99 in California. Speech: American Heart Association, Nineteenth Science Writers Forum. January 12–15, 1992.

57. Pierce JP, Evans N, Farkas AJ, Cavin SW, Berry C, Kramer M, Kealey S, Rosbrook B, Choi W, Kaplan RM. *Tobacco use in California: An evaluation of the Tobacco Control Program, 1989–1993.* La Jolla: University of California, San Diego, 1994.

58. Pierce JP, Gilpin EA, Emery SL, White M, Rosbrook B, Berry C. Has the California Tobacco Control Program reduced smoking? *JAMA* 1998;280(10).

59. Philip Morris (?). *1994 California Plan.* N.p., 1994. Bates No. 2022816070/6080.

CHAPTER 10

1. Department of Health Services. Research data shows significant drop in tobacco usage since enactment of California's tobacco education campaign. Press release, October 30, 1990.

2. Cook J. AB 75 update. Report to the Board of Directors, American Cancer Society. February 14, 1991.

3. Begay ME, Glantz SA. *Undoing Proposition 99: Political expenditures by the tobacco industry in California politics in 1991.* San Francisco: Institute for Health Policy Studies, School of Medicine, University of California, 1992 April.

4. Begay ME, Traynor M, Glantz SA. *Extinguishing Proposition 99: Political expenditures by the tobacco industry in California politics in 1991–1992.* San Francisco: Institute for Health Policy Studies, School of Medicine, University of California, San Francisco, 1992 September.

5. Scott S. Interview with Edith Balbach. September 18, 1996.

6. Beerline D. Interview with Edith Balbach. September 26, 1996.

7. Miller J, Najera T. Memo to Carolyn Martin. December 13, 1990.

8. American Lung Association, California Association of Hospitals & Health Systems, California Medical Association, California Planners and Consultants, California Schools Boards Association, County Supervisors Association of California, Service Employees International Union, Western Center for Law and Poverty. Letter to Phil Isenberg. January 7, 1991.

9. Martin C. Comments on manuscript. 1998 October.

10. Martin C, Breslow L, Dyke P, Weidmer CE, Cook J. Tobacco Education Oversight Committee press conference remarks. January 23, 1991.

11. California Medical Association. Summary of recommendations. Report to Council from the Commission on Legislation. November 10, 1990.

12. Strumpf IJ. Memo to Scientific Advisory Panel on Chest Diseases re: Resolution 213-96, Anti-Tobacco Education and Research. February 5, 1996.

13. Michael JD. Letter to Lester Breslow. January 22, 1990.

14. Plested WG. Letter to the Honorable Robert Presley. July 14, 1989.

15. Howe RK. Tobacco education and socialized medicine. *California Physician* 1989 December; 48–49.

16. Michael J. Interview with Michael Traynor. April 20, 1993.

17. California Medical Association. Minutes of the 746th Council. September 14, 1990.

18. Tobacco Institute (?). California anti-tobacco advertising program. November 1, 1990. Bates No. 50779 3734/3735.

19. State of California, Legislative Analyst's Office. *Analysis of the 1991–1992 budget*. Sacramento, February 6, 1991.

20. Skolnick A. Court orders California governor to restore antismoking media campaign funding. *JAMA* 1992;267:2721–2723.

21. State of California, Legislative Analyst's Office. *Analysis of the 1994–1995 budget bill*. Sacramento, 1994.

22. American Lung Association. AB 99 (Isenberg)—active support. *Capitol Correspondence* 1991 March 26.

23. Hagen R. Executive notice. March 21, 1991.

24. Page BI, Shapiro RY. *The rational public*. Chicago: University of Chicago Press, 1992.

25. Oglesby MB, Mozingo R. Memo to J. W. Johnston re: California antismoking advertising. January 24, 1991. Bates No. 50760 4050.

26. Verner KL. Memorandum to T. C. Griscom re: California's anti-smoking campaign funding. January 29, 1991. Bates No. 50775 5351–5354.

27. California Medical Association. Report to the Executive Committee from the Prop 99 Funding TAC (ratified by the Board of Trustees, July, 1991). June 14, 1991.

28. Gregory BM. Letter to Diane E. Watson. June 13, 1991.

29. Gregory BM. Letter to Phil Isenberg. June 27, 1991.

30. Gregory BM. Letter to Elizabeth Hill. March 10, 1992.

31. Western Center for Law and Poverty, California Medical Association, California Nurses Association, California Association of Hospitals and Health Systems. Memo to AB 99 Conference Committee staff working group. June 30, 1991.

32. American Lung Association. *Capitol Correspondence*. 1991 July.

33. Kiser D, Muraoka S, Velo T, Najera T. Memo to all interested parties, Proposition 99 Health Education Account. June 17, 1991.

34. AB 99 Conference Committee. AB 99: Budget related issues for resolution. June 30, 1991.

35. Miller J, Najera T, Adams M. Interview with Michael Traynor. June 20, 1995.

36. Weintraub D. Heat put on Wilson over anti-smoking funds. *Los Angeles Times* 1992 February 21;A3.

37. Warren J, Morain D. Bid to dilute anti-smoking effort revealed. *Los Angeles Times* 1998 January 21.

38. State of California, Office of the Governor. *Governor's budget 1992–1993*. January 1992.

39. American Cancer Society. Memo to unit executive directors from Ron Hagen. Executive notice. January 23, 1992.

40. Americans for Nonsmokers' Rights. Prop 99 $$ slashed: Media campaign killed already! Action Alert, January 22, 1992.

41. Russell S. Health director explains governor's "checkup" insurance plan. *San Francisco Chronicle* 1992 January 10;A8.

42. Cook J. Interview with Edith Balbach. March 19, 1998.

43. Lucas G. Demos assail Wilson plan to cut funds for anti-smoking drive. *San Francisco Chronicle* 1992 January 23;A15.

44. Gray T. Wilson's plan to shift funds disguises tax hike, critics say. *Sacramento Bee* 1992 January 26;A3.

45. Russell S. Anti-smoking program big hit—but governor seeks to cut it. *San Francisco Chronicle* 1992 January 15;14.

46. Coye MJ. A temporary diversion of the tobacco tax. *Sacramento Bee* 1992 February 18;B7.

47. Senate Budget and Fiscal Review Subcommittee. Agenda. March 16, 1992.

48. American Lung Association. Media campaign suit update. *Capitol Correspondence* 1992 June;1–3.

49. Malmgren KL. Memorandum to Samuel D. Chilcote, Jr. April 18, 1990. Bates No. TIMN 298437/298420W.

50. Grubb K. Smoking program. Associated Press, 1992 January 23.

51. Pierce JP. Evaluating Proposition 99 in California. Speech: American Heart Association, Nineteenth Science Writers Forum. January 12–15, 1992.

52. Winslow R. California push to cut smoking seen as success. *Wall Street Journal* 1992 January 15;B1.

53. Matthews J. Anti-smoking initiative called effective. *Washington Post* 1992 January 19.

54. Zamichow N. Anti-smoking effort working, study finds. *Los Angeles Times* 1992 January 15.

55. California smokers quitting. *USA Today* 1992 January 15;D1.

56. State set to scrap anti-smoking TV ads. *Los Angeles Times* 1992 January 16;B8.

57. State study lauds anti-smoking drive. *San Francisco Examiner* 1992 January 25;A5.

58. Duerr J. Memo to Dileep Bal. January 29, 1992.

59. Williams L. Officials: Wilson undercut TV ads on smoking. *San Francisco Examiner* 1996 December 22;A1.

60. Cook J, Velo T. Memo to Ron Hagen. February 27, 1992.

61. Cook J, Velo T. Memo to Ron Hagen, Sharen Muraoka, and George Yamasaki, Jr., Esq. April 1, 1992.

62. Skolnick A. American Heart Association seeks to delay state health department director's confirmation. *JAMA* 1992;267:2723–2726.

63. Kiser D. Testimony to California Senate Rules Committee. April 22, 1992.

64. Matthews J. Smoking ads revived. *Sacramento Bee* 1992 May 7;A3.

65. Dresslar T. Tobacco industry slashes away at tax. *San Francisco Daily Journal* 1992 May 4.

66. Najera T. Memo to Scarcnet. July 15, 1992.

67. Russell S. Battle brewing over plan for tobacco tax. *San Francisco Chronicle* 1992 July 29;A21.

68. Waters G. Letter to Tony Najera. June 23, 1992.

69. American Lung Association. *Capitol Correspondence.* July 17, 1992.

70. Schilla P. Letter to Willie Brown. August 7, 1992.

71. Najera T. Memo to the Prop 99 anti-redirection coalition. August 12, 1992.

72. Hayes TW, Hordyk D. Letter to Alquist et al. October 1, 1992.

73. Department of Health Services. Federal Financial Participation (FFP) guidelines for Maternal and Child Health (MCH) programs. Sacramento, July 1, 1993.

74. Shah R. Deposition of Rugmini Shah. Superior Court of the State of California, County of Sacramento, 1994. Case No. 379257.

75. Tobacco Education Oversight Committee. Minutes. November 16, 1992.

76. Tobacco Education Oversight Committee. Minutes. March 29, 1993.

77. Martin C, Cook J. Letter to California State Legislators. February 23, 1993.

78. Green S. Wilson taps former spokeswoman for tobacco industry as state health chief. *Sacramento Bee* 1993 November 10.

79. Cigarette tax funds grabbed. *San Francisco Examiner* 1994 March 13;B1.

80. Skolnick A. Antitobacco advocates fight "illegal" diversion of tobacco control money. *JAMA* 1994;271(18):1387–1390.

81. Begay ME, Traynor MP, Glantz SA. *The twilight of Proposition 99: Reauthorization of tobacco education programs and tobacco industry expenditures in 1993.* San Francisco: Institute for Health Policy Studies, School of Medicine, University of California, San Francisco, March 1994.

82. Hobart R. Interview with Edith Balbach. July 25, 1996.

83. Glantz SA, Bero LA. Inappropriate and appropriate selection of "peers" in grant review. *JAMA* 1994;272(2):114–116.

84. Begay ME, Glantz SA. *Political expenditures by the tobacco industry in California state politics from 1976 to 1991.* San Francisco: Institute for Health Policy Studies, School of Medicine, University of California, San Francisco, 1991 September.

85. Begay ME, Glantz SA. Tobacco industry campaign contributions are affecting tobacco control policymaking in California. *JAMA* 1994;272(15):1176–1182.

86. Foster D. The lame duck state: Term limits and the hobbling of California state government. *Harper's* 1994 February; 65–75.

87. Office of the Governor. Veto of Senate Bill No. 1088 (Bergeson). Sacramento, 1993.

88. Katz R. Interview with Edith Balbach. April 3, 1997.

89. Barinaga M. Wilson slashes spending for antismoking effort. *Science* 1992 March 13;255:1348–1349.

CHAPTER 11

1. Russell C. Letter to Stanton Glantz. June 6, 1996.

2. Pierce JP, Evans N, Farkas AJ, Cavin SW, Berry C, Kramer M, Kealey S, Rosbrook B, Choi W, Kaplan RM. *Tobacco use in California: An evaluation of the Tobacco Control Program, 1989–1993.* La Jolla: University of California, San Diego, 1994.

3. Patten C, Pierce J, Cavin S, Berry C, Kaplan R. Progress in protecting non-smokers from environmental tobacco smoke in California workplaces. *Tobacco Control* 1995;4:139–144.

4. Tobacco Control Section, California Department of Health Services. *Are Californians protected from environmental tobacco smoke? A summary of findings on worksite and household policies: California Adult Tobacco Survey.* Sacramento, 1995 September.

5. Tobacco Control Section, California Department of Health Services. *Is smoking prohibited in work areas?* Sacramento, June 11, 1996.

6. Tobacco Institute, State Activities Division. *California: A multifaceted plan to address the negative environment.* Washington, DC, January 11, 1991. Bates No. 2023012755/2944.

7. Siegel M, Carol J, Jordan J, Hobart R, Schoenmarklin S, DuMelle F, Fisher P. Preemption in tobacco control: Review of an emerging public health problem. *JAMA* 1997;278(10):858–863.

8. Macdonald HR, Glantz SA. The political realities of statewide smoking legislation. *Tobacco Control* 1997;6:41–54.

9. Kerrigan MJ. A proposed comprehensive tobacco control act in California/ RIIPP: Memo to Smokeless Tobacco Council, Committee of Counsel. June 28, 1991.

10. Lucas G. Panel defeats no-smoking bill linked to Brown. *San Francisco Chronicle* 1991 September 6.

11. Glantz SA, Begay ME. Tobacco industry campaign contributions are affecting tobacco control policymaking in California. *JAMA* 1994;272(15): 1176–1182.

12. Webb G. Speaker disguised smoking bill, memo says. *San Jose Mercury News* 1991 August 27.

13. Richardson J, Kushman R. Advice to tobacco firms admitted. *Sacramento Bee* 1991 August 30.

14. Lucas G. Health groups blast tobacco-industry bill. *San Francisco Chronicle* 1991 September 6.

15. Begay ME, Traynor MP, Glantz SA. *The twilight of Proposition 99: Reauthorization of tobacco education programs and tobacco industry expenditures in 1993.* San Francisco: Institute for Health Policy Studies, School of Medicine, University of California, San Francisco, 1994 March.

16. Friedman T. Labor chairman's bill would ban workplace smoking. Press release, February 13, 1992.

17. American Cancer Society, American Lung Association, American Heart Association. No time like the present. Memo, June 11, 1992.

18. Griffin MJ. Letter to Assembly Member Friedman. April 3, 1992.

19. Carol J. Interview with Heather Macdonald. February 15, 1994.

20. Pertschuk M. Interview with Heather Macdonald. March 10, 1994.

21. Kiser D. Rationale for support of AB 13 (Friedman) and information on Cal-Stop. Memo to Bob Doyle, Lisa Gaspard. February 16, 1993.

22. California Restaurant Association. Wake up and smell the smoke. Sacramento, 1993 May.

23. California Restaurant Association. Smoking laws: CRA position statements. Sacramento, June 5, 1990.

24. Gillam J. Panel rejects workplace smoking ban. *Los Angeles Times* 1992 June 18.

25. Thompson J-L. Letter to Assembly Member Terry Friedman. June 12, 1992.

26. Friedman T. AB 2667, as amended June 23, 1992. Sacramento, 1992.

27. Najera A. Interview with Heather Macdonald. February 18, 1994.

28. Kiser D. Interview with Heather Macdonald. January 18, 1994.

29. Du Melle F, Davis A, Ballin S. Alert on tobacco industry-initiated clean indoor air legislation and/or amendments. Memo to State Executives, State Public Issue Staff, Tobacco-Free America. February 14, 1989.

30. Friedman T. Letter to Teresa Velo. February 22, 1993.

31. Velo T. Interview with Heather Macdonald. January 18, 1994.

32. Abate B, Najera T. Clarifying Assembly Bill 13 statewide smoking ban and urging strong support by all affiliates. Memo to Affiliate Presidents, Affiliate Executive Directors, Other Interested Parties. March 1993.

33. Alvarez B. Letter to Assembly Member Terry Friedman. March 2, 1993.

34. Samuels BE, Begay ME, Hazan AR, Glantz SA. Philip Morris's failed experiment in Pittsburgh. *J Health Policy, Politics, and Law* 1992;17(2):329-351.

35. Americans for Nonsmokers' Rights. Position on AB 2667: Neutral. Position statement, June 17, 1992.

36. Ennix C, Abate B, Edmiston WA, Yamasaki G, Corlin RF. Memo to interested parties. 1993.

37. Burastero AM. Letter to Terry Friedman. April 9, 1992.

38. Assembly Committee on Labor and Employment. Committee analysis: AB 13 (T. Friedman)—As amended: February 22, 1993. March 3, 1993.

39. Sweeney JP. Wide-ranging smoking ban clears hurdles. *Santa Monica Outlook* 1993 March 10;B2.

40. Carol J, Pertschuk M. Letter to Assembly Member Friedman. December 12, 1992.

41. Blum A. Letter to Mark Pertschuk, Julia Carol, ANR Board Members. June 9, 1993.

42. McIntyre C. Letter to Assembly Member Terry Friedman. August 23, 1993.

43. Snider JR. Letter to Assembly Member Larry Bowler. March 12, 1993.

44. Friedman T. AB 13, as amended February 22, 1993. Memo to interested parties. March 18, 1993.

45. Environmental Protection Agency. *Respiratory health effects of passive smoking: Lung cancer and other disorders.* Report No. EPA 600/6-90/006F. Washington, DC, December 1992.

46. Friedman T. AB 13, as amended April 12, 1993. April 12, 1993.

47. Hunter Y. Letter to Assembly Member Terry Friedman. May 3, 1993.

48. Morain D. Legislature aims fusillade of bills at tobacco industry. *Los Angeles Times* 1993 March 10;A1.

49. American Society of Heating, Refrigeration, and Air Conditioning Engineers. *ASHRAE Standard 62-1989: Ventilation for acceptable indoor air quality.* Atlanta, GA, 1989.

50. Daynard R. What is ASHRAE and why we should care? Paper presented at a workshop on nonsmokers' rights at the 7th World Conference on Tobacco and Health, Perth, Australia, March 30, 1990 (rev. September 10, 1990). Available from Tobacco Control Resources Center, Northeastern University, Boston.

51. Forster JL, Hourigan ME, Kelder S. Locking devices on cigarette vending machines: Evaluation of a city ordinance. *Am J Pub Health* 1992;82(9): 1217–1219.

52. Kotz K, Forster J, Kloehn D. An evaluation of the Minnesota state law to restrict youth access to tobacco. Paper presented at the annual meeting of the American Public Health Association, San Francisco, 1993.

53. Miller J. Staff analysis of Assembly Bill 996 (Tucker) as amended May 4, 1993. August 4, 1993.

54. Sacramento Bee. Tucker's odorous tobacco bill. Editorial. *Sacramento Bee* 1993 April 27.

55. It's amazing what money can buy. *Petaluma Argus-Courier* 1993 June 8.

56. Scott J, Waltman N. Interview with Heather Macdonald. March 1, 1994.

57. LLA Director 5. Interview with Edith Balbach. 1998.

58. McCormick E. Tobacco money tied to smoke bill vote. *San Francisco Examiner* 1993 June 4;A21–A24.

59. Spears L. Assembly OK's bill to snuff out smoking bans. *Contra Costa Times* 1993 June 4;1.

60. Morain D. Assembly bill curbs LA's smoking ban. *Los Angeles Times* 1993 June 4.

61. Benson L. Attached economic impact study and subsequent print and electronic press coverage re: Proposed 100% smoking ban. Memo to members of the California Senate. June 16, 1993.

62. Levin M. Study halts bid to curb smoking. *Los Angeles Times* 1992 June 18.

63. Price Waterhouse. *Potential economic effects of a smoking ban in the state of California.* N.p., 1993 May.

64. Coopers & Lybrand. Letter to Stanley R. Kyker. June 29, 1993.

65. Harrison S. Assembly reverses smoke vote. *Woodland Hills Daily News* 1993 June 8.

66. Morain D. Assembly OK's tough anti-smoking bill it rejected earlier. *Los Angeles Times* 1993 June 8;A3,A27.

67. Miller J. Interview with Heather Macdonald. January 14, 1994.

68. Laufer D. E-mail to Tina Walls re: San Fran. and CA. November 1, 1993. Bates No. 2045891104.

69. Matthews J. Senate panel switches, OKs smoking limits bill. *Sacramento Bee* 1993 July 15;A3.

70. Brady DE. Battle over smoking is heating up. *Los Angeles Times* 1993 July 23, Valley edition.

71. Scott S. Is Terry Friedman giving away too much? *California Journal Weekly* 1993 September 6;3.

72. Merlo E. E-mail to David Laufer re: San Fran. and CA. November 2, 1993. Bates No. 2045891103C.

73. Merlo E. Memorandum to Geoff Bible. January 12, 1994. Bates No. 2022839335.

74. Charlton Research Company. *Philip Morris California statewide*. San Francisco, November 10, 1993. Bates No. 2023324575/4669.

75. Hyde T. Memo to Tom Griscom and Roger Mozingo re: California proposal. January 17, 1994. Bates No. 51256 8081.

76. Californians for Statewide Smoking Restrictions. California Uniform Tobacco Control Act [text of proposed initiative]. 1994.

77. Woodruff T, Rosbrook B, Pierce J, Glantz S. Lower levels of cigarette consumption found in smoke-free workplaces in California. *Archives of Internal Medicine* 1993(153):1485–1493.

78. Stillman F, Becker D, Swank R, Hantula D, Moses H, Glantz S, Waranch H. Ending smoking at the Johns Hopkins medical institutions: An evaluation of smoking prevalence and indoor air pollution. *JAMA* 1990;264:1565–1569.

79. Patten CA, Gilpin E, Cavin S, Pierce JP. Workplace smoking policy and changes in smoking behavior in California: A suggested association. *Tobacco Control* 1995;4:36–41.

80. Macdonald HR, Glantz SA. *Analysis of the smoking and tobacco products, statewide regulation initiative statute*. San Francisco: Institute for Health Policy Studies, School of Medicine, University of California, San Francisco, 1994 March.

81. Mortensen J. Letter to Philip Morris USA retailers. September 19, 1994.

82. Goebel K. Interview with Heather Macdonald. June 5, 1995.

83. Carol J. Interview with Heather Macdonald. July 11, 1995.

84. Martin C. Letter to friends. February 8, 1994.

85. Martin C. Memo to Coalition for a Healthy California (Revived). February 18, 1994.

86. Bullet Poll. *California smoking research*. Verona, NJ: Hypotenuse, Inc., March 10, 1994.

87. Dobson PH. Letter. January 28, 1994.

88. Waters G. Letter to Kathleen DaRosa. March 1, 1994.

89. Nicholl J. Memo re: Draft 100-word title and summary. February 25, 1994.

90. Attorney General. Title and summary of the chief purpose and points of the proposed measure. Sacramento, March 9, 1994.

91. Friedman T. AB 13, as amended March 7, 1994. 1994.

92. Friedman T. AB 13, as amended April 6, 1994. 1994.

93. Weintraub DM, Ingram C. Final budget bills stall as Senate tries to alter measure. *Los Angeles Times* 1993 June 29.

94. Senate Judiciary Committee. Senate Judiciary Committee Hearing. Sacramento, March 22, 1994.

95. Hunter Y. Letter to Terry Friedman. April 14, 1994.

96. American Cancer Society. Position statement. March 23, 1994.

97. American Lung Association. Oppose AB 13 (T. Friedman)—Workplace smoking. Memo, March 23, 1994.

98. Kiser D. Position statement. March 22, 1994.

99. Lucas G. State anti-cigaret bill weakened. *San Francisco Chronicle* 1994 March 23.

100. A rape in Sacramento. Editorial. *Los Angeles Times* 1994 March 27.

101. Friedman T. Statement of Assemblyman Terry Friedman on Senate attack on anti-smoking legislation. Press release, March 23, 1994.

102. Torres A. AB 13 amendments: Memo to members of the media. April 29, 1994.

103. Californians for Statewide Smoking Restrictions. Petition Response Express Pak. Voter mailer. Sacramento, 1994.

104. Hemmila D. Tobacco firm turns the ballot against foes of smoking. *Contra Costa Times* 1994 May 17.

105. Coalition for a Healthy California. Secretary of state in L.A. to inform voters of misrepresentation in tobacco industry petition drive. Press release, April 20, 1994.

106. Green S. Probe of smoking initiative's signers barred. *Sacramento Bee* 1994 June 11.

107. Wilson P. Letter to ANR member. December 21, 1994.

108. Sixth Appellate Court, State of California. *City of San Jose v. Department of Health Services et al.* H016744 (Santa Clara County Superior Court No. CV752231). August 18, 1998.

109. Hager JH. Memo to Donald S. Johnston. October 21, 1994.

110. Van Lohuizen J. Memo to Bob McAdam re: California results. July 29, 1994. Bates No. ATX05 0048753/8754.

111. Mozingo R, Hyde T. Memorandum to Tom Griscom and B. Oglesby re: Initiatives in Colorado, California, Arizona. August 4, 1994. Bates No. 51253 5293/5295.

112. Vander Jagt G. Letter to Julie Johnston. 1994.

113. V. Lance Tarrance & Associates. *Kern County smoking study.* Houston, 1982 September.

114. Roper Organization. *A study of public attitudes towards cigarette smoking and the tobacco industry.* Prepared for the Tobacco Institute. Washington, DC, 1978 May.

115. McAdam B. Memorandum to interested parties re: Weekly ballot issue update. September 22, 1994. Bates No. ATX 040540363/0366.

116. Nicholl J. Interview with Heather Macdonald. February 2, 1995.

117. Solis SE. Poll finds few voters know about fall initiatives. *San Francisco Chronicle* 1994 July 28;A17–A18.

118. Field Institute. Majorities favor Prop. 184 (three strikes) but oppose Prop. 186 (single-payer health), opinions of Prop. 188 (smoking) are evenly split. Press release, September 28, 1994.

119. Feldman P. Times Poll: 62 percent would bar services to illegal immigrants. *Los Angeles Times* 1994 September 14;A1.

120. Russell S. Interview with Heather Macdonald. *San Francisco Chronicle* 1995 May 31.

121. Morain D. Interview with Heather Macdonald. *Los Angeles Times* 1995 June 1.

122. Knepprath P. Interview with Heather Macdonald. November 29, 1994.

123. Miller J. Interview with Heather Macdonald. Senate Health Committee. June 15, 1995.

124. McElroy L. Memo to Jack Nicholl. October 6, 1994.

125. Ballin S. Interview with Heather Macdonald. December 16, 1994.

126. Mills A. Interview with Heather Macdonald. December 14, 1994.

127. Watson S. Interview with Heather Macdonald. July 17, 1995.

128. Webb G. Non-partisan ads draw partisan fire. *San Jose Mercury News* 1994 October 21.

129. Morain D. Lungren tries to avoid link of big tobacco. *Los Angeles Times* 1998 September 23;A1.

130. Russell S. Smoking initiative ad battle heats up. *San Francisco Chronicle* 1994 October 21;A4.

131. Webb G. Panel allows copycat Prop. 188 ads. *San Jose Mercury News* 1994 November 8;3B.

132. Californians for Statewide Smoking Restrictions—Yes on Proposition 188. What do people think about smoking laws? Voter contact mail, 1994.

133. Morain D. Tobacco industry abandons low profile. *Los Angeles Times* 1994 October 26;A3.

134. Frick N. Statement of Nancy Frick re: Proposition 188. October 27, 1994.

135. Levy D. California smoking initiative has tobacco industry foes fuming. *USA Today* 1994 November 4;4D.

136. Tyler J. Interview with Heather Macdonald. January 31, 1995.

137. Sohn G. Interview with Heather Macdonald. December 15, 1994.

138. Carol J. Letter to general manager. October 21, 1994.

139. Americans for Nonsmokers' Rights. Stations agreeing to use the full name of Proposition 188's sponsor. Press release, 1994.

140. Americans for Nonsmokers' Rights. Americans for Nonsmokers' Rights files FCC complaint over Prop 188 ads. October 25, 1994.

141. Carol J. Letter. October 27, 1994.

142. Coalition for a Healthy California. FCC says broadcasters must disclose tobacco ties to Pro-188 commercials. Press release, November 1, 1994.

143. McAdam B. Memo to interested parties. November 2, 1994. Bates No. ATX 04054033.

144. American Cancer Society. Bullet Poll results. Press release, November 15, 1994.

145. Hanauer P. Interview with Edith Balbach. June 4, 1998.

146. American Cancer Society, California Division, Public Issues Office. Letter to Stanton Glantz re: Proposition 188 Report. December 27, 1995.

147. Scott S. Harmonic convergence: Tobacco wars open on several fronts in 1994. *California Journal Weekly* 1994 March 28;3.

CHAPTER 12

1. Jacobs P. Ex-allies feud over use of smoking tax. *Los Angeles Times* 1994 June 27;A1.

2. State of California, Governor's Office. Governor's budget summary, 1994–1995. Sacramento, January 7, 1994.

3. Miller J. Comments on manuscript. January 31, 1999.

4. State of California, Legislative Analyst's Office. *Analysis of the 1994–1995 budget bill.* Sacramento, 1994.

5. Knepprath P, Najera T. Interview with Edith Balbach. August 16, 1996.

6. Isenberg P. Interview with Edith Balbach. April 9, 1997.

7. McNeil E. Interview with Edith Balbach. October 23, 1996.

8. State of California, Senate Rules Committee. *Tobacco surtax programs.* Sacramento, January 27, 1994.

9. Najera T, Miller J. Interview with Michael Begay. July 22, 1994.

10. California Wellness Foundation. *The future of tobacco control: California Strategic Summit.* Los Angeles, December 15–16, 1993.

11. Rutherford GW. Letter to Edward L. Baker. April 26, 1993.

12. Novotny T. *Structural evaluation: California's Proposition 99–funded Tobacco Control Program.* US Department of Health and Human Services, Public Health Service, Centers for Disease Control and Prevention, February 25, 1994.

13. Scott S. Health Services holding up report on anti-smoking program. *California Journal Weekly* 1994 February 14;5.

14. American Lung Association of California, Government Relations Office. AB 816 (Isenberg)—Reauthorization of Proposition 99. Action Alert, February 16, 1994.

15. American Lung Association of California, Government Relations Committee. Minutes. Sacramento, March 4, 1994.

16. Knepprath P. Memo to Tony Najera, John Miller, and Betty Turner. March 18, 1994.

17. Griffin M. Interview with Edith Balbach. July 22, 1996.

18. Castoreno C. Interview with Edith Balbach. July 11, 1996.

19. Hobart R. Interview with Edith Balbach. July 25, 1996.

20. Miller J. Interview with Edith Balbach. July 24, 1996.

21. American Lung Association of California, Government Relations Office. Memo to interested parties re: Reauthorization of Proposition 99. May 9, 1994.

22. Beerline D. Interview with Edith Balbach. September 26, 1996.

23. Martin C. Interview with Edith Balbach. September 4, 1996.

24. Pomer B. Letter to Phil Isenberg. June 21, 1994.

25. Pierce JP. Letter to Gordon Cumming re: Evaluation of tobacco control. May 16, 1994.

26. Jacobs P. No-smoking debate flares over funding. *Los Angeles Times* 1994 June 26;A1.

27. Glantz SA. Changes in cigarette consumption, prices, and tobacco industry revenues associated with California's Proposition 99. *Tobacco Control* 1993;2:311–314.

28. Californians for Smokers' Rights. [Analysis] of Prop 99 Funds. 1994(?)

29. California Medical Association. Some tobacco tax local anti-tobacco "Health Education." 1994 May.

30. Sanders D. Make smoke-free pork-free. *San Francisco Chronicle* 1994 March 28.

31. Heiser PF, Begay ME. The campaign to raise the tobacco tax in Massachusetts. *Am J Pub Health* 1997;87(6):968–973.

32. Koh HK. An analysis of the successful 1992 Massachusetts tobacco tax initiative. *Tobacco Control* 1996;5(3):220–225.

33. Aguinaga S, Glantz S. *Tobacco control in Arizona, 1973–1997.* San Francisco: Institute for Health Policy Studies, School of Medicine, University of California, San Francisco, 1997 October. (http://www.library.ucsf.edu/tobacco/az/)

34. Aguinaga S, Glantz SA. The use of public records acts to interfere with tobacco control. *Tobacco Control* 1995;1995(4):222–230.

35. Bialous SA, Glantz SA. Arizona's tobacco control initiative illustrates the need for continuing oversight by tobacco control advocates. *Tobacco Control* 1999;8:141–151.

36. Carol J. Interview with Edith Balbach. August 8 and September 5, 1996.

37. Hobart R. Note to Edith Balbach. August 4, 1997.

38. American Lung Association of California. Statement on lawsuit re: Prop. 99 tobacco tax revenues. Press release, April 8, 1994.

39. Martin CB. Letter to Phil Isenberg. June 28, 1994.

40. Ennix CL, Edmiston A. Letter to Jack Peltason. December 22, 1992.

41. Arditti S. Letter to the Honorable Phillip Isenberg. June 30, 1994.

42. Southwest Regional Laboratory. *California programs to prevent and reduce drug, alcohol, and tobacco use among in-school youth.* Los Alamitos, 1994 March.

43. Monardi FM, Balbach ED, Aquinaga S, Glantz SA. *Shifting allegiances: Tobacco industry political expenditures in California January 1995–March 1996.* San Francisco, Institute for Health Policy Studies, School of Medicine, University of California, San Francisco, 1996 April. (http://www.library.ucsf.edu/tobacco/sa/)

44. California Medical Association. Report to the Board of Trustees from the Executive Committee. May 13–14, 1994.

45. Foster D. The Lame Duck State: Term limits and the hobbling of California state government. *Harper's* 1994 February; 65–75.

46. Williams L. Willie Brown and the tobacco lobby. *San Francisco Examiner* 1995 September 17;B1.

47. Scott S. Interview with Edith Balbach. September 18, 1996.

48. Kennedy R. Interview with Edith Balbach. April 1, 1997.

49. Knepprath P. Save Prop. 99 Coalition: Legislators to escalate attack on administration, opponents of anti-tobacco education and research programs. Press release, June 1, 1994.

50. Knepprath P. Prop. 99 Action Alert, June 6, 1994.

51. Holsinger J. Letter to the Honorable Bill Lockyer. July 7, 1994.

52. Holsinger J. Letter to the Honorable Willie Brown. July 6, 1994.

53. Koerner S. Legislature set to kill California's historic anti-tobacco campaign. Press release, July 6, 1994.

54. American Lung Association. AB 816 Conference Report—OPPOSE. Floor Alert, July 7, 1994.

55. Thompson S, McNeil E. Memo to honorable members of the California Legislature. July 6, 1994.

56. Aguinaga S, MacDonald H, Traynor M, Begay ME, Glantz SA. *Undermining popular government: Tobacco industry political expenditures in California 1993–1994*. Institute for Health Policy Studies, School of Medicine, University of California, San Francisco, 1995 May. (http://www.library.ucsf.edu/kr/data/94.htm)

57. Los Angeles Times. A rape in Sacramento. Editorial. *Los Angeles Times* 1994 March 27.

58. Begay ME, Traynor MP, Glantz SA. *The twilight of Proposition 99: Reauthorization of tobacco education programs and tobacco industry expenditures in 1993*. San Francisco: Institute for Health Policy Studies, School of Medicine, University of California, San Francisco, 1994 March.

CHAPTER 13

1. State of California, California State Legislature. Assembly Bill 816. July 1994.

2. Bowser R. Interview with Edith D. Balbach. August 21, 1996.

3. Glynn T, Manley M. *How to help your patients stop smoking: A National Cancer Institute manual for physicians*. Bethesda, MD: National Institutes of Health, 1989. NIH Publication No. 93-3064.

4. Epps R, Manley M. *Clinical interventions to prevent tobacco use by children and adolescents: A supplement to "How to help your patients stop smoking: A National Cancer Institute guide for physicians."* Bethesda, MD: National Institutes of Health, 1991.

5. Manley M, Epps R, Husten C, Glynn T, Shopland D. Clinical interventions in tobacco control. *JAMA* 1991;266(22):3172–3173.

6. Horton A. Declaration of Ann Horton. Declaration, Superior Court of the State of California, County of Sacramento, November 8, 1994. Case No. 379257.

7. Range R. Declaration of Ruth S. Range. Declaration, Superior Court of the State of California, County of Sacramento, November 2, 1994. Case No. 379257.

8. Cumming GH. Deposition of Gordon H. Cumming. Deposition, Superior Court of the State of California, County of Sacramento, October 12, 1994. Case No. 379257.

9. Tobacco Education Oversight Committee. Minutes. December 3, 1991.

10. California Department of Health Services. *PM 160 Instructions*. Sacramento, 1992 January.

11. Manley MW. Declaration of Marc W. Manley. December 12, 1994.

12. Glynn T. Essential elements of school-based smoking prevention programs. *J School Health* 1989;59:181–188.

13. Epps RP, Manley MW. A physician's guide to preventing tobacco use during childhood and adolescence. *Pediatrics* 1991;88(1):140–144.

14. Breslow L. Declaration of Lester Breslow. Declaration. Los Angeles: University of California, Los Angeles. November 17, 1994.

15. Kennedy R. Interview with Edith Balbach. April 1, 1997.

16. Martin C. Letter to Molly Joel Coye. October 16, 1992.

17. Coye MJ. Letter to Carolyn Martin. January 22, 1993.

18. Bal D, Shah R. Memo to health officers, Maternal and Child Health directors, Tobacco Control Project directors, Local Lead Agencies. November 14, 1991.

19. Breslow L. Letter to Molly Joel Coye. October 5, 1992.

20. Kessler SW. Letter to Jennie Cook. July 26, 1993.

21. Gregory MA. CHDP Information Notice #94-C. February 10, 1994.

22. Skolnick A. Judge rules diversion of antismoking money illegal, victory for California Tobacco Control Program. *JAMA* 1995;273(8):610–611.

23. Lungren DE. Respondents' memorandum of points and authorities re: Tailoring of relief to be granted, Case No. 379257 [*American Lung Association et al. v. Pete Wilson, Governor of the State of California et al.*, Consolidated Case Nos. 379257 and 379460], Superior Court of the State of California, County of Sacramento. December 30, 1994.

24. Gregory BM. Letter to Diane E. Watson. June 13, 1991.

25. Gregory BM. Letter to Phil Isenberg. June 27, 1991.

26. Gregory BM. Letter to Elizabeth Hill. March 10, 1992.

27. Waters G, Perlite D. Petitioners' opposition memorandum re: Relief and supporting exhibits V through Y, Case No. 379257 [Consolidated Case Nos. 379257 and 379450]. January 9, 1995.

28. Glantz SA. Thoughts on the Prop. 99 lawsuit remedy. Memorandum, January 2, 1995.

29. Waters G. Memo to Tony Najera and Diane Perlite. February 23, 1995.

30. Americans for Nonsmokers' Rights. ANR Prop. 99 Lawsuit—Background. Press release, January 17, 1995.

31. Wilson P. Letter to members of the California State Legislature. June 22, 1995.

32. American Lung Association. ALAC on winning streak with Prop. 99 lawsuit. *Capitol Correspondence* 1995 June; 1.

33. Monardi FM, Balbach ED, Aquinaga S, Glantz SA. *Shifting allegiances: Tobacco industry political expenditures in California January 1995–March 1996.* San Francisco: Institute for Health Policy Studies, School of Medicine, University of California, San Francisco, 1996 April. (http://www.library.ucsf.edu/tobacco/sa/)

34. Gengler R, Donaldson R, Margolis SE, Reeve B. Letter to the Honorable Pete Wilson. June 27, 1995.

35. State of California, California State Legislature. Senate Bill 493. July 1995.

36. Hallett C. Interview with Edith Balbach. August 6, 1996.

37. Martin C. Interview with Edith Balbach. September 4, 1996.

38. American Lung Association, Government Relations Office. Proposi-

tion 99/AB 816 cigarette tax reauthorization. *Capitol Correspondence* 1994 November;4.

CHAPTER 14

1. Frost L. State launches counterattack against rise in youth smoking. Press release, September 28, 1995.

2. Knepprath P, Najera T. Interview with Edith Balbach. August 16, 1996.

3. Carol J. Interview with Edith Balbach. August 8 and September 5, 1996.

4. Scott S. Interview with Edith Balbach. September 18, 1996.

5. Adams M. Interview with Edith Balbach. July 11, 1996.

6. Hobart R. Interview with Edith Balbach. July 25, 1996.

7. Glantz SA. Interview with Edith Balbach. September 26, 1996.

8. Beerline D. Interview with Edith Balbach. September 26, 1996.

9. Miller J. Interview with Edith Balbach. July 24, 1996.

10. Lewin J. Interview with Edith Balbach. October 17, 1996.

11. Wilson P. Governor's budget summary 1996–1997. Sacramento, January 10, 1996.

12. Aguinaga S, MacDonald H, Traynor M, Begay ME, Glantz SA. *Undermining popular government: Tobacco industry political expenditures in California 1993–1994.* Institute for Health Policy Studies, School of Medicine, University of California, San Francisco, 1995 May. (http://www.library.ucsf.edu/kr/data/94.htm)

13. American Cancer Society, American Heart Association, American Lung Association. Health groups outraged by governor's budget: Announce campaign to defeat raid on Prop. 99 tobacco fund. Press release, January 11, 1996.

14. Watson D, Hayden T, Petris N. Caucus position on tobacco issues. Memo, April 24, 1996.

15. Monardi FM, Balbach ED, Aguinaga S, Glantz SA. *Shifting allegiances: Tobacco industry political expenditures in California January 1995–March 1996.* San Francisco: Institute for Health Policy Studies, School of Medicine, University of California, San Francisco, 1996 April. (http://www.library.ucsf.edu/tobacco/sa/)

16. Balbach ED, Monardi FM, Fox BJ, Glantz SA. *Holding government accountable: Tobacco policy making in California, 1995–1997.* Institute for Health Policy Studies, School of Medicine, University of California, San Francisco, 1997 June. (http://www.library.ucsf.edu/kr/data/421.htm)

17. Morain D. Tobacco lobby gaining muscle in Sacramento. *Los Angeles Times* 1996 April 22;A1.

18. Whole new pack of buddies for the cigarette industry. Editorial. *Los Angeles Times* 1996 April 23;B10.

19. Begay ME, Glantz SA. *Undoing Proposition 99: Political expenditures by the tobacco industry in California politics in 1991.* San Francisco: Institute for Health Policy Studies, School of Medicine, University of California, San Francisco, 1992 April.

20. Katz R. Interview with Edith Balbach. April 3, 1997.

21. Van Maren D. Interview with Edith Balbach. September 18, 1996.

22. Isenberg P. Interview with Edith Balbach. April 9, 1997.

23. Bowser R. Interview with Edith Balbach. August 21, 1996.

24. Miller NC. Letter to Roman Bowser. January 31, 1996.

25. Thompson SM. Letter to Roman Bowser. February 9, 1996.

26. Russell S. Tobacco tiff irks state doctors. *San Francisco Chronicle* 1996 February 14;A14.

27. McNeil E. Interview with Edith Balbach. October 23, 1996.

28. Carol J. Memo to Roman Bowser, Mary Adams, Stan Glantz, Herb Gunther, Michael Almond. March 18, 1996.

29. Gunther H. Interview with Edith Balbach. August 14, 1996.

30. Kennedy R. Interview with Edith Balbach. April 1, 1997.

31. California Medical Association. House of Delegates Resolution. March 3, 1996.

32. California Medical Association. Proposition 99 funding. April 1996.

33. Dyer J. Memo to Buffy. April 24, 1990.

34. Williams L. Memo: Candidate Wilson 'pro-tobacco.' *San Francisco Examiner* 1996 April 16;A1.

35. Levin M. Leaked memo describes Wilson as 'pro-tobacco.' *Los Angeles Times* 1996 April 16;A1.

36. Russell S. Philip Morris called Wilson 'pro-tobacco.' *San Francisco Chronicle* 1996 April 17;A13.

37. Stone PH. Our good friend, the governor. *Mother Jones* 1996 May/June; 38–39.

38. Beerline D, Martin C. Letter to Patricia Lozada-Santone and Gary O'Connell. April 29, 1996.

39. Martin C. Interview with Edith Balbach. September 4, 1996.

40. Morain D. Pringle targets anti-tobacco research, ads. *Los Angeles Times* 1996 June 27;A3.

41. Frost L. State health director responds to Proposition 99 spending plan. Press release, May 17, 1996.

42. Kennan N, Marketing and Research Counselors, Inc. An action-oriented research program for discovering and creating the best possible image for Viceroy cigarettes. Prepared for Ted Bates Advertising on behalf of Brown and Williamson Tobacco. 1975 March. FTC document AO11345. Quoted in Myers M, Iscoe C, Jennings C, Lenox W, Lenox E, Minsky E, Sacks A. *Staff report on the cigarette advertising investigation.* US Federal Trade Commission, 1991 May.

43. Coalition to Restore Prop 99. Coalition applauds additional funding, questions program changes. May 17, 1996.

44. Kerk C, Najera T. Memorandum to executive directors, communications and advocacy staff re: Proposition 99 funding proposal. May 17, 1996.

45. Smelling the smoke of governor's plan. *San Francisco Chronicle* 1996 June 3;A18.

46. Kerk C. More adults lighting up as state dismantles tobacco control programs. Press release, June 5, 1996.

47. Shuit D. Smoking rose at the end of '95, survey finds. *Los Angeles Times* 1996 June 12;A3.

48. Russell S. Small increase reported in adult smoking. *San Francisco Chronicle* 1996 June 5;A1.

49. A plan goes up in smoke. *San Francisco Examiner* 1996 January 10;A14.

50. Guthrie J. Speaker targets ads against smoking. *San Francisco Examiner* 1996 June 27;A1.

51. Russell S. Smoking foes assail limits on health ads. *San Francisco Chronicle* 1996 June 27;A16.

52. Goldman L, Glantz S. Evaluation of antismoking advertising campaigns. *JAMA* 1998;279(10):772–777.

53. Guthrie J. State bids to control UC cigarette studies. *San Francisco Examiner* 1996 July 2;A1.

54. The speaker's smoke machine. *Sacramento Bee* 1996 June 28;B6.

55. Hopper CL, Hershman LC. Letter to Kathryn Gaither and Stanley Cubanski. July 1, 1996.

56. Castoreno C. Interview with Edith Balbach. July 11, 1996.

57. State of California, California State Legislature. *1996–97 Budget.* Sacramento, 1996.

58. American Lung Association of California, Government Relations Office. Prop. 99 funding plan adopted! Action Alert, June 20, 1996.

59. Field Institute. *Statistical tabulations from a survey of Californians on Proposition 99 funding and the tobacco industry.* San Francisco, 1996 June.

60. Page BI, Shapiro RY. *The rational public.* Chicago: University of Chicago Press, 1992.

61. State of California, Office of the Governor. Veto message. Sacramento, August 21, 1998.

62. Malmgren KL. Memorandum to Samuel D. Chilcote, Jr. April 18, 1990. Bates No. TIMN 298437/298420W.

CHAPTER 15

1. Malmgren KL. Memorandum to Samuel D. Chilcote, Jr. April 18, 1990. Bates No. TIMN 298437/298420W.

2. Warren J, Morain D. Bid to dilute anti-smoking effort revealed. *Los Angeles Times* 1998 January 21.

3. Pierce JP, Gilpin EA, Emery SL, White M, Rosbrook B, Berry C. Has the California Tobacco Control Program reduced smoking? *JAMA* 1998;280(10): 893–899.

4. Nielsen, Merksamer. Memorandum to Executive Committee re: California state budget. December 15, 1988. Bates No. 50763 7136/7160.

5. Tobacco Institute, State Activities Division. *Project California proposal.* Washington, DC, February 21, 1989. Bates No. 2025848159/48192.

6. Kahan JS. Letter from Hogan & Hartson to Freedom of Information Officer at Public Health Service. November 13, 1987.

7. KRC Research & Consulting. Memo to Stanley Temko, Covington & Burling, re: California quantitative research. May 3, 1990. Bates No. TIMN 355366/355370.

8. KRC Research & Consulting. *Qualitative research report: Reaction to California's Proposition 99 and its 1990 anti-smoking media campaign*. New York (?), 1990 May. Bates No. TIMN 334989/335167.

9. Pierce JP, Gilpin EA, Emery SL, Farkas AJ, Zhu SH, Choi WS, Berry CC, Distefan JM, White MM, Soroko S, Navarro A. *Tobacco control in California: Who's winning the war?* San Diego: University of California, San Diego, June 30, 1998.

10. Johnston JW. Letter to Kimberly Belshé. October 13, 1994.

11. Glick MR, London M. Letter to Alan Nesbitt. October 6, 1994.

12. Glick MR, London M. Letter to Asher/Gould Advertising, Inc. October 6, 1994.

13. Glick MR, London M. Letter to Ms. Kim Belshé. October 6, 1994.

14. Silverman B. Letter to Ms. Valerie Quinn. October 17, 1994.

15. Russell S. Tobacco firm loses bid to yank TV ad. *San Francisco Chronicle* 1994 October 13;A26.

16. Ayres BD. Stations pull ad critical of tobacco industry. *New York Times* 1994 October 16;17.

17. Raeburn P. Ad against smoking pulled. *Sacramento Bee* 1994 October 17.

18. Jacobs P. Some TV stations drop anti-smoking ad. *Los Angeles Times* 1994 October 14.

19. Antismoking TV ads dropped after threat of suit by Reynolds. *Wall Street Journal* 1994 October 14;B14.

20. Pants on fire: Big Tobacco trots out the big lie. *Minneapolis Star Tribune* 1994 October 17;10-A.

21. Belshé SK. Letter to Martin G. Glick. October 12, 1994.

22. Stevens C. E-mail to Dileep Bal. February 1, 1995.

23. California Department of Health Services, Tobacco Education and Research Oversight Committee. *Toward a tobacco-free California: Renewing the commitment 1997–2000*. Sacramento, July 31, 1997.

24. Smoley SR. Letter to Bailey, Pertschuk, and Fung. March 7, 1997.

25. Glantz S, Slade J, Bero L, Hanauer P, Barnes L. *The cigarette papers*. Berkeley: University of California Press, 1996.

26. Pringle P. *Cornered: Big Tobacco at the bar of justice*. New York: Henry Holt, 1998.

27. Shimizu R. E-mail to Colleen Stevens. July 5, 1996.

28. Silverman BG. Letter to Dileep G. Bal. July 2, 1996.

29. Genest M. E-mail to Dileep Bal. August 23, 1996.

30. Bal D. E-mail to Mike Genest re: Media update. August 21, 1996.

31. Munso J. Memo to all deputy directors. September 16, 1996.

32. Lyman DO. E-mail to James W. Stratton. September 25, 1996.

33. Shimizu R. E-mail to Dileep Bal re: Questions regarding the media campaign strategy. October 10, 1996.

34. Bal D. E-mail to Don Lyman re: Questions regarding the media campaign strategy. October 10, 1996.

35. Bal D. E-mail to Don Lyman re: Questions regarding the media campaign strategy. October 11, 1996.

36. Bal DG, Kizer KW, Felten PG, Mozar HN, Niemeyer D. Reducing to-

bacco consumption in California: Development of a statewide anti-tobacco use campaign. *JAMA* 1990;264(12):1570–1574.

37. Cook JR. Letter to S. Kimberly Belshé. April 2, 1997.

38. Cook JR. Letter to James Stratton. December 31, 1996.

39. Tobacco Education and Research Oversight Committee, Tobacco Control Section, Department of Health Services. Minutes. February 10, 1997.

40. State of California, Department of Health Services. Standard agreement with Asher/Gould Advertising. December 1, 1996. Report No. 96-26137.

41. Stevens C. Memo to Nikki. March (?), 1997.

42. Shimizu R. E-mail to Jim Howard and Dileep Bal. January 27, 1997.

43. Friedman M. *Teen anti-smoking strategy focus groups. Summary report.* Los Angeles, 1996 November.

44. Steele C. Letter to Colleen Stevens. December 4, 1996.

45. Williams L. Cancer Society honoring tobacco favorite Brown. *San Francisco Examiner* 1996 September 15;A1.

46. Cancer Society's unlikely hero. *San Francisco Examiner* 1996 September 17.

47. Tobacco "Humanitarian." Editorial. *San Francisco Chronicle* 1996 September 17.

48. Morse R. Mayor's latest lucky strike: Top of the Mark fete for Cancer Society's favorite. *San Francisco Examiner* 1996 April 15.

49. Bailey L, Fung G, Pertschuk M. Letter to Sandra Smoley. February 4, 1997.

50. Bailey L, Fung CL, Pertschuk M. Letter to Governor Pete Wilson. April 15, 1997.

51. Haddad BA. Letter to Lisa Bailey, Gordon L. Fund, and Mark Pertschuk. May 16, 1997.

52. Cook J. Interview with Edith Balbach. March 19, 1998.

53. Morain D. Controversy flares over state's anti-tobacco efforts. *Los Angeles Times* 1997 February 11;A3.

54. Health groups rap Wilson. *Oakland Tribune* 1997 February 11.

55. Health groups say governor too soft on tobacco. *San Jose Mercury News* 1997 February 11.

56. Anti-smoking groups demand state get tougher. *Modesto Bee* 1997 February 11.

57. Bernstein D. Health groups: Anti-smoking ads stifled? *Sacramento Bee* 1997 February 11.

58. Geissinger S. Governor chided for policies on tobacco. *Contra Costa Times* 1997 February 11.

59. Gunnison RB. Wilson administration hit for hiding anti-smoking ads. *San Francisco Chronicle* 1997 February 11;A18.

60. Belshé SK. Letter to Jennie Cook. March 19, 1997.

61. Balbach E. Notes from Tobacco Education Oversight Committee meeting. March 25, 1997.

62. Matthews J. Smoking by adults increases. *Sacramento Bee* 1997 March 26.

63. Gunnison RB. More Californians are lighting up. *San Francisco Chronicle* 1997 March 26;A1.

64. Morain D. Adult smoking rises sharply in California. *Los Angeles Times* 1997 March 26;A1.

65. Steele C. Memo to Mike Genest. February 10, 1998.

66. Asher H. Memorandum to Joel Hochberg and Christine Steele. May 7, 1998.

67. Glantz S. Letter to Kimberly Belshé. August 31, 1998.

68. Asher & Partners. Response to questions for October 16th Hearing. 1998.

69. Genest M. E-mail to Jim Stratton, Jim Howard, Don Lyman, and C. Connors. March 4, 1997.

70. Ruppert B. E-mail to Dileep Bal re: TEROC meeting minutes. May 12, 1997.

71. Lyman D. E-mail to Dileep Bal re: TEROC meeting minutes. May 19, 1997.

72. Lyman D. E-mail to Dileep Bal re: TEROC agenda. May 29, 1997.

73. Shimizu R. E-mail to Jim Howard and Dileep Bal re: TEROC agenda. May 30, 1997.

74. Stratton J. E-mail to Donald Lyman, Dileep Bal, Michael Genest, re: TEROC agenda. May 30, 1997.

75. Johnson M. E-mail to Dileep Bal re: CTS data and TEROC. June 5, 1997.

76. Lyman D. E-mail to Jim Stratton re: TEROC agenda. May 30, 1997.

77. Williams L. Tobacco foe picked for state panel. *San Francisco Examiner* 1997 May 19;A6.

78. Lyman D. E-mail to Robin Shimizu re: TEROC Master Plan. July 16, 1997.

79. Macdonald HR, Glantz SA. The political realities of statewide smoking legislation. *Tobacco Control* 1997;6:41–54.

80. Hager JH. Memo to Donald S. Johnston. October 21, 1994.

81. Tobacco Control Section, Department of Health Services. *TCS AB 13 LLA smokefree bar survey results (July–September, 1996).* Sacramento, 1996.

82. Stauber J, Rampton S. *Toxic sludge is good for you.* Monroe, ME: Common Courage Press, 1995.

83. Christiansen E. *A survey on California's law for a smokefree workplace (AB 13): Attitudes after the first year of implementation.* Lincoln, NE: Gallup Organization, 1996 March.

84. Field Research Corporation. *A survey of California adults age 21 or older about smoking policies and smoke-free bars.* San Francisco, 1997 July.

85. Vellinga ML. Wilson urged to publicize bar-smoking ban. *Sacramento Bee* 1997 October 3;A3.

86. Hallett C. Interview with Sheryl Magzamen. November 16, 1998.

87. Smith S. Interview with Edith Balbach. June 24, 1998.

88. Tobacco Control Section, Department of Health Services. Policy #12 Lobbying Policy. Sacramento, 1996 April.

89. C. W. Crocker Communications, Inc. "Save a Waitress." Script for radio advertisement. Sacramento, August 19, 1997.

90. American Lung Association of California, Government Relations Office. Memo to ALAC leadership. Action Alert, August 29, 1997.

91. Roeseler A. Letter to Sue Smith. September 5, 1997.

92. American Lung Association-Sacramento-Emigrant Trails. Management meeting minutes. November 21, 1997.

93. Shimizu R. Letter to Sue Smith. December 16, 1997.

94. Ruppert B. Letter to John P. Pierce and Elizabeth Gilpin. December 8, 1997.

95. Johnson MD. Letter to John Pierce and Elizabeth Gilpin. June 15, 1998.

96. Pierce J. Memo to Evaluation Advisory Committee members for the California Tobacco Control Program. June 17, 1998.

97. Where there's smoke. Editorial. *San Diego Union-Tribune* 1998 September 25.

98. Wallack L. E-mail to Dileep Bal re: Termination of UCSD contract. August 20, 1998.

99. Cummings M. E-mail to Dileep Bal and Michael Johnson. June 22, 1998.

100. Cook JR. Letter to the Honorable Diane Watson. September 11, 1998.

101. Griffith D. State war on tobacco: Mixed results. *Sacramento Bee* 1998 September 9.

102. Monmaney T. Cuts hamper anti-smoking bid, study says. *Los Angeles Times* 1998 September 9.

103. Russell S. Cigarette firms outspend state—Fewer people quit as Tobacco Control Program is gutted. *San Francisco Chronicle* 1998 September 9;A15.

104. Williams L. AMA journal: Anti-smoking drive crippled. *San Francisco Examiner* 1998 September 9;A6.

105. LLA Director 10. Interview with Edith Balbach. 1998.

CHAPTER 16

1. Bal DG, Kizer KW, Felten PG, Mozar HN, Niemeyer D. Reducing tobacco consumption in California: Development of a statewide anti-tobacco use campaign. *JAMA* 1990;264(12):1570–1574.

2. Tobacco Education and Research Oversight Committee, California Department of Health Services. *Toward a tobacco-free California: Renewing the commitment 1997–2000.* Sacramento, July 31, 1997.

3. Glantz SA. Changes in cigarette consumption, prices, and tobacco industry revenues associated with California's Proposition 99. *Tobacco Control* 1993;2:311–314.

4. Pierce JP, Gilpin EA, Emery SL, Farkas AJ, Zhu SH, Choi WS, Berry CC, Distefan JM, White MM, Soroko S, Navarro A. *Tobacco control in California: Who's winning the war?* San Diego: University of California, San Diego, June 30, 1998.

5. Pierce JP, Gilpin EA, Emery SL, White M, Rosbrook B, Berry C. Has the California Tobacco Control Program reduced smoking? *JAMA* 1998;280(10).

6. Balbach ED, Monardi FM, Fox BJ, Glantz SA. *Holding government accountable: Tobacco policy making in California, 1995–1997.* San Francisco: Institute for Health Policy Studies, School of Medicine, University of California, San Francisco, 1997 June. (http://www.library.ucsf.edu/kr/data/421.htm)

7. Lightwood JM, Glantz SA. Short-term economic and health benefits of

smoking cessation: Myocardial infarction and stroke. *Circulation* 1997;96(4): 1089–1096.

8. Lightwood J, Phibbs C, Glantz S. Short-term health and economic benefits of smoking cessation: Low birth weight. *Pediatrics* 1999;(in press).

9. Glantz SA. Preventing tobacco use—the youth access trap. *Am J Pub Health* 1996;86(2):156–158.

10. Goldman L, Glantz S. Evaluation of antismoking advertising campaigns. *JAMA* 1998;279(10):772–777.

11. California Department of Health Services. "A Couple More Good Years." Script for television advertisement. 1990.

12. Glantz S, Slade J, Bero L, Hanauer P, Barnes L. *The cigarette papers.* Berkeley: University of California Press, 1996.

13. Martin C. Memo to Stan Glantz and Edith Balbach. October 24, 1998.

14. A-K Associates, Inc., Kinney P. *Status and campaign plan for tobacco tax initiative.* Sacramento, September 24, 1987. Bates No. 50660 9215/9232.

15. Tobacco Institute, State Activities Division. *Project California proposal.* Washington, DC, February 21, 1989. Bates No. 2025848159/48192.

16. Nielsen, Merksamer. Memorandum to Executive Committee re: California state budget. December 15, 1988. Bates No. 50763 7136/7160.

17. Wolinsky H, Brune T. *The serpent on the staff.* New York: G. P. Putnam's Sons, 1994.

18. Sharfstein J. 1996 Congressional campaign priorities of the AMA: Tackling tobacco or limiting malpractice awards? *Am J Pub Health* 1998;88:1233–1236.

19. Oliver TR, Paul-Shaheen P. Translating ideas into actions: Entrepreneurial leadership in state health care reforms. *J Health Policy, Politics, and Law* 1997;22(3):721–788.

20. Feldman M. *Order without design.* Stanford, CA: Stanford University Press, 1989.

21. Stone DA. *Policy paradox: The art of political decision making.* New York: W. W. Norton, 1997.

22. Jacobson PD, Wasserman J, Raube K. The politics of anti-smoking legislation. *J Health Policy, Politics, and Law* 1993;18(4):787–819.

23. Loveday P. Speech in Minneapolis. February 3, 1979. Bates No. 2024372711/2741.

24. Pepples E. *Campaign report—Proposition 5, California 1978.* Louisville, KY: Brown and Williamson Tobacco, January 11, 1979. Brown and Williamson Document 2302.05.

25. Taylor P. *The smoke ring.* New York: Pantheon Books, 1984.

26. Balbach ED, Glantz SA. Tobacco. In: Faigman DL, Kaye D, Saks MJ, Sanders J, eds. *Modern scientific evidence: The law and science of expert testimony.* St. Paul: West Publishing Co., 1997. pp. 453–506.

27. Allenby C. Interview with Michael Traynor. June 16, 1995.

28. Kingdon JW. *Agendas, alternatives, and public policies.* 2d ed. New York: Harper Collins, 1995.

29. Page BI, Shapiro RY. *The rational public.* Chicago: University of Chicago Press, 1992.

30. Monardi F, Glantz SA. Are tobacco industry campaign contributions influencing state legislative behavior? *Am J Pub Health* 1998;88(6):918–923.

31. Monardi FM, Balbach ED, Aguinaga S, Glantz SA. *Shifting allegiances: Tobacco industry political expenditures in California January 1995–March 1996.* San Francisco: Institute for Health Policy Studies, School of Medicine, University of California, San Francisco, 1996 April. (http://www.library.ucsf.edu/tobacco/sa/)

32. Begay ME, Glantz SA. Tobacco industry campaign contributions are affecting tobacco control policymaking in California. *JAMA* 1994;272(15): 1176–1182.

33. Charlton Research Company. *Californians speak out on medical research.* Prepared for Research!America. N.p., 1996 May.

34. Schattschneider EE. *The semisovereign people: A realist's view of democracy in America.* New York: Holt, Rinehart and Winston, 1960.

35. Scott S. Smoking out tobacco's influence. *Californian Journal* 1997 April;14–18.

36. Thompson S. Interview with Michael Traynor. June 30, 1995.

About the Authors

Stanton A. Glantz, Ph.D., is professor of medicine and member of the Institute for Health Policy Studies and the Cardiovascular Research Institute at the University of California, San Francisco. In 1983 he helped to defend the San Francisco Workplace Smoking Ordinance against a tobacco industry attempt to repeal it by referendum. The San Francisco victory represented the tobacco industry's first electoral defeat and is now viewed as a major turning point in the battle for nonsmokers' rights. He is one of the founders (with Peter Hanauer and others) of Americans for Nonsmokers' Rights. In 1982 he resurrected the film *Death in the West*, suppressed by Philip Morris, and developed a curriculum that has been used by an estimated one million students. In addition, he helped write and produce the films *Secondhand Smoke*, which concerns the health effects of involuntary smoking, and *On the Air*, which describes how to create a smoke-free workplace. In 1994, he received several thousand pages of previously secret tobacco industry documents and made them public at the UC San Francisco library. These documents formed the backbone of lawsuits that have cost the tobacco industry hundreds of billions of dollars. He is lead author of *The Cigarette Papers* (University of California Press, 1996), which explains these documents. An associate editor of the *Journal of the American College of Cardiology* and a member of the California State Scientific Review Panel on Toxic Air Contaminants, Dr. Glantz has served as a consultant to the National Institutes of Health, Environmental Protection Agency, Occupational Safety and Health Administration, National Science Foundation, and numerous scientific publications. He conducts research on cardiovascular function, passive smoking, applied biostatistics, and tobacco policy and politics, and is the author of six books, including *Primer of Biostatistics* and *Primer of Applied Regression and Analysis of Variance* (published by McGraw-Hill), two software packages, including SigmaStat (published by SPSS, Inc.), and over one hundred scientific papers, including the first major review that identified involuntary smoking as a cause of heart disease.

Edith D. Balbach, Ph.D., is the director of the Community Health Program at Tufts University in Medford, Massachusetts, and an assistant professor of family medicine and community health at the Tufts University School of Medicine in Boston. She previously worked at the Institute for Health Policy Studies at the University of California at San Francisco, where she conducted research on California tobacco policy and the implementation of California's Proposition 99. Her Ph.D. in Public Policy was earned at the University of California at Berkeley.

Index

Compositor:	G&S Typesetters, Inc.
Text:	10/13 Sabon
Display:	Sabon
Printer:	Data Reproductions
Binder:	Data Reproductions